Cloud Computing Applications for Quality Health Care Delivery

Anastasius Moumtzoglou
Hellenic Society for Quality and Safety in Healthcare, Greece & P. & A. Kyriakou Children's Hospital, Greece

Anastasia Kastania
Athens University of Economics and Business, Greece

A volume in the Advances in Healthcare
Information Systems and Administration (AHISA)
Book Series

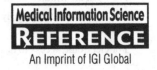

Managing Director:	Lindsay Johnston
Production Editor:	Jennifer Yoder
Development Editor:	Erin O'Dea
Acquisitions Editor:	Kayla Wolfe
Typesetter:	Kaitlyn Kulp
Cover Design:	Jason Mull

Published in the United States of America by
Medical Information Science Reference (an imprint of IGI Global)
701 E. Chocolate Avenue
Hershey PA 17033
Tel: 717-533-8845
Fax: 717-533-8661
E-mail: cust@igi-global.com
Web site: http://www.igi-global.com

Library of Congress Cataloging-in-Publication Data

Cloud computing applications for quality health care delivery / Anastasius Moumtzoglou and Anastasia Kastania, editors.
    p. ; cm.
  Includes bibliographical references and index.
  Summary: "This book focuses on cloud technologies that could affect quality in the healthcare field, with experts presenting their knowledge and contributions to the demystification of healthcare in the Cloud"--Provided by publisher.
  ISBN 978-1-4666-6118-9 (hardcover) -- ISBN 978-1-4666-6119-6 (ebook) -- ISBN 978-1-4666-6121-9 (print & perpetual access)
  I. Moumtzoglou, Anastasius, 1959- editor. II. Kastania, Anastasia, 1965- editor.
  [DNLM: 1. Medical Informatics Applications. 2. Delivery of Health Care--methods. 3. Quality Assurance, Health Care--methods. W 26.5]
  R858
  610.285--dc23
                                    2014013791

This book is published in the IGI Global book series Advances in Healthcare Information Systems and Administration (AHISA) (ISSN: 2328-1243; eISSN: 2328-126X)

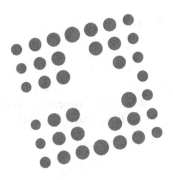

Advances in Healthcare Information Systems and Administration (AHISA) Book Series

Anastasius Moumtzoglou
Hellenic Society for Quality & Safety in Healthcare and P. & A. Kyriakou Children's Hospital, Greece
Anastasia N. Kastania
Athens University of Economics and Business, Greece

ISSN: 2328-1243
EISSN: 2328-126X

MISSION

The **Advances in Healthcare Information Systems and Administration (AHISA) Book Series** aims to provide a channel for international researchers to progress the field of study on technology and its implications on healthcare and health information systems. With the growing focus on healthcare and the importance of enhancing this industry to tend to the expanding population, the book series seeks to accelerate the awareness of technological advancements of health information systems and expand awareness and implementation.

Driven by advancing technologies and their clinical applications, the emerging field of health information systems and informatics is still searching for coherent directing frameworks to advance health care and clinical practices and research. Conducting research in these areas is both promising and challenging due to a host of factors, including rapidly evolving technologies and their application complexity. At the same time, organizational issues, including technology adoption, diffusion and acceptance as well as cost benefits and cost effectiveness of advancing health information systems and informatics applications as innovative forms of investment in healthcare are gaining attention as well. **AHISA** addresses these concepts and critical issues.

COVERAGE

- Clinical Decision Support Design, Development and Implementation
- E-Health and M-Health
- IT Applications in Physical Therapeutic Treatments
- IT Security and Privacy Issues
- Management of Emerging Health Care Technologies
- Pharmaceutical and Home Healthcare Informatics
- Rehabilitative Technologies
- Role of Informatics Specialists
- Telemedicine
- Virtual Health Technologies

IGI Global is currently accepting manuscripts for publication within this series. To submit a proposal for a volume in this series, please contact our Acquisition Editors at Acquisitions@igi-global.com or visit: http://www.igi-global.com/publish/.

Titles in this Series

For a list of additional titles in this series, please visit: www.igi-global.com

Cloud Computing Applications for Quality Health Care Delivery
Anastasius Moumtzoglou (Hellenic Society for Quality and Safety in Healthcare, Greece & P. & A. Kyriakou Children's Hospital, Greece) and Anastasia N. Kastania (Athens University of Economics and Business, Greece)
Medical Information Science Reference • copyright 2014 • 337pp • H/C (ISBN: 9781466661189) • US $245.00 (our price)

Achieving Effective Integrated E-Care Beyond the Silos
Ingo Meyer (empirica, Germany) Sonja Müller (empirica, Germany) and Lutz Kubitschke (empirica, Germany)
Medical Information Science Reference • copyright 2014 • 332pp • H/C (ISBN: 9781466661387) • US $245.00 (our price)

Social Media and Mobile Technologies for Healthcare
Mowafa Househ (College of Public Health and Health Informatics, King Saud Bin Abdulaziz University for Health Sciences, Saudi Arabia) Elizabeth Borycki (University of Victoria, Canada) and Andre Kushniruk (University of Victoria, Canada)
Medical Information Science Reference • copyright 2014 • 308pp • H/C (ISBN: 9781466661509) • US $245.00 (our price)

Advancing Medical Practice through Technology Applications for Healthcare Delivery, Management, and Quality
Joel J.P.C. Rodrigues (Instituto de Telecomunicações, University of Beira Interior, Portugal)
Medical Information Science Reference • copyright 2014 • 361pp • H/C (ISBN: 9781466646193) • US $245.00 (our price)

Handbook of Research on Patient Safety and Quality Care through Health Informatics
Vaughan Michell (University of Reading, UK) Deborah J. Rosenorn-Lanng (Royal Berkshire Hospital Foundation Trust Reading, UK) Stephen R. Gulliver (University of Reading, UK) and Wendy Currie (Audencia, Ecole de Management, Nantes, France)
Medical Information Science Reference • copyright 2014 • 486pp • H/C (ISBN: 9781466645462) • US $365.00 (our price)

Research Perspectives on the Role of Informatics in Health Policy and Management
Christo El Morr (York University, Canada)
Medical Information Science Reference • copyright 2014 • 323pp • H/C (ISBN: 9781466643215) • US $245.00 (our price)

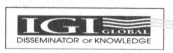

www.igi-global.com

701 E. Chocolate Ave., Hershey, PA 17033
Order online at www.igi-global.com or call 717-533-8845 x100
To place a standing order for titles released in this series, contact: cust@igi-global.com
Mon-Fri 8:00 am - 5:00 pm (est) or fax 24 hours a day 717-533-8661

This book is gratefully dedicated to my mother Maria Moumtzoglou

A.M.

In memory of my father Nikolaos M Kastanias

A.K

Editorial Advisory Board

Table of Contents

Detailed Table of Contents

Chapter 1
Rahul Ghosh, IBM, USA
Ioannis Papapanagiotou, Purdue University, USA
Keerthana Boloor, IBM TJ Watson Research Center, USA

Rahul Ghosh, Ioannis Papapanagiotou, and Keerthana Boloor provide a summary of research activities in a variety of healthcare-related Cloud initiatives. They highlight the key areas of ongoing research and describe others that require attention. Their analysis and observations can be useful to healthcare Cloud professionals, and can motivate interested researchers to initiate new efforts for better healthcare services deployed on the Cloud.

Chapter 2
Vahé A. Kazandjian, Johns Hopkins University, USA

Vahe Kazandjian explores the benefits and challenges of Cloud Computing to the amelioration of medical and healthcare services given the idiosyncrasies of medicine and healthcare. A special focus is given to the extent of readiness healthcare systems manifest to measuring their performance, sharing the findings with patients and communities, and the accountability these systems demonstrate for the promises, implicitly or explicitly, they made about quality and safety of care. The implications of these promises in shaping patient expectations leading to patient and community evaluation of the healthcare services is the chapter's central theme.

Yiannis Koumpouros argues that the era of open data in healthcare is under way. The progress in technologies along with their adoption by the healthcare providers and the maturity of the citizens has brought the healthcare industry to the tipping point. An unprecedented amount of healthcare data is being generated, and this data comes from researchers, healthcare professionals and organizations, and patients. If we can harness this data, it can help us improve our understanding of disease and pinpoint new and improved therapies more efficiently than ever before. Big Data technologies are coming to market in a rapid way. The challenges, however, are still there due to fragmented systems and databases, semantic differences, legal barriers, and others.

Yang Li, Chao Wu, Li Guo, Chun-Hsiang Lee, and Yike Guo visualize the role Cloud Computing will play in the healthcare sector by spearheading a shift in focus from offering better healthcare services only to people with problems to helping everyone achieve a healthier lifestyle. They first discuss the existing and potential barriers followed by an in-depth demonstration of a service platform named Wiki-Health that takes advantage of Cloud Computing and Internet of Things for personal well-being data management. It is a social platform that is designed and implemented for data-driven and context-specific discovery of citizen communities in the areas of health, fitness, and well-being. At the end of the chapter, they analyse a case study to illustrate how the Wiki-Health platform can be used to serve a real world personal health training application.

Luciana Cardoso, Fernando Marins, Cesar Quintas, Filipe Portela, Manuel Santos, António Abelha, and José Machado present the Agency for Integration, Diffusion, and Archiving of medical information (AIDA), a multi-agent and service-based platform that ensures interoperability among healthcare information systems. In order to increase the performance of the platform, beyond the SWOT analysis they performed, they created a system to prevent failures that may occur in the platform database. The system was implemented in the Centro Hospitalar do Porto (one of the major Portuguese hospitals), and it is now possible to define critical workload periods of AIDA, improving high availability and load balancing.

Wassim Itani, Ayman Kayssi, and Ali Chehab propose the design and implementation of an integrity-enforcement protocol for detecting malicious modification on Electronic Healthcare Records (EHRs) stored and processed in the Cloud. The proposed protocol leverages incremental cryptography premises and trusted computing building blocks to support secure integrity data structures that protect the medical records while (1) complying with the specifications of regulatory policies and recommendations, (2) highly reducing the mobile client energy consumption, (3) considerably enhancing the performance of the applied cryptographic mechanisms on the mobile client as well as on the Cloud servers, and (4) efficiently supporting dynamic data operations on the EHRs.

Chapter 7

Jonathan Sinclair, Benoit Hudzia, and Alan Stewart argue that an EHR is a modern specialisation of a Customer Relationship Management, which specifically focuses on the collection and exchange of electronic health information about individual patients between healthcare organisations. Electronic Heath Records systems hold personally identifiable information, especially that which falls under the category of sensitive personal data. As with all industries, the e-health industry sees potential in Cloud-based service offerings and the reduced infrastructure cost they imply, whilst realising the issues regarding security and privacy that may be encountered from outsourcing processing and storage to untrustworthy Cloud Service Providers (CSPs). In their chapter, they propose an approach to handle and audit data privacy requirements by leveraging a carefully designed architecture deployed for auditing data privacy in cloud ecosystems.

Chapter 8

Mauricio Paletta presents the current state and trends of Cloud Computing in healthcare, as well as a detailed collaboration model based on intelligent agents focusing on the EHR sharing subject. This model for enabling effective service in Cloud systems is based on a recent research proposal, which defines a collaboration mechanism by means of Scout Movement. The chapter also includes details on the way in which services and service providers are clearly defined in this particular system.

Jalel Akaichi proposes a Cloud Computing location-based services system able to query points of interest according to mobile users' preferences and contexts under dynamic changes of locations. The contribution consists of providing software as a service, based on Delaunay Triangulation on road (DTr), able to establish the Continuous k-Nearest Neighbors (CkNNs) on road, while taking into account the dynamic changes of locations from which queries, enhanced by users' preferences and contexts, are issued. The proposed software, implemented on a mobile Cloud and exploited by mobile physicians for healthcare institution localization and selection, considerably improves the quality of services provided for patients in critical situations by permitting real time localization of adequate resources that may contribute to save patients' lives.

Piero Giacomelli argues that the Cloud infrastructure has been one of the latest technologies in the e-health sector. However, despite many research studies focusing on the privacy of the e-health data stored on the Cloud, the ways of exchanging e-health information between client and Cloud have not yet been fully addressed. Moving from this initial consideration, the chapter evaluates the possibility of using Message-Oriented Middleware (MOMS) for exchanging data between the Cloud storage and the remote device used in telemedicine and remote monitoring software. The evaluation is done using a Cloud testing environment, low bandwidth connection modem, and a simulation of 50 patients taking a 10-minute 3Lead EGC test.

Andreas Kliem proposes a novel approach that allows sharing medical devices among different operators. This means that each operator books a medical device as long as it delivers required data and is present in the operator's network. Besides cost-effectiveness, this approach can extend traditional Cloud-based e-health systems, usually designed to share Electronic Health Records, by sharing the devices that emit the data. This mitigates judicial constraints because only the data sources and not the data itself are shared and allows for more real-time access to mission-critical data.

Abraham Pouliakis, Aris Spathis, Christine Kottaridi, Antonia Mourtzikou, Marilena Stamouli, Stavros Archondakis, Efrossyni Karakitsou, and Petros Karakitsos analyze the application of Cloud Computing technology for use in the everyday routine of BioLabs. Moreover, they provide a thorough bibliographical analysis of Cloud applications for research related to biology and biochemistry with emphasis on drug discovery, genomics, and artificial intelligence.

Abraham Pouliakis, Stavros Archondakis, Efrossyni Karakitsou, and Petros Karakitsos argue that by using Cloud applications, infrastructure, storage services, and processing power, cytopathology laboratories can avoid huge spending on maintenance of costly applications and image storage and sharing. Cloud Computing allows imaging flexibility and may be used for creating a virtual mobile office while security and privacy issues have to be addressed in order to ensure Cloud Computing wide implementation in the near future.

Roma Chauhan explains the need of the healthcare process re-engineering through the implementation of Software as a Service (SaaS). The chapter also highlights the potential and challenges of integrating SaaS-based health Cloud in the healthcare industry. Finally, it discusses the different healthcare Clouds and deployment models that can be used by the healthcare industry, illustrates SaaS-based solutions for the healthcare segment, and argues that Cloud-based healthcare and mobile healthcare can make health consultation convenient for patients across the world.

Anastasius Moumtzoglou argues that although the notion of organizational culture is now routinely invoked in organizations and management literature, it remains an elusive concept. However, in any case, it is clear that managing the culture is one path towards improving healthcare, and Cloud Computing introduces a dynamic system adaptation affecting the quality of care.

Foreword

Over the years, quality healthcare delivery has been a tantalising question for care providers, patients, and policymakers alike, but recently, it has grown in importance since the burden imposed on healthcare systems around the globe due to society's ageing has increased at an analogous rate.

Technological advances in the field of information and communication technologies found fruitful ground in care delivery. Clinical mentality has also changed, allowing for use in hard evidence-based medicine. These two factors have combined to where we finally have a tremendous amount of health-related data, generated from a plethora of special devices or registered through various Web applications, and the rising question now has been slightly transformed: How can we achieve maximum quality of healthcare delivery by efficiently managing the abundance of available data?

The "Cloud," originally a metaphor for the Internet, acquired even more nebulous characteristics after merging with the term "computing" as it implies something even bigger and maybe hazier. Grid computing in earlier days has also attempted to accommodate Information Technology's (IT) constant demand for increased capacity and new capabilities. Maybe the "Cloud" serves this purpose better.

Since the IT evangelists have decided that Cloud Computing is the next best thing to perfection, healthcare might also profit from it, but how can we judge which Cloud Computing application fits optimally in certain care provision models? This is a subject that this book intends to shed light on by providing successful paradigms of implementation from various disciplines, fields, and more importantly, cultures.

It is organised in 15 distinct chapters, each one covering a different topic. Special care was taken to include flavours of applications from various parts of the world, ranging from the USA all the way to India, but horizontal issues such as security or interoperability are also covered.

The first chapter provides an analytic review of research initiatives for healthcare clouds. Targeted mostly in the USA where there is even a federal guideline on the optimum utilisation of clouds, the authors represent, as is often the case, a combination of large corporate and academic R&D expertise (IBM and Purdue University).

The importance of coordinated data in comparison to meaningful data is the topic of the book's second chapter. Moreover, it introduces the concept of evaluation of disease and healthcare in general and discusses how Cloud Computing can further promote it in a more down-to-earth robust way. This insightful chapter is based on work undertaken for the School of Public Health, The Johns Hopkins University in USA.

The third chapter originates from Greece and more specifically from the Technological Educational Institute of Athens and its departments of Informatics. It provides important contributions in the demanding field of Big Data in healthcare, as we are witnessing a tremendous increase in volumes generated by patients and systems alike.

Imperial College London and the University of Central Lancashire, UK take over from Greece in the analysis of Big Data in healthcare. This time it is all about sensor data and efficient management as an important aspect of the Wiki-Health platform. This work is presented in the fourth of this book.

The fifth chapter touches upon a horizontal issue in all healthcare applications regardless of their technology platform, and it analyses in depth interoperability, one of the great inhibitors or facilitators of large-scale implementations. This chapter presents work carried out in Portugal by members of academic institutions in the domain of informatics (Minho University) and clinical practitioners (Centro Hospitalar, Oporto).

The sixth and seventh chapters continue with horizontal issues, this time working on the aspect of security in general but also elaborating on specific security aspects per chapter. Efficient healthcare integrity assurance via incremental cryptography and trusted computing is discussed in the sixth chapter from an academic team of the Arab and American Universities in Beirut, Lebanon. Auditing privacy for Cloud-based EHR systems is presented in the seventh chapter from a mixed team of academicians (Queen's University Belfast, Northern Ireland) and corporate IT specialists (S.A.P.A.G., Northern Ireland).

Sharing information between practitioners has always been a challenge, but especially now when they seem to be in abundance and their efficient sharing might be proven beneficial for the patient. Intelligent Agents and Cloud Computing are proposed and discussed in the eighth chapter of this book by a distinguished Latin American author coming from the academic community of Venezuela.

The ninth chapter of this book originates from ISG-University in Tunisia, and it analyses the relation between Cloud Computing location-based services and high quality healthcare services delivery.

The two following chapters (the tenth and eleventh) present results of research projects in healthcare-dedicated Cloud Computing. The tenth chapter, of an Italian non-academic origin (Spac S.P.A), discusses message-oriented middleware on the Cloud for exchanging e-health data, while the eleventh chapter discusses a cooperative and secure method for medical device sharing under the name CoSeMed (Technische Universität, Berlin).

Remaining in the European continent and more specifically in Greece and Attikon University Hospital of Athens, the twelfth and thirteenth chapters present the idiosyncratic implementation of Cloud Computing applications in the fields of BioLabs and Cytopathology.

Leaving Europe behind for Asia, India, and IILM Graduate School of Management, the fourteenth chapter presents a thorough and detailed analysis of a case study based on Health Cloud implementation from a business and managerial perspective.

Finally, the fifteenth chapter tackles another horizontal yet critical aspect of healthcare delivery in the Cloud, quality of service. Effort has been made from the Greek author representing the Hellenic Society for Quality and Safety in Healthcare to clear all ambiguities, hence providing for a demystification of the whole process.

After 15 chapters full of data and analyses, the authors and editors have provided the readers interested in the topics of Cloud Computing applications in healthcare with a powerful tool to help them pursue their ambitions in this challenging scientific field.

Dimitris-Dionisios Koutsouris
Naitonal Technical University of Athens, Greece

Dimitris-Dionisios Koutsouris *was born in Serres, Greece in 1955. He received his Diploma in Electrical Engineering in 1978 (Greece), DEA in Biomechanics in 1979 (France), Doctorat in Genie Biologie Medicale (France), Doctorat d' Etat in Biomedical Engineering 1984 (France). Since 1986, he has been research associate on the USC (Los Angeles), Renè Dèscartes (Paris), and Assoc. Professor at the Dept. of Electrical & Computers Engineering of National Technical University of Athens. He is currently Professor and Head of the Biomedical Engineering Laboratory. He has published over 150 research articles, more than 300 conference communications, and 48 chapters. He was supervisor in more than 40 PhD theses and in more than 150 undergraduate and postgraduate dissertations. In his career, he has more than 2,500 citations. Likewise, he has been reviewer for 20 international journals. Prof. Koutsouris has been the President-Elect of the Hellenic Society of Biomedical Technology, HL7 Hellas and of the IFMBE (International Federation Medical and Biological Engineering). He was the main Organiser of 4 Global Conferences and member of the Organising Committee in over 20 international conferences. In addition, he was recently appointed the position of Chairman of the Organising Committee of the E-Health Forum 2014, which is organised under the hospice of the Greek EU Presidency in cooperation with the European Commission.*

Preface

The Internet, having its roots in telephone applications in the early 1990s, is often referred to as "The Cloud." By the turn of the millennium, the Internet was referred to as broadband, and the term "in the Cloud" was highly desired. Telephone utilities were investing in "The Cloud" for switching and routing the appropriate connections for phone calls, faxes, live feeds, and signals. Then, around the middle of the decade, Computational Cloud Services, called "Cloud Computing," was firmly in the vocabulary as a way to describe what the user was doing: accessing computing services in the cloud.

At the beginning of the decade, companies began building their Websites in such a way that users could utilize their services exclusively through the use of a browser. Shortly, through the use of more powerful technologies, "in the Cloud" applications became commonplace. By the middle of the decade, most leading corporations with a strong Web presence had reasonable and reliable operation of their services exclusively "in the Cloud."

The "Cloud" represents a fundamental change in the use of IT services, which involves a shift from owning and managing the IT system to accessing IT systems as a service. The term Cloud Services, a distinct terminology from outsourced IT hosting, comes from the fact that the Internet has often been depicted as a "Cloud." Cloud Services have been defined as the services that meet the following criteria (Soman, 2011):

- Consumers neither own the hardware on which data processing and storage happens nor the software that performs the data processing.
- Consumers have the ability to access and use the service at any time over the Internet.

As a result, the definition of Cloud Services is twofold. The first part pertains to the ownership of the actual hardware and software that is used to perform data storage and data processing, while the second part refers to the client's ability to access the service remotely when needed.

On the other hand, as definitions evolved, Cloud Computing denoted the influence of Cloud, and implied the user experience moving away from personal computers to a "Cloud" of computers. In this context, the National Institute of Standards and Technology (NIST) defined Cloud Computing as "a model for enabling ubiquitous, convenient, on-demand network access to a shared pool of configurable computing resources (e.g., networks, servers, storage, applications, and services) that can be rapidly provisioned and released with minimal management effort or service provider interaction." (Mell & Grance, 2011). This cloud model is composed of five essential characteristics, three service models, and four deployment models (Mell & Grance, 2011). Essential characteristics, according to NIST, include on-demand self-service, broad network access, resource pooling, rapid elasticity, and measured service (Mell & Grance, 2011)). Service Models include Software as a Service (SaaS), Platform as a Service (PaaS), and Infrastructure as a Service (IaaS), while deployment models include the Private Cloud, the Community Cloud, the Public Cloud, and the Hybrid Cloud.

Moreover, the research firm IDC described Cloud Computing as "an emerging IT development, deployment, and distribution model, enabling real-time delivery of products, services, and solutions over the Internet." It also defined Cloud Services as "Consumer and Business products, services, and solutions that are delivered and consumed in real-time over the Internet" (GensIDC, 2008). Finally, analyst firm Gartner defined Cloud Computing as "a model of computing in which scalable and flexible IT-enabled capabilities are delivered as a service to external customers using Internet technologies" (Gartner, 2009).

As far as healthcare is concerned, the trend appears to be irreversible. Software applications and information once in the realm of the local computer server are now in the sphere of the public Internet. Private health information once confined to local networks is migrating onto the Internet. Patients voluntarily grant access to their health records, while the collection and management of this data are entirely legal. Microsoft and Google are two notable examples of companies following the accelerating likelihood of placing once restricted and private health records, "in the Cloud." Their initiatives hold the attention timing and force convergence of events if we consider the "Transforming Healthcare through IT" and "Enabling Healthcare Reform using Information Technology" initiatives.

THE CHALLENGES

Cloud services amount to three developments that are relevant to an ethical analysis (Timmermans, et al., 2010):

1. The shifting of control from technology users to the third parties servicing the Cloud.
2. The storage of data in different physical locations across multiple servers around the world.
3. The interconnection of various services across the Cloud.

These developments complement with the limitations of current e-health systems (AbuKhousa & Najati, 2012):

- High cost of implementing and maintaining health information technology as it requires investments in software, hardware, technical infrastructure, IT professionals, and training.
- Fragmentation of health information technology and poor exchange of patient data since health information technology, in most cases, exists as separate small clinical or administrative systems within different departments of the healthcare provider's organization.
- Lack of regulations mandating the use and protection of electronic healthcare data capture and dissemination.
- Lack of a Health Cloud model and development standards playing a vital role in the analysis of the following ethical issues of cloud services (Timmermans, et al., 2010).

Control

Customers or users of a Cloud service relinquish control over computation and data (Haeberlen, 2010; Kandukuri & Rakshit, 2009; Grimes, Jaeger, & Lin, 2009). The loss of control can become problematic if something goes wrong. The risks associated with Cloud services are prohibited entry, data corruption, infrastructure failure, or unavailability/outing (Paquette, Jaeger, & Wilson, 2010). As a result, if something goes wrong it can be difficult to determine who has caused the problem (Haeberlen, 2010). Contributing to this is the fact that the boundary between what is part of one's own IT infrastructure and what lies outside it is blurred. Systems can extend the boundaries of various parties and meet the security perimeters that these parties have put in place. This process is called de-perimeterisation.

Problem of Many Hands

Cloud services typically make sense in "a Service-Oriented Architecture (SOA), where all functionality consists of services which can be aggregated into larger applications performing functions to end-users" (Soman, 2011).

Self-Determination

In a world of ubiquitous and unlimited data sharing and storage among organizations, self-determination is challenged. This not only raises privacy issues but also puts at stake the confidence and trust of in today's evolving information society (Cavoukian, 2008).

Accountability

Accountability requires detailed records of actions by its users in the Cloud. It is, therefore, important to consider what is being recorded and who the record is made available to, as there can be a tension between privacy and accountability (Pearson & Charlesworth, 2009). Moreover, in a de-parameterized world, not only the periphery of the organizations' IT infrastructure blurs but also the limits of the organization's accountability become less clear.

Ownership

Besides data actively stored in the Cloud by users, the Cloud also generates information to provide accountability, to improve the services provided, or other reasons such as running or security. Although identity-based systems will provide many benefits, unknown risks and threats are emerging. As Cavoukian (2008) states, "Identity fraud and theft are the diseases of the Information Age made possible by the surfeit of personal data in circulation, along with new forms of discrimination and social engineering made possible by asymmetries of data, information, and knowledge."

Function Creep

Data collected for specific purposes over time might be used for other purposes (function creep).

Monopoly and Lock-In

If only a handful of companies are able to achieve a dominant position in the market for Cloud services, this might lead to abuse or could be harmful otherwise to the interests of the users (Nelson, 2010).

Privacy

Companies providing Cloud services save terabytes of sensitive personal information, which is then stored in data centers in countries around the world. As a result, a key factor affecting the development and adoption of Cloud services is how these companies, and the countries in which they operate, address privacy issues (Nelson, 2010).

Privacy across (Cultural) Borders

Cloud services prepare for a dialogue between different cultures by providing the infrastructure to exchange, collaborate, and communicate across cultural borders. However, different opinions on privacy are further enhanced by cultural differences.

Cultural Imperialism and Dealing with Diversity

Cloud services may lead to increasing cultural homogenization, suppressing local cultures, due to the fact that large corporations, which dominate the Cloud, implement Western values into Cloud applications (Ess, 2008).

On the other hand, healthcare services are delivered by individuals with a variety of beliefs and values. Moreover, patients come from different economic and cultural backgrounds. As a result, the opportunities for misunderstanding are numerous.

In addition, Cloud Computing can significantly reduce IT costs and complexities but enhances resources utilization and faces various technical challenges:

- Most healthcare providers require high availability of the Health Cloud services.
- The Health Cloud requires unfailing reliability for the provided services.
- Huge numbers of medical records and images related to millions of people will be stored in Health Clouds. The data may be replicated for high reliability and better access at different locations and across large geographic distances.
- Scalability requires dynamic organization and reconfiguration as well as an automatic resizing of used virtualized hardware resources.
- Health Cloud services must be flexible to meet individual healthcare requirements; they also must be easily configurable to meet with different needs.
- Services for the Health Cloud can be provided from various Cloud service providers. As a result, a good level of interoperability facilitates easy migration among different available systems.
- It is crucial to offer Cloud services, which underpin appropriate and equitable access control and authentication mechanisms to protect the transfer data to and from clients and service providers.
- Health Cloud services amplify the main concerns in e-health systems (Goldman & Hudson, 2000; Kelly, 2002).

- Health Clouds increase the complexity of network maintainability compared to an individual e-health system.
- Health Clouds require significant changes to clinical and business processes and also to the organizational boundaries in the healthcare industry.
- There are still no clear regulations and guidelines for clinical, technical, and business practices of healthcare in the e-context.
- Ownership of data in the Health Clouds is a place with no clear guidelines.

Among all the challenges listed above, trust, privacy, and security emerge as the major concerns for the Cloud. Hence, several efforts in this area strive to provide solutions to address these concerns and improve the security and privacy of the Health Cloud.

Finally, there are open issues in delivering Cloud services:

- Policy enforcement within the Health Cloud could prove extremely difficult.
- It may only be possible to verify that data processing takes place somewhere within the Cloud, and not the specific places where this takes place.
- It may be difficult to determine the processors of data.
- It may be difficult to know the evolution of the Cloud service, as Cloud Computing is subject to a paradigm shift in user requirements from traditional approaches.

SEARCHING FOR A SOLUTION

The Health Cloud has the potential to support collaborative work among different healthcare sectors through connecting healthcare applications and integrating their high volume of information sources. Dispersed healthcare professionals and hospitals will be able to build networks, collaborate, and exchange information more efficiently. Overall, collecting patients' data in a central location as the Health Cloud results in many benefits:

- The ability to provide a unified patient medical record containing patient data from all patient encounters across all operators results in improving patient care.
- The ability to take advantage of the capabilities of Cloud Computing creates a collaborative economic environment. Moreover, the flexibility to only pay for actual resource utilization shares the overhead costs among the participants resulting in reduced cost.
- The ability to overcome shortage issues in terms of information technology infrastructure and healthcare professionals ameliorates the issue of resources scarcity.
- The storage of clinical data in the cloud enables health organizations supplying related entities with information on patient safety and the quality of care.
- The Health Cloud provides an integrated platform, which hosts an impressive information repository, which can be uniformly and globally accessed, affecting research.
- The Health Cloud increases the ability to monitor the spread of infectious diseases and/or other disease outbreaks.

- Decision makers can use the Health Cloud data for planning and budgeting for healthcare services.
- The Cloud serves as a broker between healthcare providers and healthcare payers streamlining financial operations.
- The Health Cloud facilitates clinical trials since health organizations could partner with pharmaceutical companies and medical research institutions for clinical trials on new medicines.
- The sharing of data allows for the creation of specialized registries targeted for specific types of patients such as cancer and diabetes registries.

Despite all the efforts, the Health Cloud is still in its infancy. However, the models so far proposed indicate the emergence of more comprehensive approaches that will satisfy the requirements of the healthcare professionals. Moreover, although several differences exist between Cloud Computing and multi-agent systems, some common problems can be identified, and various benefits can be obtained by their combined use. Until now, the research activities in the area of Cloud Computing are primarily focused on the efficient use of the computing infrastructure, service delivery, data storage, scalable virtualization techniques, and energy efficiency. Moreover, we could say that the main focus of Cloud Computing research is on the adept use of the infrastructure at reduced cost. On the contrary, research activities in the field of agents are more focused on the intelligent aspects of agents and their use for developing complex applications. In this context, the main problems are related to issues such as a complex system simulation, adaptive systems, software-intensive applications, distributed computational intelligence, and collective learning.

In spite of these differences, Cloud Computing and multi-agent systems share issues and research topics, and overlap in the need to be investigated. In particular, Cloud Computing can provide a powerful, reliable, predictable, and scalable computing infrastructure for the implementation of multi-agent systems. On the other side, software agents can be used as critical components for implementing intelligence in Cloud Computing systems making them more adjusting, adaptable, and self-directing in resource management, service provisioning, and in running extensive applications.

In this frame of reference, the Health Cloud will evolve from being a static repository of data into an active resource that health professionals rely on throughout their daily practice. With new capabilities for accessing online expert systems and applications, Cloud Intelligence will allow tapping into information, analysis, and contextual recommendations in more integrated ways. Virtual agents will migrate to personalized support and assistance that provides information and performs useful tasks.

ORGANIZATION OF THE BOOK

In chapter 1, Rahul Ghosh, Ioannis Papapanagiotou, and Keerthana Boloor provide a summary of research activities in a variety of healthcare related Cloud initiatives. They highlight the key areas of ongoing research and describe others that require attention. Their analysis and observations can be useful to healthcare Cloud professionals, and can motivate interested researchers to initiate new efforts for better healthcare services deployed on the Cloud. In chapter 2, Vahe Kazandjian explores the benefits and challenges of Cloud Computing to the amelioration of medical and healthcare services given the idiosyncrasies of medicine and healthcare. A special focus is given to the extent of readiness healthcare systems manifest to measuring their performance, sharing the findings with patients and communities, and the accountability these systems demonstrate for the promises, implicitly or explicitly, they made about quality and safety of care. The implications of these promises in shaping patient expectations leading to patient and community evaluation of the healthcare services is the chapter's central theme. In chapter 3, Yiannis Koumpouros argues that the era of open data in healthcare is under way. The progress in technologies along with their adoption by the healthcare providers and the maturity of the citizens has brought the healthcare industry to the tipping point. An unprecedented amount of healthcare data is being generated, and this data comes from researchers, healthcare professionals and organizations, and patients. If we can harness this data, it can help us improve our understanding of disease and pinpoint new and improved therapies more efficiently than ever before. Big Data technologies are coming to market in a rapid way. The challenges, however, are still there due to fragmented systems and databases, semantic differences, legal barriers, and others. In chapter 4, Yang Li, Chao Wu, Li Guo, Chun-Hsiang Lee, and Yike Guo visualize the role Cloud Computing will play in the healthcare sector as spearheading a shift in focus from offering better healthcare services only to people with problems to helping everyone achieve a healthier lifestyle. They first discuss the existing and potential barriers followed by an in-depth demonstration of a service platform named Wiki-Health that takes advantage of Cloud Computing and Internet of Things for personal well-being data management. It is a social platform that is designed and implemented for data-driven and context-specific discovery of citizen communities in the areas of health, fitness, and well-being. At the end of the chapter, they analyse a case study to illustrate how the Wiki-Health platform can be used to serve a real world personal health training application. In chapter 5, Luciana Cardoso, Fernando Marins, Cesar Quintas, Filipe Portela, Manuel Santos, António Abelha, and José Machado present the Agency for Integration, Diffusion, and Archiving of medical information (AIDA), a multi-agent and service-based platform that ensures interoperability among healthcare information systems. In order to increase the performance of the platform, beyond the SWOT analysis they performed, they created a system to prevent failures that may occur in the platform database. The system was implemented in the Centro Hospitalar do Porto (one of the major Portuguese hospitals), and it is now possible to define critical workload periods of AIDA, improving high availability and load balancing. In chapter 6, Wassim Itani, Ayman Kayssi, and Ali Chehab propose the design and implementation of an integrity-enforcement protocol for detecting malicious modification on Electronic Healthcare Records (EHRs) stored and processed in the Cloud. The proposed protocol leverages incremental cryptography premises and trusted computing building blocks to support secure integrity data structures that protect the medical records while: (1) complying with the specifications of regulatory policies and recommendations, (2) highly reducing the mobile client energy consumption, (3) considerably enhancing the performance of the applied cryptographic mechanisms on the mobile client as well as on the Cloud servers, and (4) efficiently supporting dynamic data operations on the EHRs. In chapter 7, Jonathan Sinclair, Benoit Hudzia, and Alan Stewart argue that an EHR is a modern specialisation of a Customer Relationship Management, which specifically focuses on the collection and exchange of electronic health information about individual patients between healthcare organisations. Electronic Heath Records systems hold personally identifiable information that falls under the category of sensitive personal data. As with all industries, the e-health industry sees potential in Cloud-based service offerings and the reduced infrastructure cost they imply, whilst realising the issues regarding security and privacy that may be encountered from outsourcing processing and storage to untrustworthy Cloud Service Providers (CSPs). In their chapter, they propose an approach to handle and audit data privacy requirements by leveraging a carefully designed architecture deployed for auditing data privacy in Cloud ecosystems. In chapter 8, Mauricio Paletta presents the current state and trends of Cloud Computing in healthcare, as well as a detailed collaboration model based on intelligent agents focusing on the EHR sharing subject. This model for enabling effective service in cloud systems is based on recent research proposal, which defines a collaboration mechanism by means of Scout Movement. The chapter also includes details on the way in which services and service providers are clearly defined in this particular system. In chapter 9, Jalel Akaichi proposes a Cloud Computing location-based services system able to query points of interest, according to mobile users' preferences and contexts, under dynamic changes of locations. The contribution consists on providing software as a service, based on Delaunay Triangulation on road (DT_r), able to establish the Continuous k-Nearest Neighbors (CkNNs) on road, while taking into account the dynamic changes of locations from which queries, enhanced by users' preferences and contexts, are issued. The proposed software, implemented on a mobile Cloud and exploited by mobile physicians for healthcare institutions localization and selection, considerably improves the quality of services provided for patients in critical situations by permitting real time localization of adequate resources that may contribute to save patients' lives. In chapter 10, Piero Giacomelly argues that the Cloud infrastructure has been one of the latest technologies in the e-health sector. However, despite many research studies focusing on the privacy of the e-health data stored on the Cloud, the ways of exchanging e-health information between client and Cloud have not yet been fully addressed. Moving from this initial consideration, the chapter evaluates the possibility of using Message-Oriented Middleware (MOMS) for exchanging data between the Cloud storage and the remote device used in telemedicine and remote monitoring software. The evaluation is done using a Cloud testing environment, low bandwidth connection modem, and a simulation of 50 patients taking a ten-minute 3Lead EGC test. In chapter 11, Andreas Kliem proposes a novel approach that allows sharing medical devices among different operators. This means that each operator books a medical device as long as it delivers required data and is present in the operator's network. Besides cost-effectiveness, this approach can extend traditional Cloud-based e-health systems, usually designed to share Electronic Health Records, by sharing the devices that emit the data. This mitigates judicial constraints because only the data sources and not the data itself are shared and allows for more real-time access to mission-critical data. In chapter 12, Abraham Pouliakis, Aris Spathis, Christine Kottaridi, Antonia Mourtzikou, Marilena Stamouli, Stavros Archondakis, Efrossyni Karakitsou, and Petros Karakitsos analyze the application of Cloud Computing technology for the use in the everyday routine of BioLabs. Moreover, they provide a thorough bibliographical analysis of Cloud applications for research related to biology and biochemistry with emphasis on drug discovery, genomics, and artificial intelligence. In chapter 13, Abraham Pouliakis, Stavros Archondakis, Efrossyni Karakitsou, and Petros Karakitsos argue that using Cloud applications, infrastructure, storage services, and processing power, cytopathology laboratories can avoid huge spending on maintenance of costly applications and image storage and sharing. Cloud computing allows imaging flexibility and may be used for creating a virtual mobile office while security and privacy issues have to be addressed in order to ensure Cloud Computing wide implementation in the near future. In chapter 14, Roma Chauhan explains the need of the healthcare process re-engineering through the implementation of Software as a Service (SaaS). The chapter also highlights the potential and challenges of integrating SaaS-based Health Cloud in the healthcare industry. Finally, it discusses the different Healthcare Clouds and deployment models that can be preferred by the healthcare industry, illustrates SaaS-based solutions for the healthcare segment, and argues that Cloud-based healthcare and mobile healthcare can make health consultation convenient for the patients across the world. In chapter 15, Anastasius Moumtzoglou argues that although the notion of organizational culture is now routinely invoked in organizations and management literature, it remains an elusive concept, but, in any case, it is clear that managing the culture is one path towards improving healthcare, and Cloud Computing introduces a dynamic system adaptation, affecting the quality of care.

Conclusively, *Cloud Computing Applications for Quality Healthcare Delivery* opens new avenues for understanding research initiatives for Healthcare Clouds, exemplifies big data, arguing that data should not just be meaningful but coordinated, explores interoperability and privacy in Healthcare Clouds, and presents ways of sharing medical information. Finally, it provides insight for Cloud Computing in bio labs and cytopathology, and explains that managing the culture is one path towards improving healthcare, and Cloud Computing introduces a dynamic system adaptation, affecting the quality of care.

Anastasius Moumtzoglou
Hellenic Society for Quality and Safety in Healthcare, Greece & P. & A. Kyriakou Children's Hospital, Greece

Anastasia Kastania
Athens University of Economics and Business, Greece

REFERENCES

AbuKhousa, E., & Najati, H. A. (2012). UAE-IHC: Steps towards integrated e-health environment in UAE. In *Proceedings of the 4th e-Health and Environment Conference in the Middle East*. Dubai, UAE: Academic Press.

Cavoukian, A. (2008). Privacy in the clouds. *Identity Journal,* 89-108.

Ess, C. (2008). Culture and global networks, hope for a global ethics? In J. van den Hoven, & J. Weckert (Eds.), *Information Technology and Moral Philosophy* (pp. 195–225). New York: Cambridge University Press.

Gartner, Inc. (2009). Defining Gartner Highlights Five Attributes*highlights five attributes* of Cloud Computing*cloud computing*. Retrieved June 1, 2013, from http://www.gartner.com/it/page.jsp?newsroom/id=/1035013

Gens, F. (2008). Defining "Cloud Services" and "Cloud Computing". Retrieved June 1, 2013, from http://blogs.idc.com/ie/?p=190

Goldman, J., & Hudson, Z. (2000). Virtually exposed: Privacy and e-health. *Health Affairs, 19,* 140–148. doi:10.1377/hlthaff.19.6.140 PMID:11192397

Grimes, J. M., Jaeger, P. T., & Lin, J. (2009). *Weathering the storm: The policy implications of cloud computing*. Retrieved June 1, 2013, from http://nora.lis.uiuc.edu/images/iConferences/CloudAbstract-13109FINAL.pdf

Haeberlen, A. (2010). A case for the accountable cloud. *SIGOPS Operating Systems Review, 44,* 52–57. doi:10.1145/1773912.1773926

IDC. (2008). *IDC market analysis: IT spend on cloud services to grow to $42 billion / 25% of spend by 2012*. Retrieved June 1, 2013 from http://blogs.idc.com/ie/?p=190

Kandukuri, R., & Rakshit, A. (2009). Cloud Security Issues. In *Proceedings of the 2009 IEEE international Conference on Services Computing*, (pp. 517-520). Lincoln. NE: University of Nebraska Press.

Kelly, E. P., & Unsal, F. (2002). Health information privacy and e-healthcare. *International Journal of Healthcare Technology and Management, 4*, 41–52. doi:10.1504/IJHTM.2002.001128

Mell, P., & Grance, T. (2011). *The NIST definition of cloud computing*. Gaithersburg, MD: NIST.

Nelson, M. R. (2010). The Cloud, the Crowd, and Public Policy. *Issues in Science and Technology*. Retrieved June 1, 2013, from http://www.issues.org/25.4/nelson.html

Paquette, S., Jaeger, P. T., & Wilson, S. C. (2010). Identifying the security risks associated with governmental use of cloud computing. *Government Information Quarterly, 27*(3), 245–253. doi:10.1016/j.giq.2010.01.002

Pearson, S., & Charlesworth, A. (2009). Accountability as a way forward for privacy protection in the cloud. In M. G. Jaatun, G. Zhao, & C. Rong (Eds.), *Cloud computing* (pp. 131–144). Berlin: Springer-Verlag. doi:10.1007/978-3-642-10665-1_12

Soman, A. K. (2011). *Cloud-based solutions for healthcare IT*. Science Publishers. doi:10.1201/b10737

Timmermans, J., Ikonen, V., Stahl, B. C., & Bozdag, E. (2010). The ethics of cloud computing: A conceptual review. In Proceedings of Cloud Computing Technology and Science (CloudCom), (pp. 614-620). IEEE Press.

Acknowledgment

We would like to thank the editorial advisory board for their invaluable advice, the reviewers for the care with which they reviewed the manuscripts, and all the authors for their diverse and outstanding contributions to this book.

Anastasius Moumtzoglou
Hellenic Society for Quality and Safety in Healthcare, Greece & P. & A. Kyriakou Children's Hospital, Greece

Anastasia Kastania
Athens University of Economics and Business, Greece

Chapter 1
A Survey on Research Initiatives for Healthcare Clouds

Rahul Ghosh
IBM, USA

Ioannis Papapanagiotou
Purdue University, USA

Keerthana Boloor
IBM TJ Watson Research Center, USA

ABSTRACT

Cost reduction for hosted and managed services is one of the key promises of Cloud Computing. Healthcare is one such example of managed services that can greatly benefit by a Cloud offering. However, there are many research challenges that need to be addressed before one can deliver a mature service. This chapter provides a summary of research activities in a variety of healthcare-related Cloud initiatives. The authors highlight the key areas of ongoing research and describe others that require attention. The analysis and observations can be useful to healthcare Cloud professionals and can motivate interested researchers to initiate new efforts for better healthcare services deployed on the Cloud.

INTRODUCTION

In recent years, the healthcare (HC) industry has faced significant challenges related to limited budgets, service demands that comply with new regulations and legislation, e.g., HIPAA (HIPAA, 1996), as well as technology-savvy consumers that demand a higher level of interaction, e.g., instant access through mobile phones (Delgado, 2011). Moreover, as HC enterprises expand, their

IT infrastructure is becoming more complicated, hence requires more IT staff for maintenance (Zhang & Liu, 2010).

To address these challenges some forward-thinking health organizations are transitioning towards Cloud offerings. Cloud reduces the complexity of maintaining a dedicated infrastructure, reduces the capital expense of introducing new services, and allows experienced entities to handle their applications. At the same time, Cloud offer-

DOI: 10.4018/978-1-4666-6118-9.ch001

ings allow HC organizations to have high business agility. The HC organizations are able to identify relevant products and services in a dynamic environment. They can quickly provision applications, bring new products and services to market, and improve the customer and patient experience.

However, there are several challenges when trying to migrate an IT infrastructure to a Cloud service. This chapter tries to summarize the research activities that address some of these challenges around the HC Cloud. First, we provide a brief background on the concepts of Cloud computing and then describe in details the research trends in HC Cloud offerings. The rest of the chapter is organized as follows. Section 1 presents a background on Cloud computing and its key features. We also introduce representative examples to show how Cloud computing has been used in the HC domain and discuss potential applications. In Section 2, we talk about the research efforts in identifying the vulnerabilities and mitigation techniques in security and privacy aspects of HC applications in the Cloud. This is because a variety of privacy and security acts (e.g. HIPAA, ARRA (ARRA, 2009) etc.) dictate the compliance requirements for HC services. Therefore, it is important to understand the research challenges in the security procedures, encryption of data, and periodic usage logging in the Cloud. Section 3 describes the importance of analyzing the medical data in the Cloud. Since HC records are typical examples of Big Data, we talk about the benefits of using Cloud computing in performing data analytics. In Section 4, we analyze how Cloud can drastically reduce the cost of HC services. Since HC data is typically accessed/utilized by disparate players (HC providers, physicians, patients, insurance agencies, government agencies), HC applications are typically composed of services from more than one provider, each utilized by more than one consumer. Section 5 presents a survey of the research efforts in service composition of HC applications deployed in the Cloud. Performance aspects of the HC Cloud services are described

in Section 6. In Section 7, we highlight some of the aspects of the HC services that have not been well addressed in the current literature. These include the availability, resiliency and Service Level Agreements (SLAs) of HC services.

BACKGROUND AND CLASSIFICATION OF HEALTHCARE CLOUD SERVICES

Many health organizations have transformed their IT services into Cloud offerings, primarily because of: (i) cost reduction, (ii) management simplification, and (iii) improved service delivery. A variety of Cloud services are available to health and life science organizations that include online health and wellness tools, data and image storage and sharing, HC portals etc. Cost reduction is achieved by eliminating large capital expenditures for computing infrastructure as well as human expenses to operate it. The ability to grow and shrink IT capacity with respect to demand is another feature that avoids over provisioning of resources and hence reduces cost. For a HC service provider, understanding the characteristics of Clouds is important to ensure the platform meets all in-house IT requirements.

Cloud computing is a model of Internet based computing. It delivers access to the applications, platforms, and hardware over the Internet (Armbrust et al., 2010). More specifically, the National Institute of Standards and Technology (NIST) defines (Mell & Grance, 2011) "Cloud computing as a model for enabling convenient, on-demand network access to a shared pool of configurable computing resources (e.g. networks, servers, storage, applications, and services) that can be rapidly provisioned and released with minimal management effort or service provider interaction." In this section, we describe key characteristics, service models, and deployment models in Cloud (Liu et al., 2011).

Characteristics:

- **Standardization and Automation:** Cloud provides standardized Internet-based services. The tasks involving Cloud service discovery, consumption, and management are highly automated for easy Internet access. Historically, this is similar to: (i) use of telecom switches rather than manual operators and (ii) use of Automated Teller Machines (ATM) in banks instead of manual counters. No human interaction is needed for provisioning of computing resources in the Cloud.
- **Rapid Elasticity:** Cloud computing has the ability to quickly grow and shrink the capacity of the IT systems because of standardization and automation. Enterprises can cope with the variability in demand because of such dynamic scaling up and down of IT resources.
- **Flexibility:** Various business solutions can be composed by judiciously configuring and consolidating the shared physical and virtualized resources in Cloud. Because of such capabilities, provisioning capabilities available to a Cloud user appears to be infinite.
- **Pricing:** Through metered services, a pay-as-you-go model of computing can be

enabled in the Cloud. Thus, Cloud users can have fine grained control of cost and service.

Cloud delivery models are listed in Table 1.

We describe the Cloud delivery models in the context of HC services. As shown in Table 1, IaaS is designed for HC organizations that prefer to standardize and automate their IT infrastructure via easy deployment of computing resources. Some of the examples are small to mid-size hospital/health systems, and HC organizations that want to virtualize their IT infrastructure. This model can be beneficial for organizations that are looking at implementing EMR (Electronic Medical Record) and EHR (Electronic Health Record) that may reduce the complexity of their infrastructure (Zhang & Liu, 2010), do not want the capital expense of the new service, want to transfer large files (e.g. PACS images) and are lacking internal IT staffing.

On the other hand, in SaaS, an application provider hosts a software/service and offers the solution on-demand for a fee. In the HC settings, a hospital or clinic can pay a monthly fee for its employees to access the software system. SaaS versions for HC include EMR and EHR software and revenue and practice management software.

Table 1. Cloud delivery models

Cloud Service Model	Capability Provided	Manage Infrastructure	Manage Computing Platforms	Manage Applications
Software as a Service (SaaS)	Consume provider's applications running in Cloud	No	No	No (with limited user-specific app configurations)
Platform as a Service (PaaS)	Install/develop software / services on Cloud middleware platforms using APIs or tools provided by the provider	No	No	Yes
Infrastructure as a Service (IaaS)	Deploy fundamental computing resources (CPU, RAM, disk, network etc.) and run any OS/software.	No	Yes	Yes

This model eliminates the need for significant upfront expenses, and in many cases, it can be attractive compared to licensed-based installed software systems. This enables a HC organization to require little or no IT support. In fact even the software upgrades, and new version releases, are executed by the application provider and content is stored on or off premises.

The PaaS Cloud delivery model sits in between the aforementioned IaaS and SaaS models. This model is suitable for healthcare providers that want to avoid managing the bare-metal computing platform but are interested in allocating IT development support to manage their own applications. Examples include the hospitals that have developed on-premise software platforms on which other in-house services reside.

Deployment Models:

- **Private Cloud:** Cloud infrastructure/middleware/applications are operated solely by an organization. In the HC context, it could be managed by the HC organization or a third party and may exist on or off premise.

- **Public Cloud:** Cloud infrastructure/middleware/applications are made available to the general public. A large hospital can host its own public Cloud or may outsource the responsibilities to an organization selling Cloud services.

- **Hybrid Cloud:** Cloud infrastructure/middleware/applications are composition of more Clouds (private or public). HC organizations with private Cloud may adopt this model when service demand goes high.

Figure 1 shows an example model for HC Cloud service deployment. Different parties involved in a HC Cloud are patients, physicians, health providers and insurance providers. Each of them can access Cloud based HC services via portals which are examples of SaaS applications running on public Cloud. These applications interact with a role based access manager and provide access to only those resources for which users have permissions. All the HC related data, e.g., patient records, are stored in a backend database. Such databases are hosted on virtual machines or

Figure 1. An example model for HC Cloud service deployment

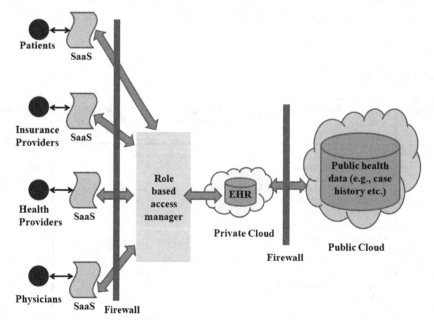

physical machines, which are examples of IaaS model of service delivery. Deployment model of such Cloud services is private when the IaaS components are maintained within an internal environment (e.g., within an enterprise). Firewalls are configured in a manner so that the internal private Cloud components can also fetch health related data from public repositories.

In this section, we introduced Cloud computing, the benefits it offers to the HC services industry and summarized the different Cloud deployment models commonly available to the HC providers.

SECURITY AND PRIVACY IN HEALTHCARE CLOUD

In HC settings, Cloud computing is fast being adopted as a platform for persisting and sharing EMRs and EHRs. EHRs containing sensitive personal health information are governed by existing security, privacy guidelines like HIPAA (HIPAA, 1996). One of the main advantages of deploying an application on the Cloud is the elasticity, i.e., the ability to quickly increase or decrease server capacity across datacenters to adapt with the dynamic changes in application demand. Data requested by end-users can be dynamically located from servers in one datacenter to another. Datacenters need not be geographically co-located. However, the elastic nature of the Cloud that improves availability and performance of applications, results in violation of medical data protection legislation in several countries. In addition, typically in public Clouds, high resource utilization is achieved by allocating multiple applications/instances of different consumers on the same physical machine (multi-tenancy). This increases the possibility of rogue applications gaining access to sensitive patient information when co-located. The above

are some examples of security loopholes that are present in HC Clouds, as well. In this section, we describe research works that focus on identifying and/or resolving security issues typically found in the HC Clouds.

Deng et al., (Deng, Petkovic, Nalin & Baroni, 2011) identify security and privacy challenges in a typical home HC system deployed in the Cloud. The authors propose additions to the architecture of Trustworthy Clouds (TClouds) (TClouds, 2011) to mitigate the risk of security breaches when hosting a home HC system. The authors identify the following security and privacy requirements for hosting a HC application/data in a Cloud:

1. **Distributed Data-Centric Protection:** Since the volume of data is large enough to warrant distributed persistence, there is a need to ensure protection of the distributed data.
2. **Timely Access to Data:** Emergency HC workers should experience low latencies, as timely access to secure data is a key to saving lives. Hence, security measures should be efficient.
3. The Cloud hosting HC applications should protect the privacy of patients, in multiple countries. Patient data, when accessed by users other than the patient's HC personnel, should be anonymized.
4. Patient-centric confidentiality has to be ensured by the Cloud by providing rule-based and role-based access control.
5. The Cloud should also ensure the integrity of the data and records of transactions performed on the patient's data.

The authors identify specific systems in the TCloud's infrastructure that are susceptible to various security and privacy threats as per the requirements elicited above and offer mitigation techniques via cryptographic technologies, attribute based encryption technologies and digital rights management.

Bracci et al., (Bracci, Corradi, & Foschini, 2012) present another example of identifying security challenges and mitigation techniques for HC systems deployed in the Cloud. The authors present a use case of a SaaS based home HC system deployed in a public Cloud. Unlike the previous example that proposes design modifications in the research prototype TCloud, the authors focus on enhancing/adding cryptographic and key management techniques to an existing deployment of a public Web/Database system to secure sensitive patient data.

The third example is from Chen et al., (Chen, & Hoang 2011) who propose a scheme for scalable, fine-grained data protection models for HC Cloud. To enable scalability and fine-grained control in addition to some of the mitigation techniques provided by the above given examples, the authors propose the adoption of "triggerable" file systems and active auditing schemes where any policy constraints can be imposed at the file/data-object level and policy violations can be reported by the auditing schemes implemented only at the data-object level. This enables decentralization of the enforcement of security and privacy policies and allows greater control by the patient (owner of the data).

Typically, medical information and images have been persisted over several years in well-established and adopted digital formats (Schaefer, Huguet, Zhu, Plassmann & Ring, 2006). DICOM (Digital Imaging and Communication in Medicine) (DICOM, 2006) is the standard file format in which medical images are stored and exchanged across multiple HC systems. PACS (Picture Archiving and Communication System) (Hood & Scott, 2006) is the commonly used implementation of the medical image exchange and persistence standard. However, PACS has traditionally been implemented in private networks and hence security issues typically seen in a multi-tenant, geo-graphically distributed network like the Cloud has not been of concern in the past. This discrepancy motivated Rostrom and Teng (2011) to propose secure communication schemes between Cloud-based PACS server and client.

Over several years, there have been several national and international regulations on recording, persistence and access of HC information, primarily EMRs. HC IT providers are required by the US law to comply with one or more of these regulations, e.g., HIPAA. Several research efforts have focused on developing techniques for compliance of these regulations in the Cloud. Wu, Ahn and Hu (2012) present a HIPAA compliant secure medical data sharing system deployed on the Cloud. The compliance management solution proposed by the authors entails creating a keyword dictionary encompassing all the words in the rules listed in HIPAA, use NLP techniques to extract rules stated in the regulation, transformation of the rules and analyzing the compliance of an EMR stored in the Cloud by leveraging logic-based reasoning techniques.

In contrast to the previous research effort, which proposes management schemes deployed in the Cloud to meet the existing HC data regulations, Delgado (2011) evaluates whether existing U.S. privacy policies are sufficient when HC systems and data migrate to the Cloud. The author states that HIPAA only provides a baseline for security and privacy protection and additional regulations need to be included in the standard to cover all possibilities of access and deployment in the Cloud. The author identifies several gaps in existing regulations:

1. Lack of access control standards, which specify that the patient is the owner of the data and any access to the data, should be dependent on the consent from the owner.
2. Regulations ensuring tracking and reporting of viewers of the data.
3. Ability to revoke consent other than for billing purposes.

The author favors the standardized security and privacy policies proposed by HITRUST Alliance (HITRUST Alliance, 2013) when HC applications are deployed in the Cloud. This comprehensive standard combines several existing, overlapping security guidelines, standards and frameworks and aims to provide specific guidelines for different scenarios without duplicating redundant controls.

In this section, we surveyed existing research efforts identifying vulnerabilities and mitigation techniques in security and privacy aspects of migrating HC applications to the Cloud. Several innovative solutions to this challenging problem have been proposed by these research initiatives. Hence, in conclusion the outlook towards improved security and privacy of HC data in the Cloud is positive.

ANALYTICS IN HEALTHCARE CLOUD

The possibility for unlimited scaling in Cloud computing has enabled the emergence of a plethora of Cloud-based data analytics applications in the HC domain. These include new applications for business intelligence, semantic Web searches, video recording, and medical image analysis. The common feature in these applications is that they are bandwidth and storage intensive. Therefore, computationally intensive applications where the computation can be decomposed into small parallel computations over a partitioned data set are the perfect match for the Map-Reduce Framework (Bhattacharya, 2012). Map-Reduce provides a simple programming model using map and reduce functions over key/value pairs that can be parallelized and executed on a large cluster of machines (Dean & Ghemawat, 2008; Ananthanarayanan, 2009).

In fact, health related data is growing faster and moving faster than HC organizations can consume it. Moreover, the majority of the medical data is unstructured, but clinically relevant. The data

resides in multiple places like EMRs, laboratory and imaging systems, physician notes, medical correspondence, claims, and CRM systems. Therefore, the challenge is to convert and combine the data to provide meaningful information, using the appropriate Business Intelligence (BI) tool for real time analysis and reporting. As Bhattacharya (2012) mentions, in order to have a good BI an appropriate infrastructure with support for the following components is required:

- Structured and unstructured data,
- Data quality and integration,
- HC data warehouse,
- HC business intelligence and analytics engine,
- HC portal.

An example of the aforementioned analytic and computation challenges can be found in Avorn and Schneeweiss (2009). The authors reveal some of the diverse challenges facing epidemiological research in the current era. Some of them are related to applying new rigorous analytical techniques to enhance the levels of confidence in observed drug safety results as well as challenges in organization politics, patient privacy and administration. Examining data after the fact to confirm a suspected drug safety problem will always be a crucial element of safety research. Powerful computation simultaneously opens up avenues for identifying issues after a drug has entered the market, but before it is in widespread use.

The huge amounts of data generated by HC transactions can benefit from distributed database systems deployed on the Cloud. A distributed database allows load balancing across multiple instances when patterns are explored in databases, and predictive models are constructed. In HC, data mining is becoming increasingly popular, if not essential. Several factors have motivated the use of data mining application in HC. The existence of medical insurance fraud and abuse, for example, has led many HC insurers to reduce their losses by finding and tracking offenders (Milley, 2000). On the other hand, data mining applications on the Cloud can benefit HC providers, such as hospitals, clinics and physicians, as well as patients, by identifying effective treatments and best practices (Koh, 2011).

Apache UIMA (Unstructured Information Management Architecture) (Apache UIMA, 2013) is an open source framework for developing analytic applications that processes unstructured information. It enables composition of analytic applications from multiple analytics providers and facilitates information extraction from unstructured sources. The UIMA framework is a popular framework to use when building analytics for HC (Mack, Mukherjea, Soffer, Uramoto, Brown, Coden, Cooper, Inokuchi, Iyer, Mass, Matsuzawa and Subramaniam, 2004). UIMA-AS (Asynchronous Scaleout) is a set of capabilities

provided in UIMA that enables the elasticity of the framework by enabling asynchronous scale out of the analytic modules deployed and provides the ability to distribute processing of unstructured text to multiple servers as shown in Figure 2. Apache UIMA thus enables HC analytics to be deployed on the Cloud.

In summary, the following are the needs for any healthcare data analytics system:

- Capability to process data in parallel and over a large number of clusters;
- Rapid execution of analytics of structured and unstructured medical data;
- Ability to work on HC record databases;
- Accelerated development and testing of new data analytics algorithms;
- Security features that both guarantee patient and personnel privacy.

Figure 2. Pictorial description of the UIMA-AS framework deployed in the Cloud

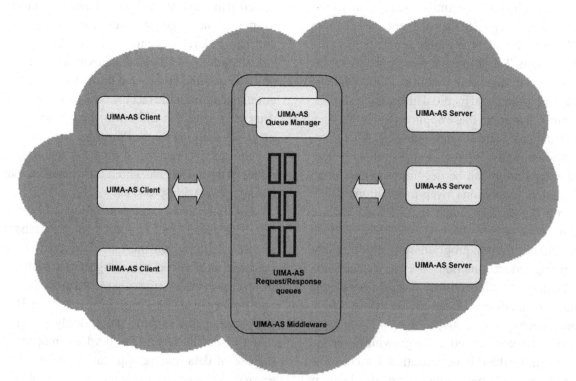

COST REDUCTION VIA HEALTHCARE CLOUD

In general, the common trend is to introduce SOA for HC service delivery. Cloud computing is typically adopted as the backend mechanism to support the infrastructure for such delivery. Such a model reduces the cost of the HC service hosting by eliminating some of the front-end infrastructure.

In Mcgregor (2011), the author presents a Cloud framework that offers HC service in a SaaS model. The key idea is to run several Cloud based Web services (e.g., clinical rules, monitoring, and analyze Web service) specifically designed for remote patient care. Compared to a traditional in-hospital HC model, such a SaaS offering can reduce the cost in various ways. When supporting medical devices are installed in patient home locations, they can save critical care unit transportation costs to the actual HC facility. From the HC provider's perspective, potentially, administrative costs can also be reduced. The author has demonstrated the working of such a prototype with an intensive care unit case study.

In Delgado (2011), the author shares his views regarding adoption of Cloud services for IT in the United States HC facilities. According to the author, ambulatory care is one of the major obstacles to achieve low cost HC services. For smaller HC facilities, Cloud computing model could reduce costs by cutting down expenditures associated with HC staffs as well as maintenance. Echoing the same opinion as the author in Mcgregor (2011), this paper also suggests that SaaS style of delivery is best suited for HC Clouds.

Another example of SaaS based HC Cloud prototype is described by Rodriguez-Martinez et al., (2012). According to the authors, monetary cost is one of the major obstacles for widespread adoption of EHR and billing systems. Interestingly, they also cite that existing HC systems in the US incur Medicare fraud, leading to a loss in billions of dollar. To reduce the costs due to fraudulent activities, they develop a novel prototype named MedBook. The developed prototype primarily accomplishes the following tasks: (1) analyze the billing patterns for patient types, provider types, procedure types etc., (2) correlate the billing system with the EHR and (3) analyze the medical history of the patient to see if the procedure was really needed. Additionally, MedBook also detects and reduces errors caused by incomplete medical information. Such incomplete information can lead to unnecessary procedures and result in high expenses. From a service delivery perspective, the prototype is really a SaaS application developed using open source technologies. Client side applications to access MedBook also support mobile platforms.

Sharing EHRs among HC providers, patients and partners is an important but costly aspect of HC Clouds. The MedCloud prototype described earlier (Sobhy, El-Sonbaty, & Abou Elnasr, 2012) also helps in reducing such costs. The main idea behind MedCloud is to create a common platform for storing and sharing EHRs. This helps in cutting down the cost of sharing and transforming variety of EHR types among multiple HC providers.

To summarize, different research efforts have developed prototypes demonstrating the cost reductions feasible in the HC Cloud. Broadly, two major types of cost reduction approaches are: (1) use of remote SaaS platforms for remote and urgent patient care (Mcgregor, 2011; Delgado, 2011), (2) use of simplified SaaS solutions for efficient billing and EHR access (Rodriguez-Martinez, Valdivia, Rivera, Seguel, & Greer, 2012; Sobhy, El-Sonbaty, & Abou Elnasr, 2012).

SERVICE COMPOSITION IN HEALTHCARE CLOUD

End users of HC services include patients, insurance agencies, emergency care providers, primary care providers, local government agencies and so on. HC services eco-systems are typically composed of multiple providers who could in-turn be consumers of other services.

An EHR belonging to a patient consists of massive amounts of data existing in different forms - text (structured/unstructured), images, videos etc. This massive information is persisted in disparate systems such as relational databases, file systems etc. Additionally, as this information exchanges "hands" between the providers and consumers previously described, it is persisted in different platforms. For example, VISTA (Veterans Health Information Systems and Technology Architecture) is the single largest medical system in the United States that caters to a quarter of the nation's population. A composition of around 168 application packages and modules form the VISTA system (Vista, 2008). This results in significant investment on IT infrastructure for the maintenance and standardized interoperability of the different services consumed and produced by the various players on the same data in a single medical system.

With Cloud based EHR systems, standardized interoperability can be achieved via SaaS based applications interacting with each other in the Cloud. The various processes in the HC ecosystem can now be streamlined via standardized tools. In this section, we discuss data interoperability issues and propose solutions in active research for the exchange of HC data between different stakeholders to achieve efficient service composition in applications deployed in HC Clouds.

Due to the requirement of HC applications to be composed of multiple services, a lot of research work has focused on interoperability standards, data modeling and enabling loosely coupled deployment of HC services. Bahga and Madisetti (2013) propose CHISTAR (Cloud Health Information Systems Technology Architecture), an Electronic Health Record (EHR) system that achieves semantic interoperability. The authors propose a reference model which defines general purpose set of data structures and an archetype model that defines the clinical data attributes. Their approach comprises of loosely coupled components that communicate asynchronously. The motivation for their work is to enable effective retrieval and processing of clinical information about a patient from different providers by prescribing to similar technical and semantic standards. CHISTAR achieves semantic interoperability by using a generic design approach. CHISTAR uses a two-level modeling approach that separates data from clinical knowledge. In CHISTAR, applications can be created using the templates that can be extended to adopt HL7 and other data formats. Standardization typically results in loss of performance. However, when the implementation of the CHISTAR model was evaluated on a public Cloud using synthetically generated data sets, the application achieved an average response time comparable to traditional deployments of tightly coupled Web-based EHR applications.

Another example is the design and implementation of an e-healthcare Web service Broker deployed in the Cloud described by Wu and Khoury (2012). The broker enables the exchange of medical records between a variety of providers and is designed to avoid data duplication, reduce medical errors and cost.

Research efforts are also focused on employing the OSGI (OSGI, 2012) framework in building Web service framework in the HC domain. OSGI by design provides flexibility and interoperability and is a well-established industry standard that can be adopted by the different participants in the HC IT ecosystem (Chih-Jen, 2008).

One of the major challenges in service composition of HC services is the validity and semantic correctness of the data since the misinterpretation of data in the HC domain can have serious, pervasive consequences. Several research areas focus on optimizing data or selection of heath care services deployed in the Cloud. Wu, Khoury and Shah (2012) propose a multi-agent Web service framework and an evolutionary algorithm for the dynamic optimization of medical data quality. Their work has two-fold focus:

1. Enable seamless extraction of data from distributed systems and optimize the data to find the best medical task sequence with a focus on improving medical data quality and support ease in medical decision making.
2. Pareto dominance evolutionary algorithm that can optimize medical data such as diagnostics and treatment process according to multi-objective QoS attributes. They use the distance ranking function to find a set of optimal solutions.

They also compare their optimization algorithm with a generic penalty-based genetic algorithm and show that they can achieve the optimal solution in lesser number of generations than the former, resulting in improved efficiency.

Another area of service composition gaining interest in the research community is automatic discovery and composition of services in HC IT. This automation of service composition is the most advantageous when HC services are deployed in third-party Clouds. Wang et al., (2009) propose a process oriented service discovery approach for dynamic HC service composition. The authors aim to dynamically discover services to match the requirements of the abstract process definition with requirements represented as semantic profiles. In their approach, any service that satisfies the semantic requirements of an activity can potentially be used to perform that specific activity in the HC process. This system adopts Web service standards such as OWL-S/UDDI, WSBPEL in the automatic discovery, composition and building of the HC workflow process. The main contribution of this work is the utilization of semantic profiles for service matching since previous research work has shown that semantic and not syntactic information in HC data is key in developing automatic/

semi-automatic service compositions in HC solutions (Della Valle, Cerizza, Bicer, Kabak, Laleci, Lausen, & DERI-Innsbruck, 2005).

Another example is the implementation of QoS based optimization algorithm in the e-healthcare Web services broker mentioned previously in this section (Wu & Khoury, 2012). The optimization algorithm implemented in the broker allows discovery and composition of medical services based on a pre-described workflow and QoS attributes of the different services.

Research efforts have long since focused on context-aware automatic service composition. One of the main areas of application of this work is in the HC domain primarily for assisted living solutions, remote health monitoring etc. Meersman et al.,(2013) propose a service value network approach to automatically match medical practice recommendations based on patient sensor data in a home care monitoring content to HC services provided by a network of providers. They automate the process by utilizing rules extracted from national medical guidelines and infer health service networks from medical benefits schedule item listings. They extract patterns in sensor readings, infer clinical diagnosis and match them with specific HC services. However, the disadvantage of this approach is that the availability of machine-readable rules is limited and hence this approach needs to be adopted in a targeted care scenario.

In the same area of context-ware HC service composition, Widya, van Beijnum and Salden (2006) investigate the use of Quality of Context in optimizing end-to-end mobile HC data delivery services in the presence of alternate delivery paths. This work focuses on the pre-establishment phase of the data delivery service. The quality of context becomes important in mobile HC as the quality of the data inferred from mobile devices would influence the service offered. The authors propose algebraic computational models for computing several quality measures. They also propose a workflow management based method to solve the problem of optimizing the selection of end-to-end workflow paths based on the multidimensional metric of computed quality dimensions. In the work, they illustrate by measuring freshness, availability and cost dimensions for a sensor based mobile health data delivery service.

In this section, we surveyed the research efforts in the space of service composition of HC applications deployed on the Cloud. We identified three major areas of active research in this area:

1. Interoperability standards, data modeling and enabling loosely coupled deployment of HC services on the Cloud.
2. Ensuring validity and semantic correctness of HC data during inter-exchange between services.
3. Automatic discovery and composition of services in HC Clouds.

PERFORMANCE ANALYSIS OF HEALTHCARE CLOUDS

While HC services running on a Cloud are gaining popularity, users will also experience predictable performance as the overall technology matures. In this section, we summarize the research efforts that investigated different performance aspects of HC Clouds.

Hanna, Mohamed, and Al-Jaroodi (2012) analyze the performance of a HC Cloud service from a holistic perspective. The performance of such services should not be measured in isolation; rather they should take into account other system-wide requirements, e.g., storage need, data integrity and authenticity. Especially, for HC Clouds, managing EHRs via efficient storage is important. Although, not mentioned directly in (Hanna, Mohamed, & Al-Jaroodi, 2012), storage performance plays a critical role in accessing and modifying those records. Interestingly, authors' analyses show that not all types of Cloud performance requirements are stringent in HC setting.

For example, scalability of virtual instances (i.e., ability to increase or decrease the number of instances based on demand) is not a high priority item for HC Clouds, unlike a generic public or private Cloud. Such distinctions are very useful during design and architectural phase of a HC Cloud.

Lomotey, Jamal, and Deters (2012) focus on using mobile platforms for accessing HC Cloud services. Performance of wireless links primarily dictates the overall of Web service quality for a HC application. The authors developed a mobile distributed infrastructure called SOPHRA that helps in fast sharing of health records from a backend server. The SOPHRA framework developed by the authors supports Wi-Fi access for SOAP and REST Web services. Under specific test cases, response time analysis shows that the SOAP Web services have slightly larger response time compared to REST services when using SOPHRA framework. Results also indicate that their framework can support order of thousand concurrent Web service requests.

Similar to the architecture described in (Lomotey, Jamal, & Deters, 2012); Lounis, Hadjidj, Bouabdallah, and Challal (2012) describe a Cloud based architecture that gathers medical data via wireless sensor networks. The key idea is to store the HC related data on a backend Cloud server and pull them in an on-demand basis. Of course, the major challenge in this work is security concerns since Cloud servers are assumed to be untrusted. While private key-based encryption technique is used, authors conduct a performance comparison between Attribute-Based Encryption (ABE) (Bethencourt, Sahai, and Waters, 2007) and their proposed encryption algorithm. Since HC platforms require complex access policies, solution proposed by the authors outperforms ABE, which is linear with the number of leaf nodes in the user access tree.

Hu, Lu, Khan, and Bai (2012) describe a middleware software as a service to share the HC data among hospitals and HC centers (e.g., primary care). Using a hosted Cloud platform they analyze the performance of the middleware service in terms of delay of sending/receiving large data. Specifically, their test case involves medical images, which is quite practical from HC perspective. Such analysis shows the limits of the hosted Cloud service in terms of image size beyond which the transfer latency becomes unbounded.

Efficient sharing of EHRs among multiple HC providers is another critical area from the performance perspective. El-Sonbaty and Elnasr (2012) address this problem and propose a HC Cloud solution named MedCloud to mitigate this issue. They identify that the core problem stems from the fact that the patients can have multiple providers as well as insurance. Hence, a common platform specifically targeted for storing and sharing EHR is of interest. MedCloud platform designed by the authors is built on three major components: (i) Hadoop for server implementation, (ii) column-oriented No-SQL databases, and (iii) RESTlet framework for Web access. As shown by the authors, key performance gain come from the No-SQL databases since they help to maintain near-constant request rate with increasing number of nodes.

In summary, there are two broad areas where performance analysis research has been focused for HC services: (1) understanding the database and storage performance is important because HC services eventually transfer bulk of data from one location to another, and (2) when designing mobile/wireless platforms for accessing HC services, reliability, throughput and the security of the underlying wireless mediums should be taken into account.

FUTURE RESEARCH DIRECTIONS

In this section, we discuss three aspects of HC service that are less investigated and may potentially open up new research directions.

Availability of HC Services

High availability is in general a strong requirement for mission critical systems and HC services are no exceptions. There are few research articles that address downtime concerns in HC settings. We envision that potentially there are two areas which require attention for providing high availability. First, availability of the software services that interact directly with the HC professionals. Although software reliability is a well-studied area, understanding the failure and recovery of databases are perhaps the most important factors in this context. These databases typically contain a large number of EHRs, loss of which can be catastrophic. To emphasize such issues, authors in Hanna, Mohamed, and Al-Jaroodi (2012) treated service availability and data availability as two different factors. Scheduled backups of database services should always be implemented along with any HC SaaS. Second, availability of back-end infrastructure is another aspect of high availability. This includes network reliability, fault-tolerance of the virtual and physical infrastructure that hosts the software and services.

From a research perspective, some of the key research questions for achieving high availability are: (1) In a generic HC service, what are the major bottlenecks (i.e, most failure probable components) that lead to higher downtime? and (2) What are the different failure and repair modes for a HC service? Answer to these questions will drive the design decisions of highly available HC service.

Resiliency of HC Services

While availability of HC services addresses the failure and recovery scenario, notion of resiliency is larger than that of availability. Resiliency of a system or service is the persistence of service delivery that can be justifiably trusted when facing changes (Laprie, 2008;Simoncini, 2009). These changes can occur beyond the normal behavior of the system. In Ghosh, Longo, Naik, and Trivedi (2010), authors quantified the resiliency of an IaaS Cloud, in terms of sudden changes in workload demand and system capacity. More research is needed for resiliency quantification in software services. For example, after an epidemic outbreak or natural disaster, hospitals and other HC services experience high load of patients. Under such circumstances, response time of the software calls needs to be part of resiliency metrics.

Key research questions for resiliency analysis in HC services are:

1. What are the systematic methods to quantify the resiliency of HC service?
2. What are the important metrics that need to be considered for such resiliency considerations?

Similar to availability analysis, understanding these issues can help to construct the design envelope while architecting a HC service.

SLA of HC Services

As the HC services are getting more mature, users will require a guarantee of service delivery in terms of SLA contracts. Understanding the system behavior and offering meaningful, comprehensive SLAs is an important problem that the HC providers would be required to solve. Typically, any Cloud service comes with a downtime SLA. However, providing a performance SLA is quite rare. Especially, for a HC service, performance SLAs are critical, e.g., guaranteed low response time, serving multiple patients at the same time without compromising the quality of service.

SLA driven capacity planning is one of interesting research questions for the providers. Given a SLA requirement, minimum number of the system or service instances need to be estimated. Such estimations should be part of cost and feasibility analysis while offering a specific SLA to customer.

Since HC services access and modify sensitive information, when deployed on the cloud, SLAs for HC services should also include several security and privacy measures (Valarmathi, Menaga, Abhirami, Uthariaraj, 2012). This requirement is unique to SLAs employed in HC services deployed on clouds.

CONCLUSION

In this chapter, we investigated the recent trends in HC Cloud services. We covered multiple topics including the security aspects, the data analytics, the cost benefits, the performance, as well as the service composition of HC applications. We also identified some research topics that have not been properly analyzed by the research community such as the availability, resiliency and SLAs of HC services. While there are many aspects of the HC Cloud service that have not been addressed in this chapter, we believe that it provides a summary of the research trends and can be useful for interested researchers looking to initiate new research efforts for better HC services around the Cloud.

REFERENCES

Alliance, H. I. T. R. U. S. T. (2013). *Common Security Framework*. Retrieved December 07, 2013, from http://www.hitrustalliance.net/commonsecurityframework/

Ananthanarayanan, R., Gupta, K., Pandey, P., Pucha, H., Sarkar, P., Shah, M., & Tewari, R. (2009). Cloud analytics: Do we really need to reinvent the storage stack. In *Proceedings of the 1st USENIX Workshop on Hot Topics in Cloud Computing (HOTCLOUD'2009)*. San Diego, CA: USENIX.

Apache UIMA. (n.d.). Retrieved September 19, 2013, from http://uima.apache.org/

Armbrust, M., Fox, A., Griffith, R., Joseph, A. D., Katz, R., & Konwinski, A. et al. (2010). A view of cloud computing. *Communications of the ACM, 53*(4), 50–58. doi:10.1145/1721654.1721672

ARRA. (2009). *American Recovery and Reinvestment Act of 2009*. Retrieved December 07, 2013, from http://www.gpo.gov/fdsys/pkg/BILLS-111hr1enr/pdf/BILLS-111hr1enr.pdf

Avorn, J., & Schneeweiss, S. (2009). Managing drug-risk information—What to do with all those new numbers. *The New England Journal of Medicine, 361*(7), 647–649. doi:10.1056/NEJMp0905466 PMID:19635948

Bahga, A., & Madisetti, V. (2013). A cloud-based approach for interoperable electronic health records (EHRS). *IEEE Journal of Biomedical and Health Informatics, 17*(5), 894–906. doi:10.1109/JBHI.2013.2257818

Bethencourt, J., Sahai, A., & Waters, B. (2007). Ciphertext-policy attribute-based encryption. In *Proceedings of Security and Privacy* (pp. 321–334). IEEE.

Bhattacharya, I. (2012). Healthcare Data Analytics on the Cloud. *Online Journal of Health and Allied Sciences, 11*(1).

Bracci, F., Corradi, A., & Foschini, L. (2012). Database security management for healthcare SaaS in the Amazon AWS Cloud. In Proceedings of Computers and Communications (ISCC), (pp. 812-819). IEEE.

Chen, L., & Hoang, D. B. (2011). Towards Scalable, Fine-Grained, Intrusion-Tolerant Data Protection Models for Healthcare Cloud. In Proceedings of Trust, Security and Privacy in Computing and Communications (TrustCom), (pp. 126-133). IEEE.

Chih-Jen, H. (2008). Telemedicine information monitoring system. In Proceedings of e-health Networking, Applications and Services, (pp. 48-50). IEEE.

Dean, J., & Ghemawat, S. (2008). MapReduce: Simplified data processing on large clusters. *Communications of the ACM, 51*(1), 107–113. doi:10.1145/1327452.1327492

Delgado, M. (2011). The evolution of health care it: Are current us privacy policies ready for the clouds? In Proceedings of Services (SERVICES), (pp. 371-378). IEEE.

Della Valle, E., Cerizza, D., Bicer, V., Kabak, Y., Laleci, G., Lausen, H., & DERI-Innsbruck, S. M. S. M. (2005). The need for semantic web service in the eHealth. In *Proceedings of W3C workshop on Frameworks for Semantics in Web Services*. Academic Press.

Deng, M., Petkovic, M., Nalin, M., & Baroni, I. (2011). A Home Healthcare System in the Cloud-Addressing Security and Privacy Challenges. In *Proceedings of Cloud Computing (CLOUD), 2011 IEEE International Conference on* (pp. 549-556). IEEE.

DICOM. (2006). *Digital Imaging and Communication in Medicine*. Retrieved December 07, 2013, from http://medical.nema.org/dicom/

Ghosh, R., Longo, F., Naik, V. K., & Trivedi, K. S. (2010). Quantifying resiliency of IaaS cloud. In *Proceedings of Reliable Distributed Systems* (pp. 343–347). IEEE.

Hanna, E. M., Mohamed, N., & Al-Jaroodi, J. (2012). The Cloud: Requirements for a Better Service. In Proceedings of Cluster, Cloud and Grid Computing (CCGrid), (pp. 787-792). IEEE.

HIPAA. (1996). *Health Insurance Portability and Accountability Act of 1996*. Retrieved from http://www.gpo.gov/fdsys/pkg/PLAW-104publ191/html/PLAW-104publ191.htm

Hood, M. N., & Scott, H. (2006). Introduction to picture archive and communication systems. *Journal of Radiology Nursing, 25*(3), 69–74. doi:10.1016/j.jradnu.2006.06.003

Hu, Y., Lu, F., Khan, I., & Bai, G. (2012). A cloud computing solution for sharing healthcare information. In *Proceedings of Internet Technology and Secured Transactions, 2012 International Conference* (pp. 465-470). IEEE.

Koh, H. C., & Tan, G. (2011). Data mining applications in healthcare. *Journal of Healthcare Information Management, 19*(2), 64. PMID:15869215

Laprie, J. C. (2008). From dependability to resilience. In *Proceedings of 38th IEEE/IFIP Int. Conf. on Dependable Systems and Networks*. IEEE.

Liu, F., Tong, J., Mao, J., Bohn, R., Messina, J., Badger, L., & Leaf, D. (2011). NIST cloud computing reference architecture. *NIST Special Publication, 500*, 292.

Lomotey, R. K., Jamal, S., & Deters, R. (2012). SOPHRA: A Mobile Web Services Hosting Infrastructure in mHealth. In Proceedings of Mobile Services (MS), (pp. 88-95). IEEE.

Lounis, A., Hadjidj, A., Bouabdallah, A., & Challal, Y. (2012). Secure and Scalable Cloud-based Architecture for e-Health Wireless sensor networks. In Proceedings of Computer Communications and Networks (ICCCN), (pp. 1-7). IEEE.

Mack, R., Mukherjea, S., Soffer, A., Uramoto, N., Brown, E., & Coden, A. et al. (2004). Text analytics for life science using the unstructured information management architecture. *IBM Systems Journal, 43*(3), 490–515. doi:10.1147/sj.433.0490

McGregor, C. (2011). A cloud computing framework for real-time rural and remote service of critical care. In *Proceedings of the 24th International Symposium on Computer-Based Medical Systems (CBMS)* (pp. 1-6). Bristol, UK: IEEE.

Meersman, D., Hadzic, F., Hughes, J., Razo-Zapata, I., & De Leenheer, P. (2013). Health Service Discovery and Composition in Ambient Assisted Living: The Australian Type 2 Diabetes Case Study. In Proceedings of System Sciences (HICSS), (pp. 1337-1346). IEEE.

Mell, P., & Grance, T. (2011). The NIST definition of cloud computing (draft). *NIST Special Publication, 800*(145), 7.

Milley, A. (2000). Healthcare and data mining. *Health Management Technology, 21*(8), 44–47.

OSGI. (2012). *OSGI Alliance*. Retrieved December 07, 2013, from http://www.osgi.org/Specifications/HomePage

Rodriguez-Martinez, M., Valdivia, H., Rivera, J., Seguel, J., & Greer, M. (2012). MedBook: A Cloud-Based Healthcare Billing and Record Management System. In *Proceedings of the 5th International Conference on Cloud Computing (CLOUD)* (pp.899-905). Honolulu, HI: IEEE Computer Society.

Rostrom, T., & Teng, C. C. (2011). Secure communications for PACS in a cloud environment. In *Proceedings of Engineering in Medicine and Biology Society* (pp. 8219–8222). IEEE. doi:10.1109/IEMBS.2011.6092027

Schaefer, G., Huguet, J., Zhu, S. Y., Plassmann, P., & Ring, F. (2006). Adopting the DICOM standard for medical infrared images. In *Proceedings of Engineering in Medicine and Biology Society* (pp. 236–239). IEEE. doi:10.1109/IEMBS.2006.259523

Simoncini, L. (2009). Resilient computing: An engineering discipline. In Proceedings of Parallel & Distributed Processing, (pp. 1-1). IEEE.

Sobhy, D., El-Sonbaty, Y., & Abou Elnasr, M. (2012). MedCloud: Healthcare cloud computing system. In Proceedings of Internet Technology and Secured Transactions, (pp. 161-166). IEEE.

TClouds. (2011). *Trustworthy Clouds*. Retrieved December 07, 2013, from http://www.tclouds-project.eu/

Valarmathi, J., Lakshmi, K., Menaga, R. S., Abirami, K. V., & Uthariaraj, V. R. (2012). SLA for a Pervasive Healthcare Environment. In *Advances in Computing and Information Technology* (pp. 141–149). Springer. doi:10.1007/978-3-642-31513-8_15

Vista Monograph. (2008, July 1). *Department of Veterans Administration*. Retrieved September 11, 2013, from http://www.va.gov/VISTA_MONOGRAPH

Wang, S., Brown, K., Capretz, M. A., Hines, P., & Boyd, J. (2009). A process oriented semantic healthcare service composition. In Proceedings of Science and Technology for Humanity (TIC-STH), (pp. 479-484). IEEE.

Widya, I., van Beijnum, B. J., & Salden, A. (2006). QoC-based Optimization of End-to-End M-Health Data Delivery Services. In *Proceedings of Quality of Service* (pp. 252–260). IEEE. doi:10.1109/IWQOS.2006.250476

Wu, C. S., & Khoury, I. (2012). E-Healthcare Web Service Broker Infrastructure in Cloud Environment. In Proceedings of Services (SERVICES), (pp. 317-322). IEEE.

Wu, R., Ahn, G. J., & Hu, H. (2012). Towards HIPAA-compliant healthcare systems. In *Proceedings of the 2nd ACM SIGHIT International Health Informatics Symposium* (pp. 593-602). ACM.

Zhang, R., & Liu, L. (2010). Security models and requirements for healthcare application clouds. In Proceedings of Cloud Computing (CLOUD), (pp. 268-275). IEEE.

KEY TERMS AND DEFINITIONS

Analytics: Is the science of analyzing large amounts of data to detect or extract meaningful patterns.

Availability: The ability of a system to perform a given task over an interval of time or at any instant of time.

Cloud Computing: The practice of using a network of remote servers hosted on the Internet to store, manage, and process data, rather than a local server or a personal computer.

Cloud Delivery Models: The style of providing different Cloud services, e.g., infrastructure, platform, and software.

Cloud Deployment Models: The location of hosting different Cloud services, e.g., public, private, and hybrid.

Cloud Provider: An entity or an organization that offers different Cloud services.

Elasticity in the Cloud: The ability to dynamically provision new instances of servers to cater to dynamic increases in volume of requests for applications hosted on the Cloud.

Performance Analysis: A quality assessment process for given system and is evaluated under some well-known metrics, e.g., throughput, response time, utilization etc.

Service Composition in the Cloud: The process of combing multiple electronic services hosted in one or more Cloud Computing Systems that interact with one another to accomplish a larger task.

Service Level Agreement: An agreement between the provider of a service and a consumer of the service. Typically, for electronic services deployed in the cloud this includes guarantees of performance, availability and security.

Chapter 2
Not Just Meaningful Data but Coordinated Data!
Can Cloud Computing Promote Down-to-Earth E-Valuation of Disease and Healthcare?

Vahé A. Kazandjian
Johns Hopkins University, USA

ABSTRACT

The era of data collection about health systems' performance is entering the new phase of timely and simultaneous access to diverse data sources in a systematic and coordinated approach. The concepts of harmonization and the measurement of the continuum of care have laid the ground for the pursuit of collecting, organizing, accessing, and sharing treatment and outcomes results. Service industries, faced with the need for access to multiple data sources, have adopted Information Technologies ranging from localized measurement of performance to regional monitoring of services, and finally into global networking via Cloud Computing. This chapter explores the benefits and challenges of Cloud Computing to the amelioration of medical and healthcare services given the idiosyncrasies of medicine and healthcare. A special focus is given to the extent of readiness healthcare systems manifest to measuring their performance, sharing the findings with patients and communities, and the accountability these systems demonstrate for the promises, implicitly or explicitly, they made about quality and safety of care. The implications of these promises in shaping patient expectations leading to patient and community evaluation of the healthcare services is a central theme running through this chapter.

INTRODUCTION

The purpose of this chapter is to discuss the critical role coordinated data about the provision of health care plays in defining the quality of that care. The title of the chapter suggests that while

data collection, analysis and evaluation is now part of medicine and healthcare, the coordination of these data requires a framework of data storage, verification, timely access, and availability to all providers of a patient's care. Cloud Computing is considered such a framework.

DOI: 10.4018/978-1-4666-6118-9.ch002

Consider the analogy of the concept of coordination with that of a film pellicule (and I propose this at the risk of hearing all those born after the 1990s say, "*Film*? What is that?") The pellicule has a length of hundreds of meters, and each frame captures a distinct aspect of what is being filmed. When the film is shot, one can inspect the frames either one by one, or, run the film and see it as a movie. I am basing this analogy on a statement made by Donabedian while teaching his class on quality of care at the University of Michigan, in 1984. He was reviewing the work of J.W. Williamson, especially his "health care accounting method" (Williamson, 1978) which not only stressed the idea of quality encompassing the continuity of care, but also indirectly that of care coordination. Donabedian said that it was like looking at the entire film pellicule, rather than single picture frames.

As I sat down to write, the memory of that class in Ann Arbor and the passing statement by Donabedian came back to me after 30 years, and I decided to build the thesis of this chapter around that imagery.

The Frame-by-Frame Inspection Mentality

The first and systematic description of the dimensions of health care quality was by Donabedian (Donabedian, 1980). His trilogy of Structure-Process-Outcome gave health services researchers, clinicians, managers and policy makers the template upon which measures of quality were tested in the past four decades. While Donabedian did introduce the continuum of care into his thinking, it was mostly as a feedback loop where he mentioned that once patient's health and disease needs are addressed, they will come back to the health care system with new needs, but also with expectations based on their previous encounters with the care system. However, the above trilogy was mostly operationalized as there distinct dimensions thru measures of structure, measures of processes, and

whenever possible measures of outcomes. Most prominent measures took the shape of ratios or indicators (Kazandjian, 1991) and were focused on quantifying aspects of care delivery processes (Arah, 2006). Often these indicators were pilot tested using *de novo* collected samples of data to assess their validity, reliability and their usefulness. Once these were assessed, large scale data collections were initiated, worldwide.

Still, and within the analogy of a film pellicule, these indicators allow only frame-by-frame inspections. They do capture what happened at a point in time during the care process, but they are just that: a point in time during a continuous process. What was needed is a new framework, where the dots are joined into a line, or the film frames played at high speed to show the movie of care! And that movie, we have learned, can have a happy ending, be a tragedy, or have a bad script wasting large amounts of resources.

The Continuum of Care and Care Coordination

Similar to original astronomical hypotheses of heliocentrism, many of the quality of care measurement approaches were *nosocomocentric*, or used the hospital as the center of the healthcare delivery system. Why? I propose three reasons relevant to the goals of this chapter:

1. The patients are "captive" in a hospital and to all that was done to address their disease needs;
2. That is where (i.e., hospitals) the doctors who used the expensive technologies practice; and
3. Emergency rooms, often used as primary care centers, are in or near hospitals.

There are certainly other reasons as well, many of them depending on the culture of a health care system. For example, a system with a well organized and accessible primary care centers and primary care physicians may use the hospitals as referral centers only minimizing the cost of healthcare. Or, a system where midwives provide prenatal care and deliver most of the babies may not need to have "Primary or Repeat Caesarean Section Rate" as one of its performance indicators. However, isn't it more exciting and "worthwhile" to study the quality of care during a hip replacement than it is to see how Otitis Media are treated by primary care doctors or nurse practitioners?

The continuum of care takes the Copernician heliocentrism (Harmonia Macrocosmica), suggested to be in part inspired from the works of Aristarchus, Philolaus and Pythagorus (Wikipedia, 2013) to the Milky Way proposed by Hubble (Wikipedia, 2013). Now we are talking about galaxies, the sun not being stationary, elliptical orbits! We are talking about a hospital existing within the orbit of public health and patient expectations. And we are rediscovering the concepts of "measures harmonization" (National Quality Forum, 2010) and introducing the concept of Care Coordination (National Quality Forum, 2012) so that the galaxy does not collapse!

But collapsing it often threatens us, especially under the weight of its skyrocketing cost and unnecessary and unjustified treatments, and for preventable diseases' unmet needs. It can also collapse if the medical profession does not see itself as part of the galaxy and an essential force for influencing the pull and push between payors, policy makers and patients. Coordination therefore becomes an abstract concept if those who play a major role in providing services do not recognize the importance of coordination. After all, they do not teach Care Coordination and harmonization across levels of care in medical school, do they?

Given the issues raised in the above paragraphs, it is important to identify behaviors which may need to be controlled for before considering their influence on the coordination of care, which immediately implies the coordination of data and their sources.

HEALTH CARE PROFESSIONALS' BEHAVIORS AND THEIR INFLUENCE ON CARE AND DATA COORDINATION

I would like to introduce four categories of behaviors and their resulting effects on our understanding of the goodness (or quality) of services. For the purposes of this chapter, healthcare is considered a social good with associated services provided by those to whom we have given explicit privileges to provide and be accountable for these services.

False Negatives

When one says "*It did not happen*" when in fact it did, there can be a number of explanations for that statement. First, a happening has to be quantifiable. One cannot say "I think the patient is now able to eat" unless there is observed and documented evidence that the patient had consumed food. Thus, a false positive may be the result of not having the recorded evidence for whatever happened.

Second, a false negative can follow the recording of incorrect data. In the above case, there may in fact be documentation that the patient did not eat food, when in fact the patient may have consumed a much appreciated hospital gourmet dinner!

Finally, a false negative may be the disturbing manifestation of people not willing to collect or share data. All three of these scenarios have implications for the existence, veracity and completeness of data collected by or about healthcare organization to assess the quality of the care they provided. Let us explore each scenario.

Scenario 1: "*There are no medical errors in our hospital.*" While I am making an inflated statement, such pronunciation was not uncommon at the start of the safety of care movement in the late 1990s (Kohn, 2000). The reason was not to mislead the public, but it was because truly, the hospital representatives had no idea what the situation was regarding errors and safety of care. There were no systematically collected data, and if there were, their reliability was unknown. So, hospitals showed their good-faith accountability through statements about quality of care based on false negatives.

Scenario 2: This category of false negatives is not a reflection of services provided or of the services consumed. Rather, it deals with the question of errors, as a general aspect of the organizational performance. There are two aspects to this kind or error. One clearly follows the incorrect recording of data. Thus, if the patients record shows that the patient did not eat when he had; or that the medication was given when it was not; or yet that the patient was discharged when still occupying a hospital bed, then the false positive is a reflection of the lack of data validation before making a statement. In other words, if the data are incorrectly recorded but the hospital used these data to make a statement, then the false negative is consequent to both the recording of the data AND their use without appropriately checking the validity of these data.

Scenario 3: *"The best way not to have nosocomial infections is not to collect them"* I once was told. It seems far-fetched in today's measure-everything world, yet this attitude may be more common than believed. It is well documented that "coding creep" occurs when a classification system is used for reimbursement (Carter, 1990). If creative coding exists and even glorified through coding improvement software, is it far-fetched to propose that if performers did not have to show how they were doing, their initial instinct would be to not quantify and show? In the same vein, if they do have to show, one may expect that organizations would have

the tendency to put their best foot forward, even if sometimes it is based on incomplete, hence potentially not representative, data.

The above three scenarios introduce the classification of organizational performance profiles into the false negatives category, where things did happen but for various reasons, were not captured or reported as true events.

False Positives

In this category fit the statements and organizational performance profiles which propose that things did happen when in fact they did not. A Taoist may say "Quality happens," but what if we do indeed say so despite it being of lesser, questionable or plainly dis-quality? Will that be misleading, unprofessional, and irresponsible? Consider a hospital that shows its patients regaining functional status, or even improving on it, following knee replacement. Was that good quality care? Perhaps. To evaluate the quality, one first needs to know if the patients needed a knee replacement. As another example, consider a hospital where cardiac stents were inserted and patients did very well afterwards. Again, the question is: did they need stents? A study from the UK's National Health System (NHS) (Walker, 2013) shows that when performance indicators are used on small samples, the power of the analysis cannot validly detect all sub-par performers, in this case surgeons. And when a sub-par performer is not identified through statistical analysis, they may incorrectly be considered as "good" performers.

These are not hypothetical examples: there is an entire literature documenting that such demonstrations of quality can be based on false positives (Wright, 1982; Lilford, 2004; Wikipedia, 2010). The question then becomes: were these false demonstrations of good quality the result of a conscientious and systematic manipulation of reality, or, were they false positives because of the incomplete or incorrect data, interpreted with an organization's market competitiveness bias?

False Accountability

The working definition of accountability is that it is a contract between two or more parties—one asks for services; a second applies to provide it, and upon completion, the first party evaluates of what was agreed to provide and achieve was indeed done (Kazandjian, 2002). We deal with accountability on a daily basis—the butcher is accountable for hormone free-meat if that is what we ask for and he says it is; the car mechanic is accountable for changing the brake pads if that is what we asked him to do; and the policeman is accountable for upholding the law and protecting us. If any one of the above "sub-contractors" says that they did what was agreed upon but in reality they did not, then they are held accountable, they will not be paid for their service, and may lose their license to practice. There is no car mechanic who can be trusted by his saying "Just trust me, I did what you expected, what we agreed upon, and I did it very well." One needs to drive the car to test.

Yet, that is exactly how healthcare and medicine have asked to define accountability – through trust. The challenge of this request is that trust is difficult to quantify via indicators of performance, outcomes, satisfaction and cost-consciousness. While the older generation of patients may still ask little and trust healthcare professionals to provide the most appropriate, timely, cost-conscious and evidence-based care, those who rely on their smartphones for all information and can check on a topic within the simultaneous stroke of two thumbs, are most likely to say "show me and tell me why."

It is through this evolution of community and patient expectations that false accountability by service providers becomes a prominent issue. If a hospital claims "*there are no medical errors in our institution*" is it because they are purposefully misleading their clientele, or is it because they really do not know all that they need to know? For the purposes of this chapter, the second explanation is most relevant. Specifically, I would propose that when false accountability occurs, it is because the organization has not measured what should be measured, nor has it measured it well. Rather, that they have measured what was possible to measure and sometimes made unwarranted extrapolations from the data.

The discussion about false negative, false positive and false accountability in the context of healthcare organizations' description of the goodness of their performance narrows our focus into the issues of data, measurement, and the harmonization across measures. These will constitute the cornerstones for the discussion of the benefits and challenges of Cloud Computing. Yet, there is one more dimension to consider for the completeness of the argument: that of True Promises.

True Promises

The medical profession has long been the keeper of the wisdom regarding treatment and healing. As the "dominant profession" (Starr, 1982) medicine not only treated illnesses but also promised to teach patients about what to expect regarding the healing process. And it is that very promise that sometimes was unachievable, unreasonable, or plainly false. Yet the keepers of the wisdom were never questioned. Why? Because the knowledge and wisdom were unevenly distributed between the providers and recipients of medical services. A patient, his family, or the community at large could not evaluate the goodness of what was done, or the avoidability (as the potential for avoidance) of an adverse outcome. It was promised to them that the hospital was safe that the surgeon was licensed and done many similar surgeries before;

that the diagnosis was solid and may not require a second opinion and that medicine deals with probabilities and bad outcomes will happen.

The game change came with the global imperative to know more on why things are done, how they are done, and what adverse events and outcomes could be avoided (Kohn, 2000; Kazandjian, 2002). The critical factor in answering any of these questions, hence not just trusting that all the right promises were made and actively pursued, was the search for the appropriate data for decision-making. The 1980s saw the first large scale quantification and medical services classification efforts in the United States with the introduction of Diagnosis Related Groups (DRG) (Wikipedia, 2011). Since then, the measurement of performance via indicators and the translation of these measures into quality (Kazandjian, 1999) has become a worldwide phenomenon leading to a transformation of what we once took for granted: that the right thing is always done in Medicine. In the 1990s, the focus on safety of care (Kohn, 2000) made the questioning of historical promises more tangible: patients and communities realized that hospitals are dangerous places if a strict strategy for safety is not in place; and that unnecessary exposure to healthcare is bad for your well-being. In other words, communities, researchers, and policy-makers revisited some of the promises implicitly or explicitly made by the healthcare systems to find out that some of these promises were false.

The immediate outcome of these external reviews and evaluations is now in the phase of indirectly defining what the true promises should be. For example that any avoidable hospitalization should be avoided, and if not, hospitals will not receive payment for the care they provide for treating the avoidable hospitalizations (Centers for Medicare & Medicaid Services, 2008). On a more systemic level, a true promise is that the hospital care is just a "stop" in the continuum of health care needs and services a patient gets. Specifically that true outcomes of care should be measured

thru health care coordination (Hofmarcher, 2007; O'Malley, 2010). This is a major new step toward a much awaited rapprochement between clinical care and public health (Kazandjian, 2002) where the true mission and performance of healthcare takes into account the entire experience of the patient in seeking medical care, complying with treatment and regimen, receiving sub-acute, rehabilitation or home care after discharge, and modifying his lifestyle to maintain or improve his health status.

And clearly, measuring and evaluating the goodness of the health care coordination requires data, specifically the coordination of multiple data sources. This is what will be discussed under Cloud Computing.

A Summary of the Categories

The four categories discussed above form the template upon which the advent of Cloud Computing into healthcare is discussed. These categories are not commonly analysed in tandem in the healthcare literature and as such, will require much more future scrutiny and development. For the purposes of this chapter, it is the interactive characteristics of the categories summarized in the Table that deserve exploring further within the context of measurement and interpretation.

Table 1. Categories of challenges affecting the measurement of performance[1] and its interpretation

False Positive	True Promises
It was not good performance but implied that it was	*We promised what we can deliver not more*
False Negative	False Accountability
It was good performance but was not measured appropriately[2]	*No contract on what to expect; just trust us*

[1]The term "Performance" is used as encompassing both quality and safety of care.

[2]Appropriateness encompasses measurement accuracy, completeness, replicability, and representativeness.

The four categories in this table are interactive during performance measurement and that interaction can determine the quality of the performance. Specifically

- False Positives and False Negatives can be indexed into a ratio, the FP/FN Ratio (Ioannidis, 2011). This statistic can be most informative when assessing if measurement of performance was through an inadequate metric or that the statement about the goodness of the performance was misleading. Consider the following ratio:

$$\text{FP/FN Ratio} = \frac{\text{It was bad performance but the measures implied that it was good}}{\text{It was good performance but could not measure it}}$$

This is a non-traditional ratio since it does not measure an actual % or gap. Rather, it provides an almost qualitative gauge to understanding if the FP or FN were due to data (inadequate data) or measurement (inappropriate indicators), or yet misleading since a statement about performance may have been made without a strategy of measurement (did not measure).

- False Accountability and True Promises also interact to build patient and community expectations. Consider the effort to measure patient and community satisfaction with the care received or the healthcare system in general. There are numerous satisfaction survey models and methods. All try to capture, thru responses to the survey, the patient's perceptions and sometimes evaluation of the services received. Most surveys have a high overall satisfaction score (Carr-Hill, 1992) although scores by categories such as amenities, care providing staff's behavior, personal-

ized caring, waiting time, room comfort, food's edibility, etc, are more telling as score breakdowns.

Once the surveys are conducted, the Human Resources and Communication departments use the findings for accountability statements and indirectly, for marketing the quality of their healthcare organization.

The challenging question is, however, "What were the expectations of patients, families and their community?" I propose that satisfaction surveys without expectation baselines ascertained first, do not provide a useful picture of satisfaction. Why? Because the quantification of satisfaction is again thru a ratio, this time the Expectation Achievement Ratio (EAR). This ratio is my construct and will not be found in the literature thru a Google search, yet the logic of it follows that of any gap analysis as follows:

$$\text{EAR} = \frac{\text{What was Expected}}{\text{What was Obtained}}$$

and

Satisfaction = the Gap between Expected and Obtained

Defined as such, the relationship between satisfaction, the expected and the obtained has a direct influence from healthcare's accountability and promises. Indeed, while it is known for patients to have unreasonable expectations, if the healthcare system's promises are factual (i.e., verifiable) and tenable (i.e., repeatedly achievable) then expectations do get adjusted over time. It is, therefore, the role of physicians, nurses, pharmacists, hospital communication specialists and the Board to act not only as providers of services, but as teachers about what can be achieved and why (Kazandjian, 2012) More importantly, patients should know what cannot be achieved and to avoid asking to fix it for as long as possible. When reasonable expectations are shared between communities, patients and their healthcare system, utilization of unnecessary services diminishes as do costs and the frequency of adverse outcomes. All three of these quantifiable observations would lead to justifiably higher satisfaction among the providers and recipients of health care services.

CLOUD COMPUTING: WHAT IS IT AND WHY IT WILL IMPROVE HEALTHCARE QUALITY?

Since collecting data follows storing these data, the astronomical amounts collected about patients' demographics, medical history, past utilization, the voluminous details about the treatment, the medications, the procedures, etc, require a "place" to store. The traditional Health Information Technologies (HIT) rely on variations of hard drives to store these data, and hard drives are physical entities that themselves take space and maintenance. Further, these HIT are physically implemented and maintained by staff at a hospital or hospital system level. In short, present-day HITs are also nosocomocentric! But since too often one HIT does not communicate with other hospitals' HITs, I would qualify them as "uncooperatively nosocomocentric"…

The pursuit of a continuum of care, its measurement and the resulting care coordination goals require a centralized storage of data from "each frame of the film" as proposed above. In fact, they require access to the library of all films. A physical space where mainframes, hard drives, optical disks and other material entities store, maintain the security, manage, update, and manipulate the massive data from the healthcare system is technically unfeasible or cost-prohibitive.

We need a non-material space to store encrypted massive amounts of data as a central repository accessible by all those authorized to access either confidential patient data, or information about evidence-based practices on a timely basis. Cloud Computing holds many of the answers and solu-tions to these requests, especially for healthcare where the data about quality have been so difficult to harmonize and use.

What is It?

Cloud computing is a method capable of pooling theoretically unlimited amounts of data and storing them in a non-conventional or cloud way. The computing abilities are thru the algorithms that can be written to access and analyze any or sets of data again with seemingly unlimited way. For these two characteristics, the sky is truly the limit for the cloud!

Is it a New Technology?

Yes to healthcare, not so for other service industries where mega companies like Google have been successfully using the cloud for their massive data storage and manipulation. For Gmail users, it should be known that all communication is through the cloud.

Who Manages the Cloud?

Cloud service providers have already established a distinctly unique technology framework, where because of lower cost of maintenance (no hardware, physical space, etc) they can build redundant systems to both enhance speed of access and use, as well as security of the stored data.

The availability of numerous service providers is also a business case for using the cloud. Since the data are in the Cloud, a hospital can evaluate which service provider can provide the safety, security and computing assistance at a lower cost. This value assessment can be done on an ongoing basis and if a provider is not accountable for the contractual agreement, a hospital can shift providers with a seamless and short transition phase without affecting the data in the cloud or access to them. Try to change an existing IT system in a hospital or hospital system: it is practically impossible, and if it is it will take years and a new infrastructure (physical space, new equipment, endless times of programming and testing among others) and added cost (new contract, new equipment, re-training of existing staff, possible additional staffing) to do so.

This is a shift of thinking paradigm for the health care system which is among the most human-power intensive industry. While this characteristic is beneficial to communities by creating jobs for them, the use of the cloud, via service providers, is a novel concept.

Are Data in the Cloud as Safe as when in a Hospital IT System?

The data are expected to be safer because of the low cost of redundant systems and the frequency of data back-up. The latter activity, vitally necessary to be systematic and timely, is often the first to be "negotiated" given its cost, the hard drives/equipment and the manpower needed. Non backed-up data, if corrupted or lost, could significantly compromise the safety of patient care. Consider the situation where a patient's medication list data gets lost or misclassified as that of another patient. If there was no back up to verify against, medication reconciliation may not be possible putting the patient at risk for allergies, anaphylactic shock, or at least constipation.

In the United States HIPPA data, with emphasis on patient data security and privacy, already uses Cloud Computing where hundreds of security checks are done continuously for each data element.

Can Cloud Computing Assist Patients to Access Health Information when They Cannot Access a Healthcare Provider?

In the era of physician shortage (especially in primary care) there is evidence that patients use the expensive setting of an Emergency Depart-

ment for primary care needs. This unnecessary use of resources not only increases healthcare cost, but deprives other patients in true need for emergency care to get access to them. Finally it also unnecessarily exposes patients and family members to the healthcare environment increasing their chances of airborne infections, falls, and of unnecessary treatment.

Cloud computing is expected to help smart phone savvy patients to use their smart phones for accessing either health care information and guidance, or reach their physician immediately and be triaged for a visit or not. This is believed to be possible the same way Google has all its "Apps" on the Cloud. Healthcare systems can participate in building a health advisory cloud database which can be accessed through "Apps-like" means. Given the total dependency of the new generation on personal digital devices for decision making, getting directions to, or socializing through digital media and networks, healthcare Apps do not seem far-fetched.

If Healthcare Apps Are the Mobile Application for Consumers, Can They Also Be for Providers?

Already mobile devices (phones, tablets, etc) are part of every physician clinic, hospital, and increasingly public health workers worldwide. While the culture is already adopted for using mobile devices for verifying a diagnosis, checking on appropriate medication dosage and regimen, and adapting an evidence-based treatment modality when available, the existing HIT are not always capable to provide access to medical records or clinical protocols.

Cloud computing is believed to build on this existing culture and provide seamless, fast, secure and accessibility to unlimited sources of data and analyses. Contrary to challenge a hospital may have to shift from its IT system to computing, a physician or an Emergency Medical Technician would continue to use their smart phone, this time with much higher effectiveness and efficiency. By decreasing the inefficiencies of today's IT, basing the treatment or intervention on evidence supported protocols, and hence increasing the effectiveness of the care, the potential contributions of Cloud Computing for quality of care are astonishing.

However, Cloud Computing is not a HIT panacea. Like any tool and technology, it will answer (well or not) to the questions of the users. When addressing questions about quality of care, the Cloud is expected to address inquiries faster, tapping into more data sources, do so at a fraction of today's health IT systems cost, maintain the safety of data, and keep patient privacy protected. But, quality of care will be explored, measured, evaluated and strategies for improvement adopted only if the users ask the appropriate and relevant question during their inquiries from the cloud's datasets.

So panacea it will not be, but the Cloud will open new horizons for exploring the dimensions of quality by helping us ask the new and relevant questions.

What are the Questions We Have Not Yet Answered and Can Better Ask through the Cloud?

Let us go back to three frameworks I used in this chapter to define the dimensions of quality:

1. Donabedian's trilogy of Structure-Process-Outcome;
2. The US Centers for Medicare and Medicaid Services (CMS) Care Coordination model; and
3. The single frame versus movie inspection mentality.

Within these frameworks, and for illustration purposes, three yet incompletely or inadequately answered questions are chosen and the Cloud's contribution to better answers is further explored.

Q1: How well do we ascertain and evaluate the relationship between processes of care and the resulting outcomes?

While Donabedian spoke about quality as the interplay between structure, process and outcome, the operationalization of the measures demonstrated that it was either structure, process or outcome that were measured via indicators, not their interrelatedness (Kazandjian, 2002). For instance, patient death is an outcome (unless measured in a culture where reincarnation is part of the continuity of life. In that case mortality may be a process). But in a Western culture, mortality as an outcome can be classified by its underlying diseases such as "diabetes," or immediate cause of death "from heart failure," or as of recently as "due to medication error." This extremely simplified example is again a point in time of or a single-frame since we do not necessarily build into that measure the patient's lifestyle (sedentary, stress levels, eating habits, smoking, alcohol use, etc) or the potentially lengthy list of medications prescribed in the past year. And one may even push the stratification by asking if we even know if the patient was appropriately adhering to the medication regimen.

The above discussion illustrates the need for linking across the domains of performance to come close to understanding quality of care. I have proposed elsewhere that the operational definition of quality can be "Quality is the evaluation of performance" (Kazandjian, 1999). In other words, performance is what we measure, at one point in time. The linking of the points (or picture frames) gives us a more encompassing view of what was done, for what, where, how and by whom. Once these are established, then comes the evaluation phase. This is when we put a "value" on the measured, in this case performance: was it good or bad? The result is a statement about the quality of the care.

Thus, the answer to Q1 is that we do know what to link, increasingly why, and often how.

But to do so requires the access to, compatibility across, and timeliness of the analysis not only to evaluate performance, but give timely feedback to the provider about what to improve and how. This is where Cloud Computing is seen as a unique technology allowing the fast and low cost linkages among and across limitless sources of data to yield evaluative results and recommendations about better practices. And the latter will be compiled and organized into the growing data sources about evidence-based practices.

While this promise and theoretical capability of cloud Computing is what healthcare has been awaiting, not all is rosy. In order for the linkages among and across data sets to happen, there has to be a common structure and language among these data sets. Needless to say that is not the case yet today although much has been done toward that goal (The National Institute of Standards and Technology, 2010). Perhaps the benefits of Cloud Computing will convince health care systems to accelerate the pace of uniformization and harmonization in the structures and languages of health IT, and, why not, create a "Equalizer App Maximus" (my term) which would harmonize across discordant IT structures and languages!

Q2: Does the patient play a role during the evaluation of the quality of care for each of the three components of Donabedian's trilogy?

The patient inputs a need to initiate the care process. That need can be justified or not, and it is the first role of the healthcare system to triage the need and decide if the care process should be started. The urgency for the patient to get medical assistance is based on either felt or assumed need. The literature on the unnecessary use of emergency rooms and the demand for a caesarean section for lifestyle reasons are among the global challenges of how does the healthcare system triage patients' "input."

Once the patient is initiated into the care process, he/she becomes either a partner in the phases of treatment and compliance with regimens (medication, diet, exercise, and self-care) or an almost passive recipient of interventions. While increasingly patients are more educated about the processes of care, their evaluation of that care remains largely based on the amenities and structures surrounding these processes.

The outcomes of care are more accessible to patients and family, as any evaluation will consider the restoration or improvement of health, lack of adverse events and complications, and a quality of life that was expected to be achieved. In the instance when all these positive outcomes are observed and experienced, the patient's trust in the healthcare system will be a positive input when the patient returns to the system with his future needs, If the outcomes were less than expected or dramatically unacceptable (medical errors, complications, harm, and deterioration of health status) the patient either will resist returning to the system even for legitimate needs, or will be a doubting partner making the future processes of care more challenging for the care providers.

Cloud Computing, through its potential and ability to synthesize across datasets, is expected to provide a more reasonable set of expectations about outcomes associated with various interventions (Kazandjian, 2010). This is a major contribution to the education of patients, their families and their communities about how they would use and evaluate their health care systems. A parallel can be seen between the concepts of Evidence-based Medicine (EBM) and evidence-based expectations (again, my terminology). While EBM provides guidance to the providers of care about better practices, evidence-based expectations provide guidance to the recipients of care services about what outcomes are reasonable to expect based on the pooling, synthesis and analysis of potentially limitless sources of data.

Today's educated patient is the one who purposefully or passively receives knowledge from the information world which surrounds us every second of our days. The Interent makes information a click away, and while it should be taken with a grain of salt, the average surfer of the Interent will be capable of self-educating himself incontestably more than our parents or grandparents ever could. The result is not only a better preparedness to become a partner in the care process, but also a more reliable evaluator of the services received. However, the Cloud's results about outcomes of care and what is reasonable to expect may not be readily understood by patients. Therefore, the new generation of outcomes data and expectations will put the direct care providers into an old but vanishing role: that of the educators.

Q3: Does the Care Coordination model equate to a true continuum of care analysis or a fragment of the continuum?

Care Coordination has been a focus of a number of national experiments, predominantly in the United States, Germany and the United Kingdom. The concept of a continuum is the consequence of the realization that care delivered in "silos" (physician office, primary care center, acute care hospitals, rehabilitation centers, home care, Long Term Care, etc) cannot describe the true picture of care. Or, within the spirit of this chapter, does not show the film of the care, rather depicts one frame of that movie.

The evaluation of the experiments has yielded mixed results. A large study involving 18,309 Medicare patients from 15 care coordination centers was supported by the Centers for Medicare and Medicaid Services (CMS) from 2002 to 2005. Patients with chronic conditions (congestive heart failure, coronary artery disease, and diabetes) were randomly assigned to treatment or control (usual care). The study results were analysed retrospectively using a case-control methodology focusing on costs, hospitalization, quality of care indicators, as well as a patient survey 7 to 12 months after enrollment (Peikes, 2009)

Upon evaluation of the practices in the 15 care coordination centers, cost savings were not clearly identified. However, there were indications that if the practice variation across the 15 care coordination centers were minimized, the intervention could be cost-neutral and can improve the health of patients.

Specifically, it was found that unless a frequent contact was established between the care providers and their patients/families, the patients may not be convinced about the importance of care coordination as integral part of the care, hence may not adhere to the regimen regarding medication, life style change, etc. As importantly, the frequent contact gave the providers timely information about patient hospitalization/hospitalizations and helped them better manage transitions and reduce short-term readmissions. The authors suggested that in addition to care coordination models resulting in cost-neutral outcomes for the system, the fragmentation of care can be minimized by providers having constant contact with patients, involving physicians at the forefront. The contacts would also yield timely data about the patients' hospitalization and treatment, helping minimize readmissions through tailoring transition care models to each patient and minimizing readmissions. A number of studies have shown that transition of care models do minimize readmission and generate cost savings to the system (Rich, 1995; Naylor, 1999; Coleman, 2006).

In 2007 the Organization for Economic Co-operation and Development (OECD) published its Health Working Paper No. 30 entitled "*Improved Health Systems Improvement through better care Coordination*" (Hofmarcher et al, 2007) with similar findings about the paucity of support for cost savings but a strong argument that care coordination can improve the quality of care and patients' well-being. Specifically, it suggested that to be successful, care coordination models require better system of care integration, specifically in the area of care transition. The silo or fragmentation of care is still a dominant aspect of many health care systems and needs to be transformed thru the concept of the continuum of care. Specifically the

OECD paper recommends that there is "scope for improving performance in coordination by "tweaking" existing health-care systems through a policy mix ranging from better organised ambulatory care to patient-centered integration of health and long-term care."

The Ultimate Benefit of Cloud Computing to Healthcare

The title of this chapter includes the words "Meaningful" and "coordinated" indicating that for data to be conducive to better practices and patient participation in the care, these data need to be linked to show a continuum of the processes. As early as 1978, Williamson had already touched on the crucial importance of the coordination by using the analogy of a film pellicule: that each frame capture a split second of the action, but that the entire episode is akin to a roll (pellicule) of film showing the progression of the individual frames. And the measurement of each step of the process (the individual film frames) were done using "accounting" indicators (Williamson, 1971; Williamson, 1978).

The past 25 years have seen a heavy emphasis on the measurement of hospital-based care. The qualities, or better, the performance indicators, have often dealt with what can be measured rather than what should be measured. The rationale is justifiable as a matter of course since the data were often available in type and in validity for certain performance aspects only leading to a tailoring of the indicators to these very data. Indeed, and staying within Donabedian's trilogy, the measures and indicators started by focusing on aspects of structures (e.g., availability of a quality committee and reports to the hospital Board) to processes (e,g., antibiotic prophylaxis protocol for surgery, waiting time in the Emergency Department) to some outcomes of care (e.g., in-hospital mortality, nosocomial infections, patient falls). The systematic focus on outcomes, under the rubric of adverse events, started in the early 1990, and

with the safety of care movement became a global health care imperative (Kohn, 2000; Hunt, 2013).

While the science of developing better indicators progressed to globally applicable measures of performance, it became clear that identifying the types of data necessary for a more complete and representative approach to measuring performance had to progress in tandem. Healthcare Information Technology (HIT) provided the medium and capability to capture a vast array of data about the diseases, patients and processes of care. Today, the shift from institution-centered measures to disease-centered and increasingly to patient-centered indicators is paving the path of the continuum of care. To illustrate, it became clear that a "successful" joint replacement was not to be only measured in lack of complications such as deep vein thrombosis, but in documenting how the patient had fared in regaining functional health status and quality of life, post discharge. Similarly, an early discharge from a hospital meant little about the efficiency of the care process if the patient was readmitted for complications. Unfortunately, many a hospital-based HIT were and still are impotent in capturing any readmissions if the patient was admitted to another hospital.

This is where Cloud Computing can be both a bridge and a path to the continuum of care and the realization of that roll of film. The groundbreaking promise of the Cloud is not in its ability to store practically limitless amounts of data, but to allow the harmonization among and synchronization across the data for each critical observation during the episode of care. That is the path we know Cloud Computing can achieve since many industries have already successfully achieved that synchronization. But since knowledge of healthcare outcomes is the critical dimension for evaluating the quality of care, Cloud Computing can also build the bridge between the processes of care and the outcomes. Evaluation, operationalised as the act of putting a value on the observed, is expected to be enhanced by Cloud Computing and its electronic and digital medium, hence

E-Valuation. And it can do so throughout the continuum of the care by incorporating aspects of care coordination with patient compliance and the associated changes in health status.

Will We Ever See a "Documentary" About the Patient Care Episode and How it Affected the Functional Status and the Quality of a Patient's Life?

That is the ultimate goal of performance evaluation and accountability. Yet, the promises of Cloud Computing are the promises of a tool when used appropriately and continuously. The critical variable remains the existing healthcare system structure (uncoordinated HIT platforms, providers not fully trained in electronic methods of data collection and sharing), the notoriously slow pace of change in any healthcare system, and the cost of re-engineering the health information collection and sharing systems. The good news is that the latter is of lesser magnitude than the existing HIT systems, since as stated at the outset, there are no new hardware or physical space requirements, nor the budgeting for extensive training of existing staff thanks to the intermediary role of Cloud vendors.

In conclusion, I cannot resist recalling an Armenian saying, dear to my grandfather *"If one puts a golden saddle on a donkey, it does not make it a horse."* The Cloud Computing is the golden saddle, but it depends on the healthcare organization and its professionals to first assess if the recipient system is a beast of burden or a Pegasus!

REFERENCES

Arah, O. A., Westery, G. P., Hurst, J., & Klazinga, N. S. (2006). A conceptual framework for the OECD Health Care Quality Indicators Project. *International Journal for Quality in Health Care*, (18): 5–13. doi:10.1093/intqhc/mzl024 PMID:16954510

Carr-Hill, R. A. (1992). The measurement of patient satisfaction. *Journal of Public Health Medicine*, *14*(3), 236–249. PMID:1419201

Carter, G. M., Newhouse, J. P., & Relles, D. A. (1990). *How Much Change in the Case Mix Index Is DRG Creep? (RAND Report #3826)*. Santa Barbara, CA: RAND.

Centers for Medicare & Medicaid Services. (2008). Retrieved July 20, 2013 from http://downloads.cms.gov/cmsgov/archived-downloads/SMDL/downloads/SMD073108.pdf

Coleman, E. A., Parry, C., Chalmers, S., & Min, S. J. (2006). The care transitions intervention: Results of a randomized controlled trial. *Archives of Internal Medicine*, *166*(17), 1822–1828. doi:10.1001/archinte.166.17.1822 PMID:17000937

Donabedian, A. (1980). *Exploration in Quality Assessment and Monitoring: The Definition of Quality and Approaches to its Management* (Vol. 1). Ann Arbor, MI: Health Administration Press.

Hofmarcher, M. M., Oxley, H., & Rusticelli, E. (2007). *Improved Health System Performance through better Care Coordination* (OECD Health Working Papers, No. 30). OECD Publishing.

Hunt, J. (2013). *The Silent Scandal of Patient Safety*. UK Government Speeches. Retrieved July 17, 2013 from https://www.gov.uk/government/speeches/the-silent-scandal-of-patient-safety

Ioannidis, J. P., Tarone, R., & McLaughlin, J. K. (2011). The false-positive to false-negative ratio in epidemiologic studies. *Epidemiology (Cambridge, Mass.)*, *22*(4), 450–456. doi:10.1097/EDE.0b013e31821b506e PMID:21490505

Kazandjian, V. A. (1991). Performance Indicators: Pointer-dogs in disguise- A commentary. *Journal of the American Medical Record Association*, *62*(9), 34–36. PMID:10112933

Kazandjian, V. A. (2002). *Accountability through Measurement: A Global Healthcare Imperative.* Milwaukee, WI: ASQ Quality Press.

Kazandjian, V. A. (2012). Quality is Not an Accident: The Planning for a Safe Journey through the Healthcare System. *International Journal of Reliable and Quality E-Healthcare, 1*(2), 1–11. doi:10.4018/ijrqeh.2012040101

Kazandjian, V. A., & Lied, T. (1999). *Healthcare Performance Measurement: Systems Design and Evaluation.* ASQC Quality Press.

Kazandjian, V. A., & Lipitz-Snyderman, A. (2010). HIT or Miss: The application of health care information technology to managing uncertainty in clinical decision making. *Journal of Evaluation in Clinical Practice, 17*(6), 1108–1113. PMID:20630010

Kohn, L. T., Corrigan, J. M., & Donaldson, M. S. (2000). *To err is human: building a safer health system.* Washington, DC: National Academy Press.

Lilford, R., Mohammed, M. A., Spiegelhalter, D., & Thomson, R. (2004). Use and misuse of process and outcome data in managing performance of acute medical care: Avoiding institutional stigma. *Lancet, 363,* 1147–1154. doi:10.1016/S0140-6736(04)15901-1 PMID:15064036

National Institute of Standards and Technology. (2010). Retrieved July 19, 2013 from http://healthcare.nist.gov/testing_infrastructure/

National Quality Forum. (2010). Retrieved July 19, 2013 from www.qualityforum.org/Projects/Measure_Harmonization.aspx

National Quality Forum. (2012). Retrieved July 17, 2013 from www.qualityforum.org/projects/care_coordination.aspx

Naylor, M. D., Brooten, D., Campbell, R., Jacobsen, B. S., Mezey, M. D., Pauly, M. V., & Schwartz, J. S. (1999). Comprehensive discharge planning and home follow-up of hospitalized elders: A randomized clinical trial. *Journal of the American Medical Association, 281*(7), 613–620. doi:10.1001/jama.281.7.613 PMID:10029122

O'Malle, A. S., Grossman, J. M., Kemper, N. M., & Pham, K. H. (2010). Are Electronic Medical Records Helpful for Care Coordination? Experiences of Physician Practices. *Journal of General Internal Medicine, 25*(3), 177–185. doi:10.1007/s11606-009-1195-2 PMID:20033621

Peikes, D., Chen, A., Schore, J., & Brown, R. (2009). Effects of Care Coordination on hospitalization, quality of care, and health care expenditures among Medicare beneficiaries 15 randomized trials. *Journal of the American Medical Association, 301*(6), 603–618. doi:10.1001/jama.2009.126 PMID:19211468

Rich, M. W., Beckman, V., Wittenberg, C., Leven, C. L., Freedland, K. E., & Carney, R. M. A. (1995). Multidisciplinary intervention to prevent the readmissions of elderly patients with congestive heart failure. *The New England Journal of Medicine, 333*(18), 1190–1195. doi:10.1056/NEJM199511023331806 PMID:7565975

Starr, P. (1982). *The social transformation of American medicine.* New York, NY: Basic Books.

Walker, K., Neuburger, J., Groene, O., Cromwell, D. A., & Vand der Mulen, J. (2013). Public Reporting of Surgeon outcomes: Low Numbers of Procedures Lead to False Complacency. *The Lancet.* http://dx.doi.org.10.1016/S0140-6736(13)61491-9

Wikipedia. (2010). Retrieved July 13, 2013 from http://hbr.org/2010/12/column-good-decisions-bad-outcomes/ar/1

Wikipedia. (2011). Retrieved July 22, 2013 from http://en.wikipedia.org/wiki/Diagnosis-related_group

Wikipedia. (2013a). Retrieved July 17, 2013 from http://en.wikipedia.org/wiki/Edwin_Hubble

Wikipedia. (2013b). Retrieved November 29, 2013 from http://en.wikipedia.org/wiki/Copernican_heliocentrism

Williamson, J. W. (1971). Evaluating quality of patient care: A strategy relating outcome and process assessment. *Journal of the American Medical Association, 218*(4), 564–569. doi:10.1001/jama.1971.03190170042009 PMID:5171005

Williamson, J. W. (1978). *Assessing and Improving Outcomes in Health Care: The Theory and Practice of Health Accounting*. Cambridge, MA: Ballinger.

Wright, D. D., & Kane, R. L. (1982). Predicting the outcome of primary care. *Medical Care, 20*(2), 180–187. doi:10.1097/00005650-198202000-00005 PMID:7078280

KEY TERMS AND DEFINITIONS

Care Coordination: The communication and synchronization of care processes across the traditional "silos" of health care that care delivered in "silos" (physician office, primary care center, acute care hospitals, rehabilitation centers, home care, Long Term Care, etc). Care coordination is based on the realization that without the concept of a continuum of services one cannot describe the true picture of care and caring for patients.

Cloud Computing: Cloud computing is a method capable of pooling theoretically unlimited amounts of data and storing them in a nonconventional or cloud way.

E-Valuation: Putting a value on the measured using reference points through the Cloud.

Evaluation: Putting a value on the measured, which à priori is a value-free statistic.

Measurement Appropriateness: An evaluation concept encompassing measurement accuracy, completeness, replicability, and representativeness.

Nosocomocentric: Performance measurement, interpretation and evaluation method focusing exclusively on hospital care.

Satisfaction: A self-reported evaluation of the gap between what was expected and what was observed.

Chapter 3
Big Data in Healthcare

Yiannis Koumpouros
Technological Educational Institute of Athens, Greece

ABSTRACT

The era of open data in healthcare is under way. The progress in technologies along with their adoption by the healthcare providers and the maturity of the citizens has brought the healthcare industry to the tipping point. An unprecedented amount of healthcare data is being generated today. This data comes from researchers, healthcare professionals and organizations, and patients. If we can harness this data, it can help us improve our understanding of disease and pinpoint new and improved therapies more efficiently than ever before. Big Data technologies are coming to market in a rapid way. The challenges, however, are still there due to fragmented systems and databases, semantic differences, legal barriers, and others. The hidden and unexploited knowledge is hindered by these barriers. The big data revolution promises a solution both to this situation, as well as to act as a catalyst to the viability of the healthcare systems. This is supported by the numerous efforts and explored in this chapter.

INTRODUCTION

Healthcare is the industry that first promotes and adopts as well the Information and Communication Technologies (ICTs) innovations (Koumpouros, 2012). The individualities and characteristics of healthcare develop a unique area that requires special care and attention in all aspects. Security, privacy, quality are only some of the concerns raised and studied for many years. Another characteristic of the healthcare domain is the production of big volumes of data and information produced every second. A patient, every time that passes through i.e. a hospital, leaves thousands of "footprints" in his/her visit. These "footprints" are either demographic data, historical data, illness related information, new or older exams, other relevant information, etc. The patient's pathway is therefore filled with a significant amount of data that have to be treated accordingly in order to have the desired outcome. On the other hand, the healthcare providers (physicians, hospitals, diagnostic centers, etc.) have to collect and store all this information for each and every patient in a proper manner and be able to reproduce and exploit it for achieving the best possible result. And this is only the one side of the coin. The same provider has also to collect and relate to each patient the appropriate data regarding his/her healthcare consumables, pharmaceutical therapy,

DOI: 10.4018/978-1-4666-6118-9.ch003

other special materials used, etc. Thinking of the number of patients multiplied by the volume of data, times the number of visits we can just imagine the huge volume of information exchanged in the healthcare industry.

Nowadays, living in the knowledge society, data and information are precious. Most of the newly established well-known successful businesses are based on these (i.e. Facebook, Google, etc.). Innovation and new business models arise, constantly utilizing data-driven discovery. One of the main needs is automatic knowledge extraction and exploitation of the produced data and information. This is true in the physical, biological and cyber world. The term Big Data is widely used recently in order to explain most of the above mentioned issues. There is no single formal definition of Big Data. However, most of them seem to coalesce around the "four Vs":

- **Volume:** The massive volumes of data produced, collected and exchanged.
- **Velocity:** The need for continuous and repeated analysis in real time.
- **Variety:** The many different forms of data that is difficult to integrate.
- **Veracity:** The issues related to uncertainty and trust.

A sea of data has been formed that becomes bigger and bigger every single day. The major problem faced in all industries and by all users is to "fish" (find and collect) the appropriate data out of this deep blue data-sea. A survival scenario is therefore needed to be rescued by this data flood. There is an immense opportunity therefore for forward-thinking leaders and researchers in every industry. To fully leverage the potential that exists within this storm of structured and unstructured data, organizations must quickly evaluate their business, needs and structure, improve and opti-

mize them targeting the right ICTs. Big data are there, but we have to find ways to exploit them and produce the desired valuable knowledge.

Healthcare is one of the leading sectors in the Big Data era. Producing enormous amounts of sensitive data every minute, healthcare has to find its way in order to utilize the generated valuable information. To this end, several methodologies and technologies have been introduced in order to deal with the Big Data. The need to derive predictive insights from this data for improved business operations and decision support is what drives Big Data analytics. This allows for predictive, contextual, agile, real-time exchange of information across silos. In the healthcare industry (Frost & Sullivan, 2012) introduced Advanced Health Analytics.

Regarding the healthcare's data we can adopt the aforementioned definition as follows:

- **Volume:** The volume of structured and unstructured health data is enormous, and becomes many times bigger if we could integrate all the data sources from the different healthcare providers.
- **Velocity:** There is an imperative need for real-time analysis of the generated data instead of working on key performance indicators. New algorithms and advanced analytics are therefore needed to conclude invaluable information.
- **Variety:** Today, health data comes from numerous heterogeneous sources and is extremely difficult to aggregate, compare or utilize them accordingly.
- **Veracity:** The unique characteristics of the data produced in the healthcare industry make them really sensitive. Data quality issues are a particular concern in healthcare. The relevance and meaningfulness of the data and their use for decision making

are some of the concepts lying under this characteristic. The main point of veracity is whether or not we can trust the collected data as well as its source to proceed further.

The objective of the chapter is to provide a clear view and understanding of the Big Data evolution that emerges nowadays in the healthcare sector. It presents the background of the healthcare industry and its unique characteristics from the point of view of all potential stakeholders (i.e. patients, healthcare professionals, pharmaceutical companies, etc.). A reference to the sector's needs arising from all involved parties follows, while revealing the great requirement for accumulated knowledge. This accumulated knowledge is extremely valuable in the specific domain, as documented by several real case scenarios and studies. The evolution of the Information and Communication Technologies can support effectively the changes that are taking place in the health industry. Big Data seems to be the key to achieve this objective. The chapter attempts a universal approach and mapping of the existing technologies and methodologies in the Big Data domain. The reader will acquire a holistic view of the technologies, tools and the market of Big Data and Big Data Analytics as well as their relation to Cloud computing. Specific paradigms by the adoption of such technologies in healthcare reveal the valuable benefits that derive. The latest research efforts worldwide and future prospects that rely on Big Data strengthen their usage and their potential in the market. Incorporating Big Data into healthcare clearly has the ability to transform the industry and improve quality of services. At the end, the reader will be in the position to understand the challenges and opportunities of Big Data in healthcare, and how they affect quality, while recognizing the key players and the most widely used technologies and methodologies in this domain.

BACKGROUND

Healthcare is one of the leading industries that face exponential growth in data volumes. The different stakeholders in healthcare interact with each other in a constant manner in order to fulfill their role (Figure 1).

All the above actors (as depicted in Figure 1) generate multiple sets of data in different formats. For example, following the patient's pathway we can collect volumes of information (personal and family history in a report format, x-rays, CTs, etc., as high resolution images, ultrasound, endoscopic exams in video format, demographic data collected in a database of a certain hospital, insurance coverage information stored in the company's database, and many others). Simultaneously, all this information is collected by different persons, in different locations, for different purposes and viewed by a different angle by each one of them. However, the physician in order to conclude in the best possible diagnosis and therapeutic scenario he/she needs as much accurate information as possible, which most of times this is not available.

Figure 1. The healthcare industry

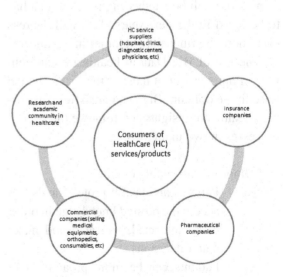

Evidence based medicine is another paradigm that is based on a large scale data sets and distributed information and has been proved a valuable "tool" for physicians (Sackett, Rosenberg, Gray, Haynes, & Richardson, 1996; Timmermans & Mauck, 2005; Elstein, 2004; Evidence-Based Medicine Working Group, 1992; Sniderman, LaChapelle, Rachon, & Furberg, 2013).

On the other hand, the case in healthcare is that in most hospitals, there are several systems within the network which are constantly changing. Vendors are also changing and typically they deliver proprietary software. Most of the times even in a single hospital the information systems (Electronic Medical Record, Laboratory Information System, Picture Archiving and Communication System, data produced in the Intensive Care Unit, prescriptions, etc.) cannot collaborate and function together.

The global financial crisis along with the proved failure of most of the health systems around the world urge for a rethinking and redesigning of the whole system or as an alternative for exploring new ways to improve it. The ageing of population (Department of Economic and Social Affairs, Population Division, 2007) (Department of Economic and Social Affairs, Population Division, 2001) will be another big problem that has to be faced in the next years. This will depress even more the financial outcomes in healthcare.

The use of Big Data in healthcare can help in the improvement of most of the issues, which arise in the domain. Big Data analytics can provide healthcare insights and improve the overall processes in two main axes:

1. Improve the quality of care
   a. Patients and health professionals can access the desired knowledge in order to be informed, educated and make better decisions.
   b. Patients can be more proactive and change their life-style on time so as to avoid any major problems.
   c. The collection and aggregation of data from different sources into one uniform and comparable way can provide insights about disease patterns, spread of illnesses, etc.
   d. The mining of multiple data sets from any possible source promotes research and accelerates the investigation of new therapies.
   e. Providers can identify high risk populations and act accordingly (i.e. offer preventive services).
   f. Will improve the patient experience.
   g. Personalize medicine and improve pharmaceutical drug design and clinical trials.
2. Improve efficiency and productivity
   a. Reduce the costs of healthcare by identifying the several "black holes" and the actors that may generate the highest costs for certain procedures.
   b. Monitor effectively the consumed resources (i.e. medications, consumables, etc.).
   c. Compare the productivity and effectiveness of health professionals against other peers.
   d. Will help to find and unearth any inconsistencies in the way the care is delivered.
   e. Facilitate evidence-based medicine and thus provide the tool to be able to pore through mountains of data.
   f. Overcome the problem of heterogeneous systems, infrastructures, databases, that have resulted in a complexity that is increasingly difficult and costly to manage.
   g. Reduce health system procurement costs by organizing them in the best possible way and through strategic sourcing.
   h. Optimize planning for healthcare capacity and workforce recruitment.

Quality of services sometimes opposes to system's financial viability. The more information is collected about a patient the best the outcome (diagnosis, treatment plan, etc.) is. On the other hand, the production of this information requires the consumption of more resources which lead to a higher cost of care. The following dilemma of course does not exist in the healthcare domain: "Which therapy or treatment is expensive enough for a patient?." The answer is only one "there is no expensive treatment even if it is based only on a limited hope for therapy." In other words, the human life is priceless. This is, however, a situation that has to be faced. As nowadays, the individualized treatments are cost-effective because they cannot be scalable or standardized. Moreover, the amount of digital content (big data that will join mobile and cloud as the next "must have" competency) around the globe, according to a forecast (Gens, 2011), totals more than 2.7 zettabytes (2.7 billion terabytes) in 2012, up 48% from 2011, and is estimated to reach 8 zettabytes by 2015. A main driving force to this, in the healthcare sector, is of course the explosion of image files both in quantity and quality, as well. (McKnight, Babineau, & Gahm, 2011) report that the data managed by a hospital will likely grow to 665 terabytes in 2015 (from 168 terabytes in 2010). Another main driver to this situation is the use of electronic health records from more hospitals. Moreover, the waves of immigrants around the world and the mobility of the population make decision making and planning for a treatment for a specific patient even harder. To this end, data are distributed across hospitals, diagnostic centers and physicians' offices, in different formats, using different architectures, in different locations or even countries.

Big Data analytics gives a great boost to leverage the benefits of the nowadays chaotic environment in healthcare. The opportunities opened are many. Using these new techniques it is easier to develop new therapies or products. This can be done by comparing and assessing similar products, designing the right criteria for clinical trials, utilizing predictive models on virtual trials, identifying the appropriate target group of patients for recruitment, as well as identifying contraindications. By analyzing epidemiology trends and treatment patterns, we can easily characterize patient population and identify disease management opportunities. By comparing the effectiveness of different models in healthcare delivery and services and assessing health economics, we can conclude in the best possible design of the next generation health system. The same analysis can be used to redesign or develop new healthcare solutions in order to optimize the use of hospitals and other healthcare infrastructures in combination with the latest telematics solutions and other IT technologies (i.e. telemedicine, e-health, etc.). Moreover, Big Data analytics can be very useful also to the insurance companies and providers in order to collate health data from the various sources and give appropriate incentives to "good" customers.

Another critical point is that all the different involved stakeholders in healthcare (i.e. clinicians, hospitals, insurance companies, etc.) analyze the collected data from a different point of views and have different or even opposing interests. This leads to the situation that a clear business case of how to use the Big Data is still missing.

Although the Big Data challenge is daunting, the opportunities ahead are compelling. Worldwide research and efforts are taking place to promote open data. This new approach of open data was inspired by the open source software movement. What actually "open data" means is that data should be freely available to everyone in order to use and republish them as they wish, without restrictions from copyright, patents or other mechanisms of control (CORDIS, n.d.). The challenges, legal, technical, social and market related are numerous, but the benefits are significant and immediately transferred to citizens, patients and the health system as well.

A recent study (Manyika, et al., 2011) reveals the opportunities to generate significant financial value in the US healthcare sector by big data applications. Healthcare costs are continuously increasing (Figure 2).

In most OECD countries, health spending grew enough between 2000 and 2009. The average share of GDP allocated to health across OECD countries climbed to 9.6% up from 7.8% in 2000. This ratio dropped slightly to 9.5% of GDP in 2010. This decrease appeared mainly due to the economic crises. Many countries, including Greece, Iceland, Estonia and Ireland implemented measures to reduce government health spending as part of broader efforts to reduce large budgetary deficits and public debt. In 2010, the share of GDP allocated to health was the largest by far in the United States (17.6%), followed by the Netherlands (12.0%), France and Germany (11.6%). A more detailed analysis of the public expenditure on health in OECD is presented in Figure 3.

As depicted in the above figure, reductions in public spending on health in many OECD countries have typically been made across the board. Pharmaceutical spending has been a prime target.

Many countries decided to cut their spending on prevention and public health. Some governments also tried to contain the growth in hospital spending by cutting wages, reducing hospital staff and beds, and increasing co-payments for patients.

The rising costs of healthcare along with the global aging urge for a solution. According to (Department of Economic and Social Affairs, Population Division, 2001) the average of the population being older than 60 years is steadily growing from 10% to 21% by 2050. EU will be the first one to face such conditions. This, combined with the changes in lifestyle (more smoking, physical inactivity, etc.), is expected to increase the risk of chronic diseases and thus more healthcare resources will be needed. Another significant issue is that almost all the healthcare systems have been designed many years ago, focusing basically on the treatment of a disease. Nowadays, it seems that monitoring, preventing and new forms of healthcare delivery are required for a viable health system. Home care and tele-health can be used to ease the healthcare burden from hospitals and other facilities. Being able to analyze the produced datasets may improve this

Figure 2. Public and private expenditure on health (% of GDP, 2010 or latest available year)
Source: OECD

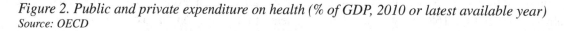
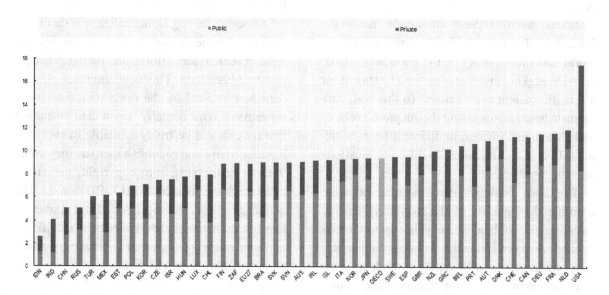

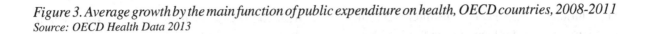

Figure 3. Average growth by the main function of public expenditure on health, OECD countries, 2008-2011
Source: *OECD Health Data 2013*

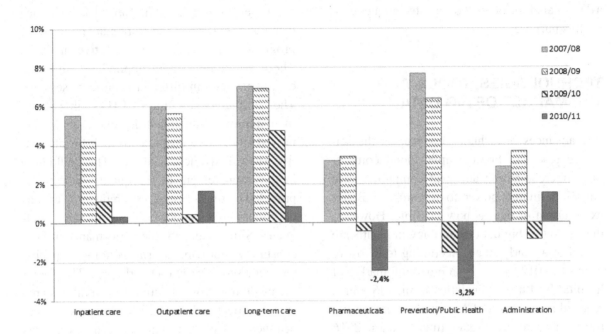

situation. According to a study (Manyika, et al., 2011), it is estimated that in ten years' time is possible for the US government to capture more than $300 billion annually in new value, with two thirds of that in the form of reductions to national healthcare expenditures. Moreover, it predicts data explosion that reaches 35 zettabytes by 2020 with a 44-fold increase from 2009.

Another report (MarketsAndMarkets, 2011) predicts that the world healthcare IT market is expected to grow from $99.6 billion in 2010 to $162.2 billion in 2015, at a CAGR of 10.2% from 2010 to 2015. There is an obvious need to cut healthcare costs, enhance clinical and administrative workflow of hospitals, as well as to have an error-free, efficient healthcare delivery, on time and at the point of need. Several initiatives have been taken for the adoption of IT healthcare solutions globally. Electronic Medical Records is expected to the highest growing market with a

CAGR of 16.7% from 2010 to 2015. Computerized physician order entry (CPOE) is also growing fast with a CAGR of 16.5% from 2010 to 2015. Point of care information systems, specialty care information systems (cardiovascular information systems, oncology information systems), and surgical and intensive care information systems are expected to have a combined CAGR of 15.1% from 2010 to 2015.

Preventive healthcare, remote patient monitoring, telemedicine, and home healthcare is the future. Healthcare IT solutions are used as a cost effective solution for augmenting the clinical and administrative workflow of healthcare providers. As the need for error-free personalized diagnosis is emerging, PACS, EMR and CPOE are adopted by many health providers. These solutions, however, produce big numbers of datasets. So, the problem is how to exploit these mountains of datasets effectively. Big Data analytics provide low cost

IT solutions, while facing the interoperability problems, and is the focus of the top healthcare IT solution providers. The next section presents a deeper analysis of the tools and techniques used for this purpose.

TECHNOLOGIES, TOOLS, AND THE MARKET OF BIG DATA

The advances in technologies support the scientific research. For example, cloud computing, supercomputing and grid computing gave almost unlimited power to researchers. Better exploitation of data is now possible. However, the market of big data technology in healthcare is still in an early stage. According to (Frost & Sullivan, 2012), there is an emerging market of hospital health data analytics in the US which reached a saturation of 14% with an increasing trend. The same study guesstimates that in 2016 almost every US hospital (95%) will use Electronic Health Records (EHRs). In respect to 2011, this represents an increase of 171% and a CAGR of 22%. The adoption of EHRs by the hospitals is of course a prerequisite as well as a driving force to the adoption of health data analytics. This leads to investments in EHRs prior investing in health data analytics. It is estimated that in 2016 50% of the US hospitals will have implemented data analytics solutions in comparison to 10% that exists in 2011, concluding in a 400% increase and a CAGR of 37.9%.

Another study (*Healthcare IT Q1 2013 Funding and M&A Report*, n.d.) reveals that venture capital (VC) in the health IT sector continue to accelerate. In the first quarter of 2013, the number of venture capital investments in health IT firms jumped to 104 from 51 in the previous quarter and raised $493 million, compared with $1.2 billion for all of last year (Terry, 2013). Most of the VCs invest in mobile health, telehealth, personal health, social health, and scheduling, rating, etc. It appears that a huge market exists in consumer-focused health solutions utilizing big data.

The increased use of electronic health records is further forcing growth. New data analytics techniques emerge to the market able to provide progressive real-time and predictive analysis. These solutions can be applied on disparate data distributed in different healthcare settings. The continuous adoption of EHRs, along with their improved functionalities and their almost proved ROI, drive hospitals to look for alternative ways of advanced analytics. This could help in the improvement of the quality of services provided by the hospitals, cost reduction, etc., as traditional tools cannot face the emerging challenges. Simultaneously, the performance of IT is constantly improving in terms of storage capacity, computation power and network speed. This allows the modeling and simulation in several research areas in order to achieve targeted and personalized healthcare. Collaboration between researchers and among peers is now possible, which enhance the scientific excellence and competition in the industry. GÉANT is a living paradigm. This is the largest communication network for educators and researchers, running in multi-gigabit speed. This network is widely adopted and connects 34 National Research and Education Networks (NRENs). It connects over 50 million users at 10,000 institutions across Europe. Operating at speeds of up to 500Gbps it offers unrivalled geographical coverage. GÉANT remains the most advanced research network in the world (GÉANT, n.d.). E-science grids are devoted to subjects such as bioinformatics and many others. EGEE (Enabling Grids for E-sciencE) is another paradigm that operates a multi-disciplinary grid with over 80,000 computers on 300 sites in 50 countries worldwide. It is obvious that data necessitates new tools and methods. To this end several efforts are made to build supercomputer infrastructures in order to meet the wide socio-economic challenges in the healthcare sector.

Data-centric science is mainly focused to improve access to scientific information. Europe formed in 2002 the ESFRI (European Strategy Forum on Research Infrastructures) initiative at the behest of the European Council as a strategic instrument to develop the scientific integration of Europe and to strengthen its international outreach. It aims to achieve peta-flop performance by 2010 and move towards exa-scale computing in 2020. Since then, research and development in software and hardware was intensified so as to implement supercomputers (European Commission, 2013).

According to (Frost & Sullivan, 2012; Manyika, et al., 2011; Groves, Kayyali, Knott, & Van Kuiken, 2013) the market of big data is continuously increasing. Since 2010 more than 200 companies working in the health data analytics sector have emerged. This market becomes highly competitive, and companies present innovative solutions to deal with big data. This justifies the fact that healthcare is technology-intensive and technology-driven. Big Data is about both infrastructures and analytics, as well. The Big Data ecosystem comprises several discrete areas (NASSCOM, 2012). The Big Data storage and management include the required storage infrastructures, as well as the continuous monitoring, administration and management of the data. After this has been achieved specific tools and technologies are used for Big Data analytics purposes, in order to generate insight from the collected data. In the next step, the insights have to work in business intelligence of the organization using the appropriate applications. Finally, the Big Data framework has to be embedded into the organization's business intelligence infrastructure. It is obvious that before someone decides on what solution to use he/she has to lay out strategies that lead to the deployment of a sophisticated big data platform and analytics. One option could be to find a solution that allows the different products to be integrated together into one concrete platform. However, several solutions exist today with dif-

ferent advantages and disadvantage each one. As in the rest software industry, the Big Data domain has also two main paths for someone to follow: the open source solution or the commercial one. A brief presentation of the major solutions provided nowadays follows.

One of the well-known companies, IBM, developed and provides the Info Sphere big data platform. Some of its key products are: (i) the Hadoop-based analytics (able to analyze any data type across server clusters), (ii) the data warehouse for improved operational insights, and (iii) a specific stream computing software for real time analysis of huge volumes of streaming data. It also includes a set of supporting applications services – such as accelerators, and application development, integration, information, governance and system management tools – as well as business intelligence and analytic tools (IBM).

Open platforms have some critical privileges. They allow users to use any type of tool they need for data analytics. The main problem in open source solutions, however, is that they require a lot of work to make them ready to use. The final platform, in either case, has to handle data ingestion, processing, and store and querying capabilities, as well as the deployment of data analytics. Apache Hadoop framework was a pioneer in this category, followed by NoSQL databases such as Cassandra and MongoDB that can handle massive amounts of data. Hadoop is an open-source framework to support applications that enable analysis of xetabyte data (both structured and unstructured). Red Hat tries to exploit big data through a platform (Red Hat Enterprise Linux) that allows capturing, processing, and integrating of big data. This platform comprises the Red Hat software-defined storage, a middleware and the OpenStack hybrid cloud.

Cisco, presented the Cisco Common Big Data Platform that integrates big data with traditional applications and systems. This platform relies on

Cisco's Unified Computing System, and integrates compute, networking and storage capabilities onto a single integrated platform, and works with a slew of vendor offerings, including Datasta, Hortonworks, Cloudera, Oracle, SAP Hanna, Intel, and Pivotal.

Some of the most common platforms and vendors for Big Data are presented below. Cloudera, 10Gen and Amazon are the ones that supported at the beginning Hadoop and NoSQL technologies. Several others appeared recently, like Hortonworks, Platfora, Amazon, DataStax, 10Gen, CouchBase and Neo Technologies. These are the major ones that support NoSQL solutions (i.e. MongoDB, DynamoDB, CouchBase, Cassandra and Neo4j). Among the pioneers in Big Data analytics, we could include Hadapt, Platfora, Splunk, Datameer, and Karmasphere.

10Gen is the developer and commercial support provider of the open source MongoDB. MongoDB seems to lead the way of the NoSQL databases. Some others that are widely used include HBase, Cassandra, DynamoDB, Neo Technologies and CouchBase. MongoDB is capable to handle semi-structured information encoded in JSON (Java Script Object Notation), XML or any other document formats. As stated in the official site, MongoDB is an open-source document database that provides high performance, high availability, and automatic scaling (www.mongodb.com). MongoDB has several exceptional features (i.e. it is flexible, easy to use and offers great speed) and characteristics (i.e. automatic sharding, support of the JSON data model, use of indexes for efficient resolution of queries, text search facility, aggregation operations that examine and perform calculations on the data sets, a connector for Hadoop, etc). CouchBase (www.couchbase.com) is one of the main competitors of MongoDB, using a flexible JSON model in order for users to be able to modify their applications without the constraints of a fixed database schema. As stated, sub millisecond, high-throughput reads and writes are included in its pros, along with its

easy scalability and support of topology changes with no downtime. Consistent, high throughput makes possible to serve more users with fewer servers, and data and workload are equally spread across all servers. Couchbase Server requires no fixed schema and, therefore, records can have a different structure, and can be changed any time, without modification to other documents in the used database.

Amazon is a leading big data services providers and users. One of its main products is the Elastic MapReduce (EMR) which is based on Hadoop. Amazon Web Services (AWS) recently included the option to choose MapR M7 on its EMR, and announced two more services (a NoSQL database service called Amazon DynamoDB and a data warehousing service called Amazon RedShift). MapR M7 is a high performance platform, which, according to the official site (aws.amazon.com), delivers ease of use, dependability and performance for HBase and Hadoop. Amazon EMR makes it easy to provision and manage Hadoop in the AWS Cloud. M7 can scale horizontally to thousands of nodes per cluster. The MapR platform supports a broad set of mission-critical and real-time production uses and claims to bring dependability, ease of use and high speeds to Hadoop, NoSQL, database and streaming applications in one unified big data platform. Amazon Redshift is a petabyte-scale data warehouse service for analyzing the organization's data using the existing business intelligence tools. It can work for datasets from a few hundred gigabytes to a petabyte or more. It uses columnar storage technology and parallelizing and distributing queries across multiple nodes for fast queries. In 2007, Amazon developed Dynamo, a NoSQL database, where DynamoDB is based on. This was initially used to run big parts of its massive consumer Website. DynamoDB is a NoSQL database service in order to store and retrieve any amount of data, which can serve any request traffic. Using local secondary indexes, it adds flexibility to the queries. It also utilizes cryptographic methods to securely authenticate users and prevent unauthorized data access. The three services are Amazon's flagship, along with the Elastic Compute Cloud (Amazon EC2) which is a Web service for resizable compute capacity in the cloud.

Cloudera (www.cloudera.com) is the leader provider of Apache Hadoop-based software and services. It enables data driven enterprises to easily derive business value from all their structured and unstructured data. Hadoop is an open source software that couples elastic and versatile distributed storage with parallel processing of varied, multi-structured data using industry standard servers. It is also supported by a wide range of useful tools and applications. However, Hadoop's main disadvantage is the slow, batch-oriented nature of MapReduce processing. In order to overcome this problem, Cloudera introduced another product, called Impala. This is an interactive-speed SQL query engine that runs on the existing Hadoop infrastructure. According to its developers, Cloudera Impala is a real-time query engine that allows users to query data stored in Hadoop Distributed File System (HDFS) and Apache HBase database tables in seconds via an SQL interface. It leverages the metadata, SQL syntax, ODBC driver, and Hue user interface from Hive (http://hive.apache.org). Impala is not dependent on MapReduce, and uses its own processing framework to execute queries. Thus, it should have improved performance and enables interactive data exploration. The Enterprise edition of Cloudera (http://www.cloudera.com/content/cloudera/en/products-and-services/cloudera-enterprise.html) provides insights through iterative, real-time queries and serving; usability with low-latency query engines and powerful SQL-based interfaces and ODBC/JDBC connectors; discovery and governance by using common metadata and security frameworks; data fidelity and optimization resulting from local data and compute proximity that brings analysis to "on read" data where needed.

Datameer (www.datameer.com) provides an analytics platform based on Hadoop. It uses the Hadoop Distributed File System (HDFS) to import, export, store and manage data. It utilizes a spreadsheet-style data analysis environment and a development-and-authoring environment for creating dashboards and data visualizations with ease. There are many analytics functions implemented to make predictive analysis even easier. Datameer facilitates custom MapReduce jobs using concepts like the Datameer Data Links and the REST API.

DataStax (www.datastax.com) is promoting the Apache Cassandra database as an alternative to Oracle. The Apache Cassandra open source NoSQL database provides scalability and high availability. It can manage large amounts of structured, semi-structured, and unstructured data across multiple data centers and the cloud. As stated in its official site, some of Cassandra's data model features include column indexes with the performance of log-structured updates, strong support for denormalization and materialized views, and powerful built-in caching. DataStax Enterprise can combine Apache Cassandra with Apache Hadoop analytics and Apache Solr search for a more powerful result. It is designed to use Hadoop for analyzing line-of-business data stored in a distributed Cassandra database cluster. It separates analytic operations from transactional workloads in order no conflict to exist between each other for data management resources. Apache Solr, being a Java-based open source search engine, provides robust full-text search and hit highlighting, faceted search (i.e. by manufacturer, brand, type, size, or price), appropriate document handling (i.e. HTML, Word, PDF, RTF, email, .zip files, and audio and video formats), as well as geospatial search (i.e. combining location information with data, etc.). Moreover, the use of the Cassandra Query Language (CQL) along with the JDBC driver provided for CQL enables SQL-like querying and ODBC-like data access.

Hadapt (www.hadapt.com) provides an Adaptive Analytical Platform, able to support native implementation of SQL to the Apache Hadoop open-source project. It combines the Hadoop's architecture with a hybrid storage layer that incorporates a relational data store. Thus, it allows interactive SQL-based analysis of the collected data sets. It enables all types of analysis, like SQL, MapReduce, and full text search. In its Hadapt 2.0 version, it offers the Hadapt Interactive Query for SQL-based analysis, the Hadapt Development Kit (HDK) for custom analytics, as well as integration with Tableau software for visual analytics (www. tableausoftware.com).

Hortonworks (www.hortonworks.com) founded in 2011 as a spinoff of Yahoo!. It released the Hortonworks Data Platform (HDP) that is an entirely open source Apache Hadoop data platform. Its latest product, HDP 2.0, contains all the services in order someone to be able to implement Hadoop, and packages all the recent innovations around YARN, HDFS2, Security and High Availability. Apache Hadoop YARN separates the resource management and processing components. YARN is actually the acronym of "Yet Another Resource Negotiator" and achieves to overcome the dependency of Hadoop based environments on MapReduce. This way it effectively makes Hadoop a general purpose multi use platform that enables all kind of processing (stream, online, interactive, etc.). Moreover, the Hortonworks Data Platform provides a new version in order to be able to integrate with the Microsoft Windows Server.

Karmasphere (www.karmasphere.com) provides a homonym solution/platform for reporting, analyzing and visualizing Big Data based on Hadoop. It can be installed on a physical or virtual Linux server and cloud server environments and can be accessed via any Web browser. It also works with Amazon Web Services and Rackspace and supports most of the Hadoop distributions, including Cloudera, Hortonworks and MapR. Karmasphere offers the Karmasphere Studio (a graphical environment for developers) and the Karmasphere Analyst (a collaborative workspace for data analysts) for Hadoop. It runs on Hive,

providing entry to structured, semi-structured or even unstructured data through SQL-like languages (i.e. HQL-Hive Query Language, or others). The Karmasphere Studio Analyst, apart from the above, includes full syntax checking and detailed diagnostics, enhanced schema browser with Hive specific support, fully JDBC4 compliant. Karmasphere is also integrating with Cloudera Impala framework for faster queries and real time interactive analysis.

MapR (www.mapr.com) released the MapR M7 solution for NoSQL and Apache Hadoop applications. MapR M7 provides scale, strong consistency, reliability and continuous low latency. MapR uses the Network File System (NFS) instead of HDFS in order to enhance the availability and reliability. Using the NFS it supports faster data streaming utilizing messaging software from Informatica. M7 delivers high-performance Hadoop and HBase (Apache HBase is the original Hadoop database) in one deployment. According to its official provided information, M7 may have two times faster performance than HBase running on standard Hadoop architectures. This is based on the fact that there are no region servers, additional processes, or any redundant layer between the application and the data residing in the cluster.

Neo Technology (www.neotechnology.com) introduced Neo4j (www.neo4j.com), an open source graph database technology. According to (Robinson, Webber, & Eifrem, 2013) a graph database is an online database management system that exposes a graph data model. Graph databases are built for use with transactional (OLTP) systems. Some graph databases use native graph storage that is optimized and designed for storing and managing graphs, while some others serialize the graph data into conditional databases (i.e. relational, object-oriented, etc). The Neo4j uses a Property Graph for storing data. The main features of a Property Graph are: (i) each vertex and edge have some properties, (ii) multiple properties may be associated with each vertex and/or edge, (iii) the edges have directionality, (iv) there may exist several types of relationships between vertices. Graph databases, unlike relational databases, are designed to store interconnected data that is not purely hierarchic. This gives them more flexibility because they do not require intermediate indexing at every run. Moreover, graph databases can depict more accurately real world situations (i.e. social networking, relationships, behaviors, etc.). Neo4j is also suitable to manage and query social graphs, as well as for recommendation engine apps. It can handle the transaction processing or analytics, and it is compatible with most development platforms, like Java, Groovy, Ruby, Python, etc.

Platfora (www.platfora.com) announced the release of its new platform (Platfora Big Data Analytics 3.0) designed to empower the fact-based enterprise. It will be available in the first quarter of 2014 and will provide the tools to analyze big data collected from multiple touch points and surfacing insights and facts in a short time. Platfora Big Data Analytics 3.0 runs on top of Hadoop. This new platform utilizes the Platfora Event Series Analytics in order to allow the analysis of the behavior and actions of the targeted group independently of the mean used (i.e. Web clicks, mobile application access, call center records, etc.) over a single timeline. The Platfora Iterative Segmentation can easily create segments of customers by the behaviors they had exhibited when they interact with the organizations' touch point, like the patterns of Web visits and tweets that occurred before a purchase, their demographic data, etc. Thus, it can provide the requested insights. The Platfora Entity-Centric Data Catalog allows the organization of raw data around any entity (i.e. customers, products, etc.) and provides access to relevant analysis, segments, and data. Platfora Dynamic Lenses allow access to all the raw data stored in Hadoop, while organizing them into an optimized structure for analysis. According to the latest announcement, Platfora Big Data Analytics 3.0 will have several enhanced features for Self Service Visualiza-

tions, Collaboration and Sharing, Security, Data Acceleration, and Ecosystem Integration (open interoperability with the Hadoop ecosystem and support for Cloudera, Pivotal, Amazon EMR, Hortonworks and MapR).

Splunk (www.splunk.com) produced the homonymous software for searching, monitoring, and analyzing machine-generated big data, via a Web-style interface. It captures, indexes and correlates real-time data (structured and unstructured) in a searchable repository from which it can generate appropriate graphs, reports, alerts, dashboards and visualizations. Splunk employs SPL (a search processing language) for managing machine-generated big data. SPL was designed by Splunk for use with Splunk software. Its syntax was originally based upon the Unix pipeline and SQL. The scope of SPL includes data searching, filtering, modification, manipulation, insertion, and deletion. The wide adoption of Hadoop drove Splunk to provide Hunk. Hunk enables the detection of patterns while it can easily find anomalies across terabytes or petabytes of raw data in Hadoop without specialized skill sets, fixed schemas, etc. Hunk allows access data in remote Hadoop clusters via virtual indexes while using the Splunk Processing Language to analyze the stored data utilizing the full power of Hadoop. Hunk enables the process of large amounts of any kind of data and can run combined reports on Hadoop data and data from the Splunk Enterprise indexes.

FUTURE RESEARCH DIRECTIONS

Healthcare organizations are increasingly turning to new architectures and tools to help make sense of the Big Data phenomenon. Many companies arose in this new era of Big Data to provide solutions for better and immediate access to statistics and figures that are effectively translated into actionable insight aiding organizations in clinical and financial decision making. The storage and effective and timely processing of the massive data sets in healthcare are one of the biggest challenges in order all involved interested parties (i.e. stakeholders, managers, doctors, researchers, etc.) get the required insights.

Big Data technologies, as presented in the previous sections, evolve every day. Many new companies are trying to leverage prior experiences to provide a better solution. The paradigms in the healthcare sector for both the need as well as the adoption of Big Data solutions are numerous. Some of them are presented in the following paragraphs.

The National Institute of Health (NIH) in USA is highly involved in Big Data by its BD2K program. The NIH Big Data to Knowledge (BD2K) initiative is focused on biomedical research. It tries to capitalize the huge datasets generated by the research communities of biomedical scientists (http://bd2k.nih.gov). BD2K aims to combine the strengths of government agencies, private organizations and stakeholders in the research community to develop new software, methods, tools, standards and competencies that will enhance the use of the produced biomedical Big Data. As biomedical research is highly data-intensive it generates complex, multidimensional, structured and unstructured data. However, today the ability to exploit them efficiently is very limited. There is a great need to locate, integrate and analyze them accordingly apart from the place or the way they were produced. To this end, BD2K formed Centers of Excellence in order to develop new approaches and tools to overcome these obstacles. These Centers form a BD2K Center Consortium that may collaborate with other centers in the consortium or with other domestic or international efforts in Big Data science. These Centers work in developing tools and solutions that will be generic in order to be able to meet the needs of the broader biomedical research community. As stated in its official site, the main challenges to using biomedical Big Data include locating data and software tools, gaining access to data and software tools,

standardizing data and metadata, extending policies and practices for data and software sharing, organizing, managing, and processing biomedical Big Data, developing new methods for analyzing biomedical Big Data, and training researchers for analyzing and for designing tools for analyzing biomedical Big Data effectively. The overall scope of B2K is, therefore: (i) to provide access to shareable biomedical data, (ii) to develop appropriate algorithms and tools for data processing, storage, analysis, integration, and visualization, (iii) to develop appropriate protection mechanisms for privacy and intellectual property, (iv) to have researchers skilled in the science of Big Data and elevate their general competencies in data usage and analysis.

The tranSMART Foundation (http://transmart-foundation.org/) is a global non for profit organization that offers the tranSMART knowledge management platform. This open-source and open-data community promote translational biomedical research by enabling effective sharing, integration, standardization and analysis of heterogeneous data from collaborative research across organizations, pharmaceutical and biotechnology companies and individuals in the world. Translational research requires massive amounts of research data in order to ignite scientific discoveries. Thus, it designed a repository of open-access, open-source data to enable collaboration across disciplines, specialties worldwide. This repository offers access to clinical observations, patient demographics, clinical trial outcomes, adverse events, metabolism data, etc. tranSMART makes possible for scientists to assess their research outcomes (i.e. any correlations between phenotypic and genetic data, etc.) based on the available published literature. It is designed for any interested party involved in the development and discovery of new drugs. According to the official information, through its usage scientists can: (1) look for multiple data sets for potential drug targets, pathways and biomarkers, (2) compare data from proteomics, metabolomics and other "omics" studies, (3) contrast patterns of gene expression in healthy and diseased individuals and in human tissue samples, (4) investigate correlations between genotype and phenotype in a clinical trial data, (5) mine pre-clinical data for insights into the biology of human disease, (6) study genetic and environmental factors involved in human disease, (7) display data visually using a graphical interface, as well as (8) stratify clinical data into molecular subtypes of a specific disease.

The Institute for Health Metrics and Evaluation (IHME) (http://www.healthmetricsandevaluation.org) is an independent research center at the University of Washington, USA. It developed and maintains a data catalog named Global Health Data Exchange (GHDx) in order to gather large amounts of distributed datasets from around the globe related to health. Anyone interested in the improvement of the health of the world's population can use GHDx in order to find and share relevant information. It collects health measurement data, from different sources, including surveys, vital statistics, disease registries, hospital records, censuses, etc. Thus, it tries to evaluate strategies, to measure health status, to find ways to maximize health system impact, and to develop innovative measurement systems. The gathered information is freely available to policymakers and other interested parties, in order to make appropriate decisions. GHDx delivers citations to encourage appropriate acknowledgement of data owners' contributions. The current version of GHDx uses the Drupal 7 (https://drupal.org/drupal-7.0) open source content management system and the Apache SOLR (http://lucene.apache.org/solr/) for searching.

Healthx (www.healthx.com) developed and provides a cloud-based solution for healthcare companies. It is focused on enrollments, claims management and business intelligence. Nowadays, many payers across the USA use this Web-based platform for their members and providers. The Healthx client base is comprised of Medicare, Medicaid, TPAs, commercial health plans and commercial carriers. Healthx converts data brought from disparate systems in order to be imported and displayed to the Web portal. It gathers and process several data, like claims, prescription information, physicians, explanation of benefits, payments, disease management, etc., using the Apache Cassandra with Hadoop.

The National Human Genome Research Institute (NHGRI) is an organization that funds research large-scale efforts around USA that investigate critical genomic information. The participating research centers are organized into a wider network, being monitored by NGHRI and LSAC (Large-Scale Genome Sequencing and Analysis Centers), which acts as scientific advisors. NHGRI for several years tracked the costs associated with DNA sequencing for benchmarking purposes and for assessing improvements in DNA sequencing technologies and for establishing the DNA sequencing capacity of the NHGRI Genome Sequencing Program (GSP). According to (Wetterstrand, 2013) the cost to sequence one genome reaches almost US$10,000 (as of 2001) using standard technology, generating about 100GB of compressed data. Using Apache Hadoop the aforementioned cost of sequencing a genome became less than US$100 (Healthcare & Life Sciences). This gives an impression of the remarkable improvements in DNA sequencing technologies and data-production pipelines in recent years along with the exploitation of the Big Data technologies.

Explorys (www.explorys.com) is a spinoff from Cleveland Clinic addressing issues related to exploit the power of Big Data in the improvement of the delivered care. It offers a cloud-based performance management platform and one of the largest healthcare databases worldwide. This database contains a huge amount of records related to medical, financial and operational data from diverse systems. The Explorys EPM (Enterprise Performance Management) Suite is a set of Software-as-a-Service (SaaS) based applications enabling rapid population management, performance measurement, and effective engagement and outreach to patients and providers. Among its clients (14 integrated healthcare systems) are Cleveland Clinic, Trinity Health, St. Joseph Health System, MedStar and Catholic Health Partners. The company relies on the services of Cloudera. Explorys solution allows providers to search across patient populations and care venues to help identify disease trends, to coordinate rules-driven patient registries, and view performance metrics. As stated by its founders, the collaboration with the Catholic Health Partners in Cincinnati, helped increase pneumonia vaccination rates by 14%, breast cancer screenings by 13% and increased HbA1c testing of diabetics by 3%. Another study (Kaelber, Foster, Gilder, Love, & Jain, 2012) reports that with the right clinical research informatics tools and EHR data, some types of very large cohort studies can be completed with minimal resources. This research used Explorys to look at EHR-generated patient data from 959,030 patients from several different healthcare systems. This helped clinicians pinpoint, in only 125 hours, those most at risk for blood clots in the extremities and lungs. The same project would take years to perform using traditional research methods.

Humedica (www.humedica.com) provides a cloud-based solution for healthcare providers, life sciences and research organizations to make better decisions by getting insights from several distributed unstructured data. It has one of the most complete clinical databases (data from 25 million patients from 30 states), which allows retrospective analysis and comparison against a large sample of the population. The collected data cover most of the desired areas (ambulatory patients and inpatients) along the time in order to be able to generate longitudinal view of patient care. Humedica gathers clinical data related to medications, lab results, vital signs, demographics, hospitalizations and outpatient visits, physician notes, etc. Some paradigms of using Humedica's analytics platform include the Cornerstone Health Care and Mid-Hudson Medical Group. Cornerstone Health Care is a group of

more than 300 physicians and other health professionals representing a wide range of specialties in more than 80 locations in North Carolina. It tries to achieve patient centered medical home (PCMH) recognition from the National Committee for Quality Assurance (NCQA). Cornerstone uses Humedica MinedShare clinical analytics to direct outreach to at-risk diabetes patients and identifies the clinical cohort for follow-up. Mid-Hudson Medical Group, on the other hand, is a 125-physician medical group with sixteen locations in the Hudson River Valley in New York. This group offers its patients team-based care led by a personal physician who provides continuous and coordinated care throughout a patient's lifetime to optimize health outcomes. In order to advance its PCMH initiative, Mid-Hudson requires more information relevant to the comparable care process and outcomes against best practices. To this end, it used Humedica MinedShare to support population health management and continuous quality and cost improvement for all the patients it serves, including those managed through its PCMH. It achieved to gain access to comprehensive longitudinal data which is continually refreshed from its electronic medical record and other systems. As a result, it extracted data on its diabetic patients to determine which patients had a HgA1c reading above 7% on their last visit and who had not been seen by a physician for the last 12 months. Mid-Hudson achieved level 3 recognition by the National Committee on Quality (NCQA).

The University of Pittsburgh Medical Center (UPMC) invested US$100 million to create a comprehensive data warehouse that brings together almost 3.2 petabytes of data from more than 200 sources across UPMC, UPMC Health Plan and other affiliated entities (UPMC'S 'Big Data' Technology Shows Promise in Breast Cancer Research, 2013). For this purpose, it utilizes a combination of the Oracle Exadata Database Machine (a high-performance database platform), the Oracle Enterprise Healthcare Analytics and Oracle Health Sciences Network, other Oracle tools

(Oracle Fusion Analytics, etc.), the IBM's Cognos software for business intelligence and financial management, the Informatica's data integration platform and the dbMotion's SOA-based interoperability platform (to integrate patient records from healthcare organizations and health information exchanges). One of its main objectives is related to patients with kidney problems that may lead to kidney failure. To this end, it monitors any minor changes in the lab results. Another effort concerns patients with breast cancer, where it tries to identify the most appropriate treatment plan based on the available genetic and clinical information of each specific patient. Researchers are using the analytics tools on the already collected both genomic and EHR data for those patients. The University of California runs a US$10.5 million project for a data repository of cancer genomes that holds biomedical information in order to allow scientists to characterize molecules of cancer. University of Ontario Institute of Technology (UOIT) uses IBM big data solutions to gather and analyze real-time data from medical monitors, alerting hospital staff to potential health problems before patients demonstrate clinical signs of infection or other issues. Harvard Medical School researchers use IBM's big data tools for drug safety and effectiveness studies. Another effort is the joint venture of IBM and Memorial Sloan-Kettering Cancer Center (MSKCC) in New York in order to use the Watson supercomputer's big data capabilities to help oncologists provide better care for MSKCC patients. Watson combines natural language processing, machine learning, and hypothesis generation and evaluation to provide responses. Watson can analyze millions of pages of unstructured text in patient records and the medical literature to locate the most relevant answers to diagnostic and treatment-related questions. It can find meaning to clinicians' questions and relates them to the theoretical background by using temporal, statistical paraphrasing and geospatial algorithms. The vision of this collaboration is to build an intelligence engine to provide specific

diagnostic test and treatment recommendations. The University of Texas MD Anderson Cancer Center is also based on Watson's capabilities to help patients by providing the tools to physicians to discover insights from the hospital's valuable patient and research databases.

A European funded project called NEWMEDS-Novel Methods leading to New Medications in Depression and Schizophrenia (http://www.newmeds-europe.com), researches new methods for drug development related to depression and schizophrenia. It set up one of the largest collaboration projects with parties involved both from the academic and the industry sectors as well. Partners from nineteen institutions from nine European countries, as well as Iceland, Switzerland Israel, are participating in this project. Among the partners are included the most well-known biopharmaceutical companies, like AstraZeneca, Eli Lilly, Janssen Pharmaceutica, Lundbeck A/S, Novartis, Orion, Pfizer, Roche, Servier and Abbott. Some of the academic institutions involved are the King's College London, the Karolinska Institutet, the University of Cambridge, the Central Institute of Mental Health (Mannheim), the Instituto de Investigaciones Biomedicas de Barcelona, the University of Manchester and the Bar Ilan University. Additionally, two pharmaceutical small and medium-sized enterprises, deCODE (Reykjavik) and Psynova (Cambridge) contribute to the project along with a GABO:mi, a German SME. The project in order to research new drugs for schizophrenia focuses on developing new animal models, utilizing appropriate behavioral tests and brain recordings. To this end, it investigates also analysis techniques to apply PET and fMRI brain imaging to drug development. It also examines the influence of the latest genetic findings (duplication and deletion or changes in genes) on the response to various drugs in order to finally produce personalized drugs.

PharmaCog (http://www.imi.europa.eu/content/pharma-cog), another research project, tries to leverage big data to accelerate drug discovery for

Alzheimer's disease. It comprises a consortium of 33 partners coming from 10 different EU member states. It is funded by IMI (Innovative Medicines Initiative) with a budget of 27.7 million euros. IMI is based on a PPP (public-private partnership) model between the EU and the EFPIA. The project investigates the prediction of cognitive properties of new potential drugs for neurodegenerative diseases in early clinical development. On the same domain, the Global CEO Initiative (CEOi) on Alzheimer's Disease (an organization of private-sector companies who have joined together to research solutions for the fight against Alzheimer's disease) has joined forces with Sage Bionetworks and IBM to initiate "AD#1," a computational challenge to better identify predictors of AD risk in pre-clinical populations. To achieve this, it utilizes "gamifying" and "crowdsourcing" data analysis. AD#1 exploits data from the Alzheimer's Disease Neuroimaging Initiative (ADNI), including cognitive, imaging, biological and whole genome sequencing data on cohorts of volunteers with dementia.

CancerLinQ is another project run by the American Society of Clinical Oncology in order to gain knowledge through all clinical trials in the specific health domain. CancerLinQ is a learning computer network that tries to unlock huge quantities of information on patient experiences that are now lost to distributed files and servers. It is foreseen to be funded with US$80 million over the next five years.

The National Institute of Health (NIH), IBM Research, Sutter Health and Geisinger Health System are funded with US2$ million to develop new methods for early detection of heart disease. This will be achieved by exploiting the latest data analytics technologies. This collaboration researches practical and cost-effective early detection methods to use in primary care practices with an electronic health record system.

The development of new treatments depends highly on the participation of patients in clinical trials. Thus, Novartis, Pfizer and Eli Lilly collaborate to provide a platform in order to improve access to information about clinical trials. This platform will provide detailed and patient-friendly information about the trials, including a machine readable "target health profile" to improve the ability of healthcare software to match individual health profiles to applicable clinical trials. The platform is planned to be launched in 2014. The partners will enrich at the beginning the formed database with 50 clinical research studies.

Stanford University, SAP and the National Center for Tumor Diseases in Heidelberg are using SAP's HANA Healthcare Platform in order to deliver to all interesting parties (researchers, hospitals, pharmaceutical and insurance companies) biological, lifestyle and clinical data for real-time personalized medicine. In this way, they try to offer personalized prevention and treatment, as well as to map drug development more precisely to the biology of disease. SAP HANA is a memory-based storage made from SAP. Its characteristic is to organize a system optimized to analysis tasks, such as OLAP. The same platform is used by the Stanford School of Medicine to achieve real-time analytics in order to uncover genetic variants that contribute to population health and disease. Stanford's work is intended to lead to new treatments targeted for autism and cardiovascular disease. The National Center for Tumor Diseases (NCT) in Heidelberg, Germany is also utilizing SAP HANA Healthcare Platform in a Medical Explorer tool, in order researchers to analyze clinical and genomic data in real-time for patient breakthroughs in cancer diagnostics and treatment options.

The State University of New York in collaboration with the Rutgers University and other industry partners run a Quantitative Tissue Assessment project. This project tries to research new methods for the effective evaluation of spleen, liver and other similar diseases (i.e. sarcopenia, etc). A private company, BioClinica, supports the Center for Dynamic Data Analytics (CDDA) in order to design innovative algorithms for the assessment of new therapies that will directly affect the health of the ageing population.

A city network in Columbia district, DC-NET, along with the Capital Area Advanced Research and Education Network (CAAREN) and the Medical Center's Division of Genomic Medicine, both owned by the George Washington University, are working on the next-generation genomic sequencing. They are trying to exploit the power of the terabytes of the gathered raw data. This way, based on the appropriate analysis of the collected DNA and RNA sequences, it will be possible to identify biomarkers and new potential targets for therapies of i.e. heart diseases or cancer.

Another effort tries to leverage big data to predict pandemics before they occur. To achieve this, Office of Science and Technology Policy's (OSTP) is promoting collaboration between communities of interest from government departments and agencies, non-governmental organizations, academic institutions, industry partners and others. To this end, it exploits appropriate sensor technologies and observation networks to enhance identification and fusion of new and existing data sets, to enable development of big data analytics.

MedRed and BT are working together to create the MedRed BT Health Cloud (MBHC) in order to enable the integration and dissemination of open health data.

CONCLUSION

We are living in the era of data, where huge amounts of data sets emerge from sensors, social networks, mobile devices, enterprise software solutions, data centers, etc. In 2012 about 2.5 quintillion bytes of data were created on a daily basis. Nowadays, two of the biggest problems are to find and locate the right data and to be able to process them accordingly. The storage, processing and management of these mountains of datasets are becoming extremely challenging both for the interesting end users and technologies

as well. This situation is currently referred as "Big Data," meaning that it is difficult for someone to unlock the valuable information out of these data volumes. The significance of Big Data in all sectors is obvious. Recently, the White House Office of Science and Technology Policy (OSTP) and Networking and Information Technology R&D program (NITRD), recognizing the values of Big Data, announced numerous collaboration projects in order to enhance the private sector's interest on federal data. The "Data to Knowledge Action" event pointed the niche target markets that vary from economics to medicine and from linguistics to geointelligence. These new projects follow the Obama Administration's Big Data Initiative, announced in March 2012. An estimated 4.4 million jobs are being created between now and 2015 to support big-data projects. In the same way, the EU current health information system recognized that it does not always provide a consistently high-quality and fully comparable information. Thus, the EU is heading to better health reporting mechanisms. It also produced guidelines and recommendations for improving quality and access to health information (European Commission, Improving health reporting mechanisms, 2013).

The Big Data phenomenon is widely faced in the healthcare sector where mountains of data are generated every second from multiple sources (electronic medical records, medical exams, prescriptions, medical histories, public health data, research activities in genes and other domains, etc.) and in different formats (video, images, text, audio), both structured and unstructured. Moreover, the produced data in healthcare differ in volume, velocity, variety and value. This is aligned with the definition of Big Data, as reported at the beginning of this chapter.

On the other hand, policy makers in every level (physicians, ministry of health, and others) covet a tool that would give them the possibility to have a clear and in real-time view of the current situation in order to take informative-wised decisions. As the outcome of every effort depends on the input (data) and its accuracy, the need for timely aggregation, retrieval and analysis is becoming mandatory. While the potential benefits of Big Data are obvious, and some initial efforts have already been appeared with significant results, there remain many technical challenges that must be addressed to fully realize this potential. The heterogeneity of the data, along with the scalability and timeliness issues are some of the major ones. As volume increases, the longer it takes to analyze them. Not to mention another huge concern in healthcare, the privacy and security issues. According to the HIPAA-HITECH regulation any healthcare provider has to carefully choose its business associate (a third party cloud provider) in order to avoid any awkward circumstances. Cloud providers have to sign therefore a business associate agreement and follow the HIPAA-HITECH regulations. Cloud computing is one of the technological achievements that helped a lot in managing Big Data, due to their nature and the fact that they require massively scalable compute and data storage. The Cloud Computing model is a perfect match for big data since cloud computing provides unlimited resources on demand. This technology allows the aggregation of multiple disparate workloads with varying performance goals into very large clusters. This kind of sharing of course requires new ways of determining how to execute data processing jobs in a cost-effective way, as well as dealing with possible system failures and other important issues.

Cloud computing services are increasingly moving into the future in health care. According to market researchers (www.marketsandmarkets. com) the healthcare industry will invest US$5.4 billion in Cloud Computing by 2017. Another study (MarketsAndMarkets, 2012), that analyzes the major market drivers, restraints, and opportunities in North America, Europe, Asia, and Rest of the World, estimates that last year at least 4% of total healthcare are changed into the cloud. This

year, this share is expected to grow to 20.5%. The cloud market provides three main discrete service models: SaaS (Software as a Service), IaaS (Infrastructure as a Service) and PaaS (Platform as a Service). Nowadays, SaaS is dominating the healthcare market. Some paradigms of SaaS providers are the CareCloud, Carestream Health, Merge Healthcare, from the USA and the GE Healthcare, and Agfa Healthcare form the EU.

Electronic Health Records (EHRs) and Electronic Medical Records (EMRs) are now prevalent. In the USA the Health Information Technology for Economic and Clinical Health Act – HITECH offers financial incentives to healthcare providers who demonstrate meaningful use of Electronic Health Records ("HITECH Act," n.d.). To keep up with all of this data, many healthcare providers are making the switch to cloud computing. When healthcare providers choose to leverage the cloud, they are able to store data on servers using the latest technology, and only pay for the computing power that they use. The ability to leverage huge amounts of computing power and data unlocks great potential. However, healthcare providers must be sure that all protected health information (PHI) is stored and handled according to the Health Insurance Portability and Accountability Act – HIPAA (http://www.hhs.gov/ocr/privacy/) and the recent HITECH Act.

Big Data technology promises many opportunities, like hunting for useful data, immediate use, better insights, handling any data structure, etc. Moreover, social medicine, mobile medicine, evidence based medicine are only some of the healthcare opportunities of the next years that can benefit by the use of Big Data applications. In any case, the huge amount of data have to be efficiently processed in a way that does not compromise end-users' Quality of Service (QoS). Even though technology progress every day, this remains a real challenge for most of the provided solutions. There is a great need therefore for new techniques to be developed. However, cloud computing solutions and platforms, like the Microsoft Azure, Amazon, and others, along with the achievements in machine learning algorithms, the semantic Web, the QoS optimization techniques, etc., promise a quick step forward to the Big Analytics improvement.

In order to confront with the huge problem of ageing and the rising costs of the health systems new solutions are needed. There is not only the need for collecting, aggregating and securing health data, but also for processing and apply them accordingly to improve treatment and the provided health services in general (i.e. cost reduction, etc.). In this direction, the PCMH (Patient-Centered Medical Home) model tries to deal with the rising costs of healthcare delivery, proposing a new way to deliver primary care. PCMH focuses on the engagement of patients in their own health and the coordination of care for those facing chronic health problems. Incorporating Big Data into healthcare clearly has the ability to transform the industry. In the future, a patient will likely be able to walk into a hospital and receive customized care immediately. The appropriate information will "follow" the patient wherever and whenever needed. Diagnoses will be faster and far more accurate thanks to the vast amount of data mining that will advance medical research. Personalized medicines and early monitoring and diagnosis are also expected due to the appropriate analysis of big data. The application of Big Data techniques and technologies can provide valuable help in most of the healthcare domains, such as the effectiveness of research activities, the clinical decision support, the clinical operation intelligence, the public health analytics, the patients' engagement, and others. Concluding, we can support the idea that by exploiting Big Data and Cloud Computing technologies and techniques there is a great potential to manage healthcare data in the ecosystem while reducing costs and complexities.

REFERENCES

CORDIS. (n.d.). Big data at your service. In *Digital agenda for Europe*. European Commission. Retrieved November 26, 2013, from http://ec.europa.eu/digital-agenda/en/news/big-data-your-service

Department of Economic and Social Affairs. Population Division. (2001). World Population Ageing: 1950-2050. New York: United Nations.

Department of Economic and Social Affairs. Population Division. (2007). World Population Ageing 2007. New York: United Nations.

Elstein, A. S. (2004). On the origins and development of evidence-based medicine and medical decision making. *Inflammation Research*, *53*(Suppl 2), S184–S189. doi:10.1007/s00011-004-0357-2 PMID:15338074

European Commission. (2013a). ESFRI. *Research & Innovation Infrastructures*. Retrieved December 1, 2013, from http://ec.europa.eu/research/infrastructures/index_en.cfm?pg=esfri

European Commission. (2013b). Improving health reporting mechanisms. *Public Health*. Retrieved December 22, 2013, from http://ec.europa.eu/health/data_collection/tools/mechanisms/index_en.htm

Evidence-Based Medicine Working Group. (1992). Evidence-based medicine: A new approach to teaching the practice of medicine. *Journal of the American Medical Association*, *268*(17), 2420–2425. doi:10.1001/jama.1992.03490170092032 PMID:1404801

Frost & Sullivan. (2012). *U.S. Hospital Health Data Analytics Market: Growing EHR Adoption Fuels A New Era in Analytics*. Retrieved November 18, 2013, from http://www.frost.com/c/10046/sublib/display-report.do?id=NA03-01-00-00-00

GÉANT. (n.d.). Retrieved December 5, 2013, from http://www.geant.net

Gens, F. (2011). Top 10 Predictions. In IDC Predictions 2012: Competing for 2020. IDC.

Groves, P., Kayyali, B., Knott, D., & Van Kuiken, S. (2013). *The 'big data' revolution in healthcare: Accelerating value and innovation*. McKinsey & Company.

Healthcare & Life Sciences. (n.d.). Retrieved November 28, 2013, from http://www.cloudera. com/content/cloudera/en/solutions/industries/ healthcare-life-sciences.html

Healthcare IT Q1 2013 Funding and M&A Report. (n.d.). MERCOM Capital Group.

HITECH. Act, (n.d.). *HealthIT.gov*. Retrieved November 18, 2013, from http://www.healthit.gov/ policy-researchers-implementers/hitech-act-0

IBM. (n.d.). *InfoSphere Platform*. Retrieved December 4, 2013, from http://www-01.ibm.com/ software/data/infosphere/

Kaelber, D. C., Foster, W., Gilder, J., Love, T. E., & Jain, A. K. (2012). Patient characteristics associated with venous thromboembolic events: a cohort study using pooled electronic health record data. *Journal of the American Medical Informatics Association*, *19*(6), 965–972. doi:10.1136/ amiajnl-2011-000782 PMID:22759621

Koumpouros, I. (2012). *Information and Communication Technologies & Society*. Athens, Greece: New Technologies Publications.

Manyika, J., Chui, M., Brown, B., Bughin, J., Dobbs, R., & Roxburgh, C. et al. (2011). *Big data: The next frontier for innovation, competition, and productivity*. McKinsey Global Institute.

MarketsAndMarkets. (2011). *World Healthcare IT (Provider and Payor) Market - Clinical (EMR, PACS, RIS, CPOE, LIS) & Non-Clinical (RCM, Billing, Claims) Information systems Trends, opportunities & Forecast till 2015*. Retrieved November 28, 2013, from http://www.market-sandmarkets.com/Market-Reports/healthcare-information-technology-market-136.html

MarketsAndMarkets. (2012). *Healthcare Cloud Computing (Clinical, EMR, SaaS, Private, Public, Hybrid) Market – Global Trends, Challenges, Opportunities & Forecasts (2012 – 2017)*. Retrieved November 28, 2013, from http://www. marketsandmarkets.com/Market-Reports/cloud-computing-healthcare-market-347.html

McKnight, J., Babineau, B., & Gahm, J. (2011). *North American Health Care Provider Information Market Size & Forecast*. ESG-Enterprise Strategy Group.

NASSCOM. (2012). *Big Data: The Next Big Thing*. New Delhi, India: NASSCOM.

Robinson, I., Webber, J., & Eifrem, E. (2013). *Graph Databases*. Sebastopol, CA: O'Reilly.

Sackett, D., Rosenberg, W., Gray, J., Haynes, R., & Richardson, W. (1996). Evidence based medicine: What it is and what it isn't. *BMJ (Clinical Research Ed.)*, *312*(7023), 71–72. doi:10.1136/ bmj.312.7023.71 PMID:8555924

Sniderman, A. D., LaChapelle, K. J., Rachon, N. A., & Furberg, C. D. (2013). The Nessecity for Clinical Reasoning in the Era of Evidence-Based Medicine. *Mayo Clinic Proceedings*, *88*(10), 1108–1114. doi:10.1016/j.mayocp.2013.07.012 PMID:24079680

Terry, K. (2013). *Health IT Startups Make VCs Swoon*. Retrieved December 2, 2013, from http://www.informationweek.com/health-care/leadership/health-it-startups-make-vcs-swoon/240147655

Timmermans, S., & Mauck, A. (2005). The promises and pitfalls of evidence-based medicine. *Health Affairs*, 24(1), 18–28. doi:10.1377/hlthaff.24.1.18 PMID:15647212

UPMC'S 'Big Data' Technology Shows Promise in Breast Cancer Research. (2013, June 19). Retrieved November 22, 2013, from http://www.upmc.com/media/newsreleases/2013/pages/upmc-big-data-tech-breast-cancer-research.aspx

Wetterstrand, K. (2013). *DNA Sequencing Costs*. National Human Genome Reserach Institute. Retrieved December 1, 2013, from: http://www.genome.gov/sequencingcosts/

KEY TERMS AND DEFINITIONS

Big Data Analytics: Alternative ways and technologies in order to gain value from big data. Big Data Analytics deals with the need to derive predictive and actionable insights from the stored big data for improved business operations and better decision making. It implies the use of automated algorithms for advanced analytics to analyze large datasets in order to solve problems that can reveal data-driven insights. Big Data Analytics may be used for example to identify specific patterns, to produce forecasts, or to reveal insights hidden previously by data too costly to process and not possible to perform without such technical means.

Big Data: Datasets that exceed the ability and processing capacity of conventional database software tools and systems to capture, store, manage, and analyze them. The term signifies exceptionally large bundles of semi-structured or unstructured data in multiple formats, which pose problems for traditional storage and analytical platforms.

Cloud Computing: An alternative way to obtain and implement technology services, infrastructure and applications. It is the delivery of IT infrastructure assets, such as server capacity and software applications, over the Internet on a utility basis. It is considered the next generation's computer infrastructure. The term is a form of virtualization that shares infrastructures (i.e. server hardware and data storage, networks, etc) and/or software (to access applications and services) remotely located at the service provider data center. In this way, it offers access to a shared pool of computing resources. Thus, the customers just hire the services they need, which implies economical savings for the management of the electronic resources and could therefore almost eliminate the need for companies to have an IT department. According to the needs of the customer, these resources are highly scalable and are provided as a service through a network, often offered at lower prices than those required to install on one's own computers. Instead of buying and maintaining servers and applications someone can gain access to the desired resource power and functionalities at a size that reflects the needs of the organization today. These services and applications are paid according to their usage.

Infrastructure-as-a-Service (IaaS): One of the service models of cloud computing. IaaS provides access to computing resource in a virtualized environment over a network (i.e. the Internet). The computing infrastructure provided comprises of servers, hardware, networking components (i.e. bandwidth, IP addresses, etc.), virtual server space, etc. The end users typically have to pay on a per-use basis according to how much resource they use. Infrastructure is dynamically scalable as needed. The hardware resources are pulled from a multitude of servers and networks usually distributed across numerous data centers, all of which the cloud provider is responsible for maintaining. Thus, the complexities and expenses of managing the underlying hardware are outsourced to the cloud provider.

Open Data: The notion that data should be available to anyone without any restrictions. These data can be used, shared, reused, republished and distributed without any copyright or other barrier.

Personalized Care: A holistic approach that considers physical, mental, and spiritual well-being.

Personalized Medicine: The science of individualized prevention and therapy.

Platform-as-a-Service (PaaS): A sub-category of cloud computing. It refers to an application platform or environment provided as a service in order the customer to be able to build, deploy and manage custom applications. PaaS services are hosted in the cloud and accessed by users via their Web browser. The platform comprises of the needed software (i.e., operating system, middleware and other required software, protocol stack, etc.) that enables applications to run on the cloud. Security, management, scalability and other issues related to the PaaS are taken care by the provider. The end users can subscribe to preconfigured features that exactly meet their own needs.

Service Quality and Availability: One of the most critical considerations when choosing cloud computer services. It is related to the service level agreements (SLAs) that are offered by providers. SLA is an agreement or a "contract" between the service provider and the customer. This details a common understanding about services, priorities, responsibilities, guarantees, and warranties and specifies the levels of availability, serviceability, performance, etc. In practice, the term SLA is sometimes used to refer to the contracted delivery time (of the service or performance), where in most situations is between 99% to 99.9% uptime availability, meaning that an interruption of the provided services from 8.7 to 87 hours/year could be presented without any penalty.

Software-as-a-Service (SaaS): End-user applications provided as a service, not stored on local devices or on customer enterprise resources. It describes any cloud service where consumers are able to access software applications over the Internet. The needed software runs in data centers owned by the SaaS service providers. SaaS most often is sold on a monthly or annual subscription. The end users access the SaaS via a Web browser, and are not involved in running the software or hardware related to the application.

Chapter 4
Wiki–Health:
A Big Data Platform for Health Sensor Data Management

Yang Li
Imperial College London, UK

Li Guo
University of Central Lancashire, UK

Chao Wu
Imperial College London, UK

Chun-Hsiang Lee
Imperial College London, UK

Yike Guo
Imperial College London, UK

ABSTRACT

Quickly evolving modern technologies such as cloud computing, Internet of things, and intelligent data analysis have created great opportunities for better living. The authors visualize the role these technological innovations will play in the healthcare sector as they spearhead a shift in focus from offering better healthcare services only to people with problems to helping everyone achieve a healthier lifestyle. In this chapter, the authors first discuss the existing and potential barriers followed by an in-depth demonstration of a service platform named Wiki-Health that takes advantage of cloud computing and Internet of things for personal well-being data management. It is a social platform, which is designed and implemented for data-driven and context-specific discovery of citizen communities in the areas of health, fitness, and well-being. At the end of the chapter, the authors analyse a case study to illustrate how the Wiki-Health platform can be used to serve a real world personal health training application.

INTRODUCTION

Recent developments in modern technologies such as cloud computing, wearable sensor devices and big data have significantly impacted people's daily lives, and offer great potential for an Internet-wide, people-centric ecosystem that will considerably extend human capabilities in acquiring, consuming and sharing personal information. In particular, these new capabilities will address a vital aspect of living – the practice and implementation of personal health care and well-being. Humans are actually becoming super organisms with support from this ecosystem. For

DOI: 10.4018/978-1-4666-6118-9.ch004

instance, with the latest mobile devices we will be able to see and review our personal health status through backend analysis services using continuously collected data from those wearable body sensors; we could make complex decisions using our computing-aided "brains."

People have always been searching for the most accurate information to empower themselves for a healthier life. Social media has changed the nature of interactions among people and organizations. According to PwC's consumer survey of 1,060 U.S. adults, about one-third of consumers are using the social space as a natural forum for health discussions (Admins, 2011). We share our lives and thoughts with the social community or the public. We depend on our networks to help us make many decisions. We seek connection and access. However, the health and wellbeing industry has been slow to embrace social media due to often insurmountable issues of privacy, data protection, but now is beginning to see the benefits.

Meanwhile, the rapidly growing popularity of smartphones and tablets globally has created many opportunities for growth within the health care and wellbeing sector. These devices provide new ways to gather information, both manually and automatically, over wide areas. Many current smart phones come with a number of embedded sensors such as microphones, cameras, gyroscopes, accelerometers, compasses, proximity sensors, GPS and ambient light. The newer generation of professional wearable medical sensors can easily connect with the smart phones and transfer the sensing results directly. This has provided a more efficient and convenient way to collect personal health information like blood pressure, oxygen saturation, blood glucose level, pulse, Electrocardiogram (ECG), Electroencephalogram (EEG) and electrocardiography (EKG). A future in which we are all equipped with devices and sensors that passively collect and interpret our health and activity data is not too far off. The scale and richness of mobile sensor data being collected and analysed are rapidly expanding. This massive growth creates both data manageability and collaboration challenges.

Traditional sensor network systems increasingly face many issues and challenges regarding their communication and resources management including data storage, data query, data processing, privacy control, and data sharing. The emergence of cloud computing is seen as a remedy for these issues and challenges. Implementing cloud computing technologies appropriately can help healthcare providers improve the quality of medical services and the efficiency of operations, share information, improve collaboration, and manage expenditures.

In this chapter, we present our work – a service platform named Wiki-Health that takes advantage of cloud computing and Internet of things for personal well-being data management. Wiki-Health is a social platform for data-driven and context-specific discovery of citizen communities in the areas of health, fitness and well-being. Wiki-Health provides new ways of storing, tagging, retrieving, analysing, comparing and searching health sensor data. It makes health-related knowledge discovery available to individual users at a massive scale. Wiki-Health is based on the concept of the wiki and mass collaboration, according to which aggregated user-contributed content is collectively curated to produce unprecedented volumes of knowledge in a multi-perspective and socially engaging way. One of key research points for Wiki-Health is to deliver novel algorithms for data-driven community discovery in large health datasets.

BACKGROUND

The growing global popularity of smartphones and tablets has resulted in new ways to gather information, both manually and automatically by means of an array of embedded sensors. Professional wearable biosensors easily connect to smart phones and can track significant physiological parameters. Existing wearable fitness sensors such as the ("Fitbit,"), ("Zephyr,"), ("NIKE+ FUEL-BAND,") and ("Withings,") have already been on the market for a while, letting users automatically collect data on their walking steps, activity levels, food intake, blood pressure and heart rate. The result is a more efficient and convenient way of collecting information about person's health and well-being. However, there is currently no standardized format for these data and it is difficult for users to reclaim, manage or remix that data in their preferred ways. From the provider's point of view, such massive growth of these big health sensor data creates both data manageability and collaboration challenges.

People have always been searching for the best knowledge to empower themselves for a healthier life. We share our lives and thoughts with the social community or the public through social media and enjoy connection with and access to a wide variety of sources for personal fulfilment. Despite often insurmountable issues of privacy and data protection facing the health and wellbeing industry, the benefits of embracing social media have begun to emerge. Today more and more patients are participating actively in all aspects of personal health information. At Sarasota Memorial Hospital (Fulmer) in Florida patients "tweet" their doctors when they have questions about their care. At Chicago's Rush University Medical Centre physicians keep connected with patients through Facebook and Twitter so that they are notified of their recovery Rush University Medical Center (Liu, Han, Zhong, Han, & He, 2009). During a real-time brain surgery in March 2009, doctors at Detroit's Henry Ford Hospital answered questions via "tweets," broadcasting to more than 6000 followers Detroit's Henry Ford Hospital (Schmuck & Haskin, 2002). Other healthcare connector sites include PatientsLikeMe.com, which incorporates patient education with online peer-to-peer communication, using information sharing

about conditions, symptoms, and treatments to link patients together. Doximity (Held, Wolfe, & Crowder, 1974) and Sermo (Berkelaar, Eikland, & Notebaert, 2004) are Web and mobile based social networking platforms where physicians can share insights about medicine and specific cases. People are now becoming very interested in using data-sharing social platforms for healthcare to communicate with other people with common needs and to learn more about themselves.

Sensor networks (Akyildiz, Su, Sankarasubramaniam, & Cayirci, 2002a, 2002b; Pantelopoulos & Bourbakis, 2010; Xu, 2002) provide infrastructure through which we obtain data about the physical environment, social systems and health data by means of sensing devices. They are being widely used in areas like healthcare and fitness. There are many existing sensor network systems such as Aurora (Abadi et al., 2003) and COUGAR (Yao & Gehrke, 2002) focused on storing and querying the sensor data. The Discovery Net system (AlSairafi et al., 2003) provides an example in which different users can develop their own data collection workflows specifying how sensor data can be processed before storing it in a centralized data warehouse. It also enabled them to develop analysis workflows for integrating the data with data collected from other data sources. Users of the system could thus share the same data and also derive new views and analysis results through sharing. The CitySense (Murty et al., 2008) project deployed a system allowing the general public to provide feedback on pollutants using mobile devices. This demonstrates how the system supports enriching the information from the users and allowing users to comment on the operation and trustworthiness of the sensors.

The aforementioned systems support a limited form of collaboration while operating on a fixed set of sensors. However, the drive toward the pervasive use of mobile and the rising adoption of sensing devices enabling everyone to collect data at any time or place is leading to a torrent of sensor data. Traditional sensor network systems face many challenges in managing this volume of data, and the emergence of cloud computing is seen as a remedy.

Cloud computing has been widely discussed in the past few years as it shows great potential to shape the development, maintenance and distribution of both computing hardware and software resources. With this computing paradigm, the actual provision of resources is only a concern at run time for specific application requirements, and so is the case for software resources as they can also be used in an on demand and pay-per-use fashion. Cloud storage takes sharing hardware one step further: unlike local storage, cloud storage relieves end users of the task of upgrading their storage devices constantly. Cloud storage services enable inexpensive, secure, fast, reliable and highly scalable data storage solutions over the Internet. Many enterprises and personal users with limited budgets and IT resources are now outsourcing storage to cloud storage service providers, in an attempt to leverage the manifold benefits associated with cloud services. Leading cloud storage vendors, such as Amazon S3 (Amazon) and Google Cloud Storage (Google), provide clients with highly available, low cost and pay-as-you-go based cloud storage services with no upfront cost. A variety of companies have outsourced at least a portion of their storage infrastructure to Amazon AWS, including SmugMug (Szalay, Bunn, Gray, Foster, & Raicu, 2006), ElephantDrive ("ElephantDrive,"), Jungle Disk ("AWS Case Study: Jungle Disk,") and 37signals(Szalay et al., 2006). Amazon announced that as of June, 2012 it holds more than a trillion objects, and the service has so far been growing exponentially (Amazon, 2012). Even so, many enterprises and scientists are still unable to shift into the cloud environment due to privacy, data protection and vendor lock-in issues. An Amazon S3 storage service outage in 2008 left many businesses that rely on the service offline

for several hours and resulted in the permanent loss of customer data (aDam LeVenthaL, 2008; Kim, Gurumurthi, & Sivasubramaniam, 2006) - an incident that led many to question the S3's "secret" architecture.

Implementing cloud computing technologies appropriately can aid healthcare providers in improving the quality of medical services and the efficiency of operations, sharing information, improving collaboration, and managing expenditures. Sensor-Cloud infrastructure (Yuriyama & Kushida, 2010) enables the sensor management capability of cloud computing by virtualizing a physical sensor. Commercial sensor network platforms such as Xively ("Xively,")(formerly known as Cosm) have taken off in recent years. They provide an online scalable sensor data management platform that allows developers to connect devices and applications through a Web-based API. However, neither the architecture nor the implementation of this type of platform has yet been made public. There is still a need for a scalable data storage and high-performance computing infrastructure for efficiently storing, processing and sharing of health sensor data as well as collaboration to allow users to create, share, reuse and remix data analysis models. The knowledge of how to provide such big data sensor management service for system architecture, storage, querying and sharing mechanisms, data labelling and analysis frameworks as well as how to utilise all the resources, reduce storage consumption and costs, and improve the latency analytics against high velocity streaming data, remains untapped.

In order to examine the knowledge behind healthcare data management services and tackle the above challenges we propose the Wiki-Health platform, a cloud-based health data management system that provides new ways of storing, tagging, retrieving, analysing and searching health sensor data. In this chapter, we discuss the system design and implementation of Wiki-Health in detail. We also demonstrate a brain training prototype for ADHD (Barkley, 1997) as a use case that will help us show the proof of concept of our platform.

SYSTEM DESIGN

There is an exponential increase in the number of sensors and devices giving us data, from the personal level to environmental and global levels. These sensors and devices have their own characteristics such as sample rate, number of channels and power consumption value. These characteristics imply that such sensor data is multi-resolution. For example, most EEG devices have very high temporal resolution, typically at sampling rates between 250 and 2000 Hz in clinical and research settings, while GPS location readings are taken

and stored every few minutes. When such data are aggregated and/or integrated for use in a new application the user is very quickly faced with the multi-resolution nature of that data. Moreover, users of the data will have their own conceptual multi-scale levels of abstraction in their models. To address all these issues, we designed Wiki-Health not only to solve the problems of managing and storing such high volume, velocity and variety of data, but to offer support tools for users to create application and analysis so they can make use of the data whilst lowering the complexity of dealing with its diversity.

Figure 1 illustrates the overall architecture of Wiki-Health. The Wiki-Health system is designed in three logical layers: application, query and analysis, and data storage.

Figure 1. The architecture of Wiki-Health system

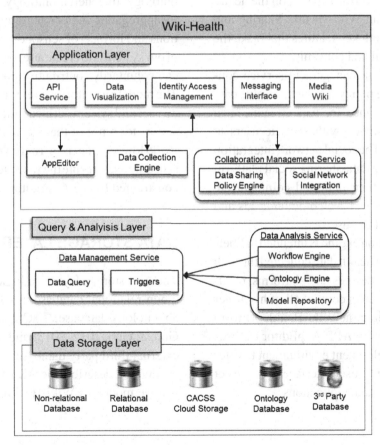

APPLICATION LAYER

The application layer comprises all of the components required for managing data access, data collection, security, data sharing and other features that support online collaboration. The API service offers a Web-based interface for access to all of the functionalities of Wiki-Health. The identity access management component is a separate service that provides authorization and access control of all requests. The messaging interface is used to connect Wiki-Health to external third party API and services. The data visualization module incorporates several charting libraries, such as HighChart ("HighCharts JS,") and Google Charts ("Google Charts,") to generate different graphical representations of raw sensor data as well as processed data. Media Wiki provides a collaborative way of allowing users to add, edit and publish content relating to data analysis models, methods and workflows, based on the health sensor data stored in Wiki-Health. Sharing and collaboration are both key features that make the cloud storage useful and convenient.

The collaboration management service contains a data sharing policy engine to resolve data sharing policies defined for data streams, such that data can be shared with specific users at prerequisite times. The social network integration component creates a data-sharing social platform for users to share their data and communicate with other people who have common needs and to learn more about themselves.

The data collection engine is intended to liberate a user's personal health data collected through different providers, devices and platforms, by allowing a user to create a copy of all of his or her data and maintain it in the Wiki-Health platform through the third party API. AppEditor exposes an application development environment to offer developers a graphical user interface to construct their health sensor data applications.

QUERY AND ANALYSIS LAYER

The query and analysis layer has two main purposes: data management and data analysis. The data management service handles all of the generic data access to different data sources in the data storage layer and triggers event actions under defined conditions. The data analysis service contains the workflow engine, ontology engine and model repository. The ontology engine component manages and queries the ontology via an API that supports the SPARQL language (Prud'Hommeaux & Seaborne, 2008). We adopt ontology in the system for two main reasons: first, ontology is used to describe the data source, and provide the semantic substrate to manipulate various health data sources, such as flexible query, data validation and etc. Second, ontology provides the basis for our data federation and fusion. For multiple data sources, we fuse them with common upper ontology. In general, ontology makes it possible for aggregating and/or integrating different resolutions and formats of sensor data. One of the goals of our system is to create an ecosystem where users can voluntarily contribute their data and models. The model repository serves this purpose; it stores all user and system defined functions, models and scripts for reuse of the data and knowledge. The workflow engine is a runtime environment to schedule and execute the workflows and processes constructed by the AppEditor.

DATA STORAGE LAYER

The data storage layer is a logical tier that hosts a non-relational database, a relational database, an ontology database, CACSS cloud storage (Li, Guo, & Guo, 2012, 2013) and data sources from external third party databases.

Figure 2 describes the Wiki-Health hybrid data storage model. In Wiki-Health, sensor metadata

Figure 2. The hybrid data storage model

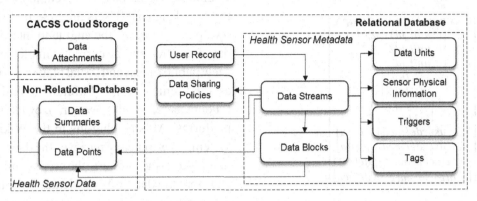

and sensor data are completely separate. The system uses a relational database to store all user information, in addition to sensor metadata such as sample rate, data format, sensor type and other Wiki-Health structured data. All sensor readings and other sensor data are stored in a non-relational (NoSQL) database and CACSS Cloud Storage System. The motivation behind this hybrid approach arises from sensor systems possessing common features such as the storage and processing of large amounts of data. Health sensor devices such as EEG and ECG employ a number of data channels and possess significantly higher temporal resolution than common environmental sensors like temperature and humidity. Such health sensor data, therefore, demands a scalable, fast and efficient system in order for it to be stored and processed. Traditional relational databases are designed for efficient transaction processing of small amounts of information in a large database. The data sets stored in these databases have no pre-defined notion of time unless timestamp attributes are explicitly added. Non-relational databases, such as HBase (HBase; Khetrapal & Ganesh, 2006), MongoDB (Chodorow, 2013; "MongoDB,") and Cassandra (Lakshman & Malik, 2010), store data in a key-value structure. They use looser consistency models than traditional relational databases, thus providing higher scalability and better perfor-

mance (Cattell, 2011; Leavitt, 2010; Stonebraker, 2010; Varley, Aziz, Aziz, & Miranker, 2009). Cloud storage is another service that helps users reduce the costs, complexities and risks in managing large data growth. Wiki-Heath uses such a hybrid approach to achieve high performance in data access and operations.

In Wiki-Health's sensor data storage model, each data stream maps and holds all the information of the actual health sensor device. A single data stream can have many data units. Such data unit is useful for health devices that provide multiple channel readings at the same time. Data points contains sensor reading data, data attachment index, tag mappings, block mappings and other user defined data, they are stored as a collection of blocks addressed by an index using data stream ID together with a timestamp (as shown in Figure 3). Data blocks and tags are designed and implemented for developers and users to be able to add more dimensions to the data so that required data can be found more easily and accurately. Data summaries can be used for storing summary or intermediate analysis result to improve the response time on retrieving certain analysis and query results. A data stream can have multiple triggers. Triggers holds action and condition information, they are used to perform actions when a defined condition is reached. For

Figure 3. Data points storage format

$$
\begin{bmatrix}
streamid - timestampX \\
\begin{bmatrix} v\colon unit\_id1 & 2.0 \\ v\colon unit\_id2 & 6.2 \\ v\colon unit\_id3 & 1.6 \end{bmatrix} \\
\begin{bmatrix} t\colon tag1 \\ t\colon tag2 \end{bmatrix} \\
\begin{bmatrix} b\colon blockid1 \\ b\colon blockid2 \end{bmatrix} \\
\begin{bmatrix} ud\colon userdefined1 & data \\ ud\colon userdefined2 & data \end{bmatrix} \\
\begin{bmatrix} a\colon attachment1 & fileloc1 \\ a\colon attachment2 & fileloc2 \end{bmatrix}
\end{bmatrix}
$$

example, such action can be an alert to inform a caregiver when a certain threshold or unusual reading is discovered.

IMPLEMENTATION AND DETAILS

In this section, we will discuss more details about each component and its implementation. We also demonstrate how Wiki-Health adapts existing storage technologies to provide efficient and scalable services.

After considerable research and experimentation, we chose HBase as the foundational non-relational database storage for the sensor data. It is designed to provide fast real time read/write data access. Some research has already been done to evaluate the performance of HBase (Carstoiu, Cernian, & Olteanu, 2010; Khetrapal & Ganesh, 2006). Its column-orientation design confers exceptional flexibility in the storing of data. We use the CACSS cloud storage system (Li et al., 2012, 2013) to store additional unstructured data as attachments to the sensor data. We chose MYSQL as the relational database for storing sensor metadata and other related information. A data sharing policy engine is implemented using Drool tools ("DROOL,"). Drools is a business rule management system (BRMS) with a forward chaining inference based rules engine, tailored for the Java language. Users are able to write their own policy rules for the engine to interpret. The data collection engine currently implements over a few public fitness and social platform APIs such as ("Endomondo,"), ("Fitbit,"), ("Withings,"), ("Foursquare,") and ("Twitter,"), by taking those platforms' APIs as plug-ins in the Wiki-Health system. It periodically retrieves the data stores on those systems according to the user's configuration and store the data in Wiki-Health for future use. The user can specify what kind of data to collect and how often they are collected. The media wiki component uses the open source PHP script from ("MediaWiki,"). Wiki-Health interacts with the wiki component through MediaWiki's API to insert and update contents.

ONTOLOGY MANAGEMENT

The implementation of Wiki-Health ontology management is depicted in Figure 4. ("Virtuoso,") is used to store and manage ontologies. Virtuoso is a "universal server" enabling a single multi-threaded server process that implements multiple protocols such as RDF data, XML and Linked data Management. The ("dotNetRdf library,") is used to communicate with the Virtuoso server. The Wiki-Health ontology engine invokes the functionalities of the dotNetRDF library and communicates with the Virtuoso server. A successful ontology submission will output a unique ontology identity. This identity will be required in order for the user to link the data stream with the ontology schema. Submitted ontology schemas are stored in the Virtuoso ontology repository. Data querying involves the user submitting a query either in SQL format or SPARQL and the system returning a result set. The user has the option to obtain the query output as either XML or RDF.

Figure 4. The implementation for ontology support

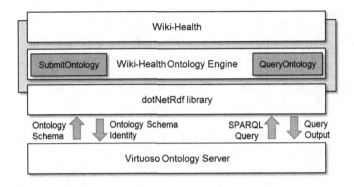

MODEL REPOSITORY

The model repository provides an environment to store analysis model and do model training. The repository is currently built on a distributed R platform on top of IC-Cloud (Y.-K. Guo & Guo, 2011). R is an open source software programming language and a software environment for statistical computing and graphics. R provides a wide variety of statistical models and graphical techniques, and is highly extensible. It has been used among statisticians and data miners for developing statistical software and data analysis (Gentleman, 2008; "R Project," ; Warnes et al., 2009). The model repository consists with the following components:

- **Model Source Storage:** The submitted models are stored as R source file in a file storage system.
- **Web Portal for R:** A Web front-end portal (as an example shown in Figure 6) for R is provided based on R-Node, to connect to the R runtime environment, and interact

Figure 5. Web portal for R (data visualization)

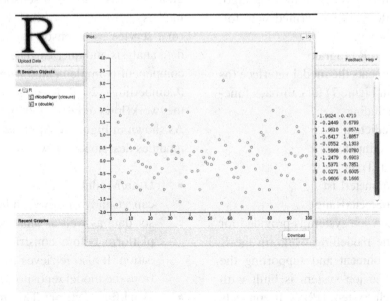

Figure 6. Web portal for R (data upload)

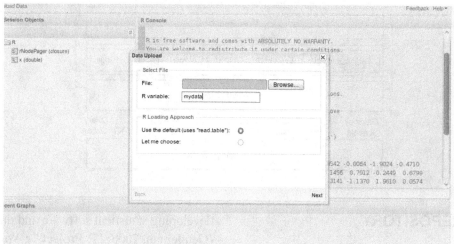

with it through the R console. Users can upload training data, view their scripts for model, and check the visualization of the runtime status and result.

- **API Package for R (Wiki-R):** Defines the interface between the R application and the environment, so that functions can be called back for actions like model training, parameter reflection, etc. When users submit a training algorithm for a model to the system via these cases, the training algorithm submitted will be verified with following conditions:
  - It's a valid R program
  - It implements the model interface (as shown in Figure 7) for call-back functions including:
    - Prediction
    - DataInput
    - DataTrain
    - ParameterList
    - ParameterRange
- **Job System:** A job system is provided for scheduling the modelling works in the R runtime environment and supporting the operations. The job system is built with Portable Batch System (PBS). It connects to a set of data sources or a query. Once

all the validations are passed, a model is successfully submitted, and a job is created for model training. A job ID is returned to the user.

APPEDITOR AND WORKFLOWS

AppEditor is an online development environment, which provides a graphical user interface to integrate data from different sensors, apply analytic models, construct the workflow, and publish the final service as a sensor application for future data analysis and queries. The workflow engine component is implemented using JBOSS jBPM (Cumberlidge, 2007; Koenig, 2004). It executes the workflows constructed by the AppEditor. As shown in Figure 8, AppEditor comprises the modules described below.

- **Data/Models Explorer:** The developers can visually discover and browse the sensor data as well as analytic models in our platform before constructing their application. It also retrieves the lists of models from the model repository.
- **Workflow Editor:** This module provides an efficient tool to assist developers to build

Figure 7. Model Interface for the Job System

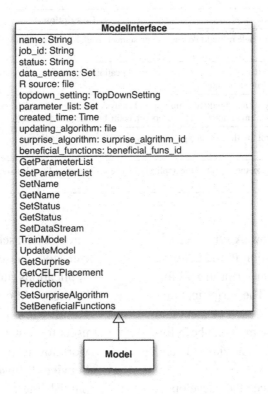

ModelInterface
name: String
job_id: String
status: String
data_streams: Set
R source: file
topdown_setting: TopDownSetting
parameter_list: Set
created_time: Time
updating_algorithm: file
surprise_algorithm: surprise_algrithm_id
beneficial_functions: beneficial_funs_id
GetParameterList
SetParameterList
SetName
GetName
SetStatus
GetStatus
SetDataStream
TrainModel
UpdateModel
GetSurprise
GetCELFPlacement
Prediction
SetSurpriseAlgorithm
SetBeneficialFunctions

Model

data applications. It is a workflow-like environment where developers can couple available elements shown in Table 1. The elements and links between them, including data and models which are listed in the tree structure by categories, can be added into a design diagram by drag-and-drop. The settings of each element, like the parameters for a model and data connection string of one data source, are edited direct-

Figure 8. Wiki-Health Analysis Framework Overview

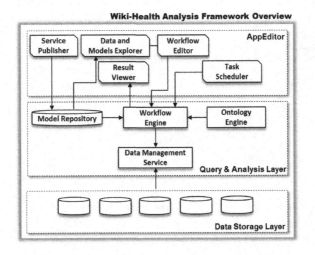

Table 1. Available elements in the AppEditor

Element (Shape)	Description
Data Source (circle)	Select single or multiple sensor data sources available in the platform
Filter (diamond)	Query the data source (e.g. query with location, time, values, etc.), undertake data fusion operations (e.g. aggregateValue, union, etc.)
Model (rectangle)	Apply various prediction, mining and analysis models on data. The system has a model repository and runtime environment where users can contribute their own models.
Connector (triangle)	Control the flow of the application, such as loops and conditions.
Visualizer (square)	Visualize the output of the application. The visualization libraries are also user-contributed.

ly in the property window. After the developers create an application in the editor, a corresponding execution script in xml format will be generated. The script includes the detail information of each element and the relations between them. It can be delivered to the workflow engine via APIs and stored to the model repository.

- **Task Scheduler:** Once the developers have done the design of their sensor application products, the developers can control the execution process of the application through task scheduler. The developers can run, stop, pause or check the status of their applications running via the APIs provided by the workflow engine.

- **Result Viewer:** The Results Viewer allows users to view the results of executing their workflow using various visualization tools.

- **Service Publisher:** Developers can finally publish the application as a Web service to allow other users to reuse the analysis methods, workflows and results (as shown in Figure 9). Some social functions like

Figure 9. An example of fMRI image analysis application composed by AppEditor

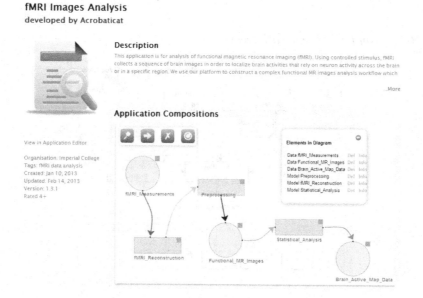

rating and comments are also provided. Such list of application would be further developed towards sensor application marketplaces.

Figure 10 shows the Web-based GUI of the Wiki-Health health data browser. All the data displayed are retrieved through the Web interface API of Wiki-Health. All the system components above described are deployed across different virtual machines on top of IC-Cloud (L. Guo, Guo, & Tian, 2010; Y.-K. Guo & Guo, 2011). IC-Cloud is a generic IaaS cloud computing infrastructure. It allows us to design and quickly compose a cloud computing environment in a flexible manner.

CASE STUDY

The recording of brain activity via EEG provides a way of measuring the state of the brain and of specific brain functions, offering the potential for safe neurofeedback treatments for ADHD (Arns, de Ridder, Strehl, Breteler, & Coenen, 2009; Barkley, 1997; Fuchs, Birbaumer, Lutzenberger, Gruzelier, & Kaiser, 2003; Lubar, Swartwood, Swartwood, & O'Donnell, 1995). Real-time measurement of concentration levels has been used in the development of video games designed to improve focus levels of patients through neurofeedback training over a period of time. In this case study, a cloud-based neurofeedback prototype system

Figure 10. GUI of Wiki-Health Web-based health data browser

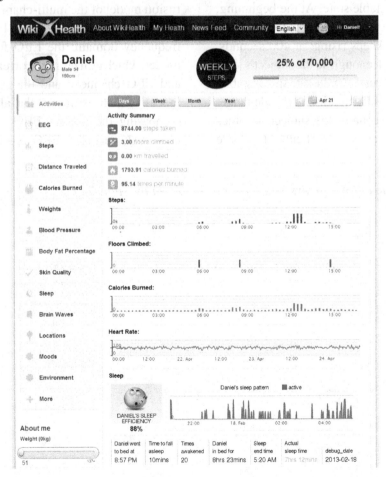

is built on top of Wiki-Health platform and by aiding the integration of models and data together using AppEditor (shown in Figure 11). One of the analysis models is used by this prototype is a k-nearest neighbour (kNN) approach to classify level of alertness (concentration) using a pre-created profile for the individual as training data.

The prototype system also includes a table tennis brain training game for evaluating the result. The real-time alertness level of the subject is calculated in order to adjust the difficulty of the game. If the subject is alert, the game difficulty is reduced; if the subject is relaxed, the game difficultly is increased. In our experiments, six subjects are tested with the table tennis braining training game. Figure 12 shows the result of the alertness level and the difficulty level during the game play. We found the game successfully guides the subject into a stable state. At the beginning, the difficulty is very low, so subject feels relaxed and the difficulty keeps rising; at 400 seconds, the difficulty is high enough so the subject's state becomes alertness, but the brain state still unstable, the alertness level is fluctuating in a wide range. After about 1000 seconds, the subject becomes fully stable; alertness and difficulty level are

stable in a small range. The purpose of the brain training games is to improve the player's ability to concentrate and put the brain into a stable and relaxed state at the same time. Typically, the game difficulty should increase if patient is not alert and decrease if patient is alert, through this feedback, the difficulty will be adjusted to a degree which allows the user to keep focus on playing game, but not tense. Therefore, this kind of brain training games can potentially be used for ADHD treatment.

Managing the large amount of growing biomedical data is always a challenge for many researchers. Especially if there is a requirement for real time access to all of the stored data. In this case study, all of the collected EEG signal data is stored and processed in Wiki-Health. We first define all of the data analysis models: the data fusion model of the multi-channel EEG data; the FFT model, which transforms EEG data into the frequency domain; the EEG feature extraction model, which utilizes high correlation parameters and EEG channels; and the data classification model, which estimates the alertness level by comparing the present EEG features with the previously recorded EEG profile. We then use

Figure 11. Example of EEG analysis application composed by AppEditor

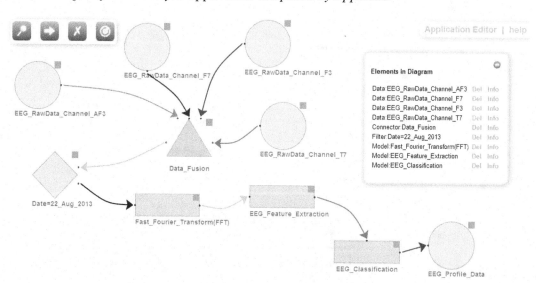

Figure 12. Experiment results of the averaged alertness values and the difficulty values at different times (100s, 200s, 400s, 800s, 1000s, 1000+s). Alertness: positive means alert, negative means relaxed. Difficulty: the higher the harder.

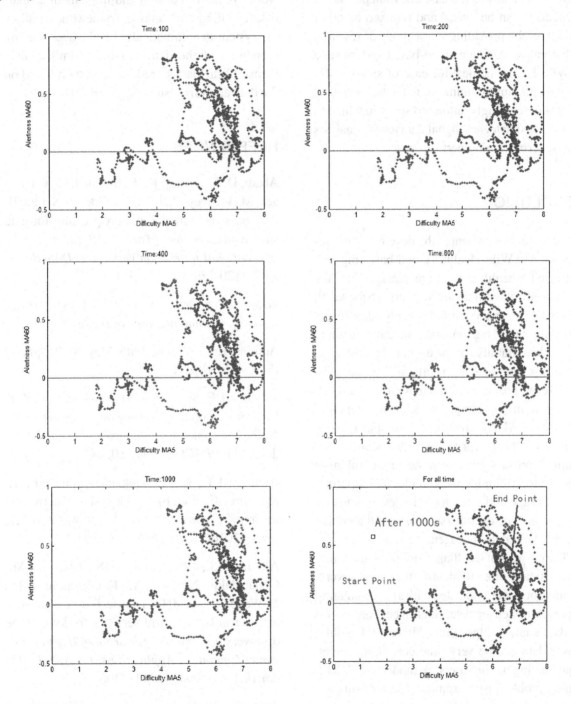

AppEditor to design and compose the application workflow, in order to connect all of the data sources and analysis models. The final published application can be reused and remixed by other users, thereby providing a new mode of research collaboration. Using a cloud-based system such as Wiki-Health is ideal for ease of storage of a growing amount of online signal data, as well as providing seemingly unlimited space in which to store extensive legacy signal data for the analysis of long term training performances.

CONCLUSION

This chapter has presented the design and implementation of Wiki-Health, a cloud-based big data platform for health sensor data management. We introduced a new collaborative approach for health sensor data management that not only allows users to collect, label, tag, annotate, update and share sensor data, but also allow users to create, reuse and remix data analysis results and models. To validate our proposed platform we have also built a brain training prototype which can potentially be used for ADHD treatment. The approach we propose offers enterprises and the research community considerable advantage in combining existing technologies such as cloud computing, cloud storage and other tools in developing and extend our work towards a successful collaborative health sensor data management system.

The purpose of labelling, tagging or annotating sensor data is often to identify the correct event, stimulus or cause associated with a corresponding sequence of sensor data. Such labels are useful for data analysis algorithms. However, labelling sensor data can be very time consuming, often requiring input from users. A fundamental data-mining problem is to examine data for "similar" items. Researchers are always interested in finding "similar" data with factors such as correlation and causality across different sets of individuals, groups or entire populations. For our future work, we plan to design and implement a smart data labelling and linking framework to allow the system to automatically label corresponding sequences of the data and link "similar" data across all the data stored in the system based on the data analysis results obtained.

REFERENCES

Abadi, D. J., Carney, D., Çetintemel, U., Cherniack, M., Convey, C., Lee, S.,... Zdonik, S. (2003). Aurora: A new model and architecture for data stream management. *The VLDB Journal—The International Journal on Very Large Data Bases, 12*(2), 120-139.

aDam LeVenthaL, B. (2008). Flash storage memory. *Communications of the ACM, 51*(7).

Admins, R. (2011). Reddit's May 2010. *State of the Servers Report, 11.*

Akyildiz, I. F., Su, W., Sankarasubramaniam, Y., & Cayirci, E. (2002a). A survey on sensor networks. *IEEE Communications Magazine, 40*(8), 102–114. doi:10.1109/MCOM.2002.1024422

Akyildiz, I. F., Su, W., Sankarasubramaniam, Y., & Cayirci, E. (2002b). Wireless sensor networks: a survey. *Computer Networks, 38*(4), 393–422. doi:10.1016/S1389-1286(01)00302-4

AlSairafi, S., Emmanouil, F.-S., Ghanem, M., Giannadakis, N., Guo, Y., Kalaitzopoulos, D., & Wendel, P. (2003). The design of discovery net: Towards open grid services for knowledge discovery. *International Journal of High Performance Computing Applications, 17*(3), 297–315. doi:10.1177/1094342003173003

Amazon. (2012). *Amazon S3 - The First Trillion Objects*. Author.

Amazon. (n.d.). *Amazon Simple Storage Service (S3)*. Retrieved from http://aws.amazon.com/s3/

Arns, M., de Ridder, S., Strehl, U., Breteler, M., & Coenen, A. (2009). Efficacy of neurofeedback treatment in ADHD: The effects on inattention, impulsivity and hyperactivity: A meta-analysis. *Clinical EEG and Neuroscience*, *40*(3), 180–189. doi:10.1177/155005940904000311 PMID:19715181

Barkley, R. A. (1997). Behavioral inhibition, sustained attention, and executive functions: Constructing a unifying theory of ADHD. *Psychological Bulletin*, *121*(1), 65. doi:10.1037/0033-2909.121.1.65 PMID:9000892

Berkelaar, M., Eikland, K., & Notebaert, P. (2004). *lpsolve: Open source (mixed-integer) linear programming system*. Eindhoven University of Technology.

Carstoiu, D., Cernian, A., & Olteanu, A. (2010). *Hadoop Hbase-0.20.2 performance evaluation*. Paper presented at the New Trends in Information Science and Service Science (NISS). New York, NY.

Cattell, R. (2011). Scalable SQL and NoSQL data stores. *SIGMOD Record*, *39*(4), 12–27. doi:10.1145/1978915.1978919

Chodorow, K. (2013). *MongoDB: the definitive guide*. Sebastopol, CA: O'Reilly.

Cumberlidge, M. (2007). *Business Process Management with JBoss JBPM: A Practical Guide for Business Analysts, Develop Business Process Models for Implementation in a Business Process Management Sytem*. Packt Publishing.

dotNetRdf library. (n.d.). Retrieved from http://www.dotnetrdf.org

DROOL. (n.d.). Retrieved from http://www.jboss.org/drools/

ElephantDrive. (n.d.). Retrieved from http://aws.amazon.com/solutions/case-studies/elephant-drive/

Endomondo. (n.d.). Retrieved from http://www.endomondo.com/

Fitbit. (n.d.). Retrieved from http://www.fitbit.com/

Foursquare. (n.d.). Retrieved from https://foursquare.com

Fuchs, T., Birbaumer, N., Lutzenberger, W., Gruzelier, J. H., & Kaiser, J. (2003). Neurofeedback treatment for attention-deficit/hyperactivity disorder in children: A comparison with methylphenidate. *Applied Psychophysiology and Biofeedback*, *28*(1), 1–12. doi:10.1023/A:1022353731579 PMID:12737092

Fulmer, J. (n.d.). *Siege HTTP regression testing and benchmarking utility*. Retrieved from http://www.joedog.org/JoeDog/Siege

Gentleman, R. (2008). *R programming for bioinformatics*. Boca Raton, FL: CRC Press. doi:10.1201/9781420063684

Google. (n.d.). *Google Cloud Storage Service*. Retrieved from http://code.google.com/apis/storage/

Google Charts. (n.d.). Retrieved from https://developers.google.com/chart/

Guo, L., Guo, Y., & Tian, X. (2010). *IC cloud: A design space for composable cloud computing*. Paper presented at the Cloud Computing (CLOUD). New York, NY.

Guo, Y.-K., & Guo, L. (2011). IC cloud: Enabling compositional cloud. *International Journal of Automation and Computing*, *8*(3), 269–279. doi:10.1007/s11633-011-0582-4

HBase. (n.d.). Retrieved from http://hbase.apache.org/

Held, M., Wolfe, P., & Crowder, H. P. (1974). Validation of subgradient optimization. *Mathematical Programming, 6*(1), 62–88. doi:10.1007/BF01580223

HighCharts JS. (n.d.). Retrieved from http://www.highcharts.com/

Khetrapal, A., & Ganesh, V. (2006). *HBase and Hypertable for large scale distributed storage systems*. Dept. of Computer Science, Purdue University.

Kim, Y., Gurumurthi, S., & Sivasubramaniam, A. (2006). *Understanding the performance-temperature interactions in disk I/O of server workloads*. Paper presented at the High-Performance Computer Architecture. New York, NY.

Koenig, J. (2004). *JBoss jBPM white paper*. JBoss Labs.

Lakshman, A., & Malik, P. (2010). Cassandra: A decentralized structured storage system. *SIGOPS Oper. Syst. Rev., 44*(2), 35–40. doi:10.1145/1773912.1773922

Leavitt, N. (2010). Will NoSQL databases live up to their promise? *Computer, 43*(2), 12–14. doi:10.1109/MC.2010.58

Lee, C. H., Birch, D., Wu, C., Silva, D., Tsinalis, O., Li, Y., & Guo, Y. (2013). Building a generic platform for big sensor data application. In *Proceedings of Big Data* (pp. 94–102). IEEE. doi:10.1109/BigData.2013.6691559

Li, Y., Guo, L., & Guo, Y. (2012). *CACSS: Towards a Generic Cloud Storage Service*. Paper presented at the CLOSER. New York, NY. Retrieved from http://dblp.uni-trier.de/db/conf/closer/closer2012.html#LiGG12

Li, Y., Guo, L., & Guo, Y. (2013). An Efficient and Performance-Aware Big Data Storage System. In *Cloud Computing and Services Science* (pp. 102–116). Springer. doi:10.1007/978-3-319-04519-1_7

Liu, X., Han, J., Zhong, Y., Han, C., & He, X. (2009). *Implementing WebGIS on Hadoop: A case study of improving small file I/O performance on HDFS*. Paper presented at the Cluster Computing and Workshops. New York, NY.

Lubar, J. F., Swartwood, M. O., Swartwood, J. N., & O'Donnell, P. H. (1995). Evaluation of the effectiveness of EEG neurofeedback training for ADHD in a clinical setting as measured by changes in TOVA scores, behavioral ratings, and WISC-R performance. *Biofeedback and Self-Regulation, 20*(1), 83–99. doi:10.1007/BF01712768 PMID:7786929

MediaWiki. (n.d.). Retrieved from http://www.mediawiki.org

MongoDB. (n.d.). Retrieved from http://www.mongodb.org

Murty, R. N., Mainland, G., Rose, I., Chowdhury, A. R., Gosain, A., Bers, J., & Welsh, M. (2008). *Citysense: An urban-scale wireless sensor network and testbed*. Paper presented at the Technologies for Homeland Security. New York, NY.

NIKE+ FUELBAND. (n.d.). Retrieved from http://www.nike.com/

Pantelopoulos, A., & Bourbakis, N. G. (2010). A survey on wearable sensor-based systems for health monitoring and prognosis. *IEEE Transactions on Systems, Man and Cybernetics. Part C, Applications and Reviews, 40*(1), 1–12. doi:10.1109/TSMCC.2009.2032660

Prud'Hommeaux, E., & Seaborne, A. (2008). SPARQL query language for RDF. *W3C Recommendation, 15*.

R Project. (n.d.). Retrieved from http://www.r-project.org/

Schmuck, F. B., & Haskin, R. L. (2002). *GPFS: A Shared-Disk File System for Large Computing Clusters*. Paper presented at the FAST. New York, NY.

Stonebraker, M. (2010). SQL databases v. NoSQL databases. *Communications of the ACM, 53*(4), 10–11. doi:10.1145/1721654.1721659

Szalay, A., Bunn, A., Gray, J., Foster, I., & Raicu, I. (2006). *The importance of data locality in distributed computing applications.* Paper presented at the NSF Workflow Workshop. New York, NY.

Twitter. (n.d.). Retrieved from https://twitter.com

Varley, I. T., Aziz, A., Aziz, C.-S. A., & Miranker, D. (2009). *No relation: The mixed blessings of non-relational databases.* Academic Press.

Virtuoso. (n.d.). Retrieved from http://virtuoso.openlinksw.com

Warnes, G. R., Bolker, B., Bonebakker, L., Gentleman, R., Huber, W., Liaw, A.,... Moeller, S. (2009). Gplots: Various R programming tools for plotting data. *R Package Version, 2*(4).

Withings. (n.d.). Retrieved from www.withings.com

Xively. (n.d.). Retrieved from https://xively.com/

Xu, N. (2002). A survey of sensor network applications. *IEEE Communications Magazine, 40*(8), 102–114. doi:10.1109/MCOM.2002.1024422

Yao, Y., & Gehrke, J. (2002). The cougar approach to in-network query processing in sensor networks. *SIGMOD Record, 31*(3), 9–18. doi:10.1145/601858.601861

Yuriyama, M., & Kushida, T. (2010). *Sensor-cloud infrastructure-physical sensor management with virtualized sensors on cloud computing.* Paper presented at the Network-Based Information Systems (NBiS). New York, NY.

Zephyr. (n.d.). Retrieved from http://www.zephyranywhere.com/

KEY TERMS AND DEFINITIONS

AppEditor: A graphical user interface to allow users and developers to construct workflows and health sensor data applications.

Collaboration Management Service: This service integrates social network features and manages data sharing policies for health sensor data.

Data Collection Engine: This engine collects health data from different service providers, devices and platforms through 3rd party APIs on the behalf of the user.

Model Repository: A storage space to store all user and system defined functions, models and scripts for reuse of the data and knowledge.

Ontology Engine: This engine provides the basis for the health sensor data and schema validation, federation and fusion.

Triggers: An approach to store action and condition information. It allow certain actions to be performed when defined conditions are reached.

Wiki-Health System: A technology takes advantage of cloud computing and Internet of Things for social and personal well-being data management.

Workflow Engine: This engine executes workflows and processes constructed by the AppEditor.

Chapter 5
Interoperability in Healthcare

Luciana Cardoso
Minho University, Portugal

Filipe Portela
Minho University, Portugal

Fernando Marins
Minho University, Portugal

Manuel Santos
Minho University, Portugal

César Quintas
Centro Hospitalar do Porto, Portugal

António Abelha
Minho University, Portugal

José Machado
Minho University, Portugal

ABSTRACT

With the advancement of technology, patient information has been being computerized in order to facilitate the work of healthcare professionals and improve the quality of healthcare delivery. However, there are many heterogeneous information systems that need to communicate, sharing information and making it available when and where it is needed. To respond to this requirement the Agency for Integration, Diffusion, and Archiving of medical information (AIDA) was created, a multi-agent and service-based platform that ensures interoperability among healthcare information systems. In order to improve the performance of the platform, beyond the SWOT analysis performed, a system to prevent failures that may occur in the platform database and also in machines where the agents are executed was created. The system has been implemented in the Centro Hospitalar do Porto (one of the major Portuguese hospitals), and it is now possible to define critical workload periods of AIDA, improving high availability and load balancing. This is explored in this chapter.

INTRODUCTION

In healthcare, information systems have been growing, and consequently the volume, complexity and criticism of data become more and more difficult to manage. However, despite these systems contribute increasing the quality of healthcare delivery, information sources are distributed, ubiquitous, heterogeneous, large and complex and the Health Information Systems (HIS) need to communicate in order to share information and to make it available at any place at any time. Data are stored in multiple independent structures. Therefore it emerges the need to create a global system

DOI: 10.4018/978-1-4666-6118-9.ch005

that brings together all the islands of information shared between services. It is necessary to develop a solid and efficient process of integration and interoperation that must take into consideration scalability, flexibility, portability and security.

Several methodologies presently exist to implement interoperable information systems in healthcare; it results in several common communication architectures and mainstream standards such as Health Level 7 (HL7). However, several concerns regarding the distribution, fault tolerance, standards, communication and tightly bound systems still exist broadly throughout the healthcare area. The multi-agent paradigm has been an interesting technology in the area of *interoperability*; it addresses many of such limitations (Miranda et al., 2012; Miranda, Machado, Abelha, & Neves, 2013).

The homogeneity of clinical, medical and administrative systems is not possible due to financial and technical restrictions, as well as functional needs. The solution is to integrate, diffuse and archive this information under a dynamic framework, in order to share this knowledge with every information system that needs it. So *AIDA – Agency for Interoperation, diffusion and Archive of Medical Information* is presented. AIDA is an agency that supplies intelligent electronic workers called proactive agents, in charge of some tasks, such as communicating with the heterogeneous systems, sending and receiving information (e.g., medical or clinical reports, images, collections of data, prescriptions), managing and saving the information and answering to information requests (J Machado et al., 2010; Miranda, Duarte, Abelha, Machado, & Neves, 2010; Peixoto, Santos, Abelha, & Machado, 2012).

With the growing importance of HIS, databases became indispensable tools for day-to-day tasks in healthcare units. They store important and confidential information about patient's clinical status and about the other hospital services. Thus,

they must be permanently available, reliable and at high performance. In many healthcare units, fault tolerant systems are used. They ensure the availability, reliability and disaster recovery of data. However, these mechanisms do not allow the prediction or prevention of faults. In this context, the necessity of developing a *fault forecasting* system emerges. It is necessary to monitor database performance to verify the normal workload and adapt a forecasting model used in medicine into the database context. Based on percentiles a scale to represent the severity of situations was created (Silva et al., 2012).

The AIDA was implemented at Centro Hospitalar do Porto (CHP), in Portugal, and was subjected to Strengths, Weaknesses, Opportunities, and Threats (SWOT) analysis in order to ascertain what can be change to improve the system. This analysis can reveal what are the great strengths of the system as well as its major pitfalls. In addition, the opportunities than can be taken as advantages are highlighted and the key threats to the system are alerted (Pereira, Salazar, Abelha, & Machado, 2013).

The main goal of this chapter is to explain the importance of interoperability in the context of the quality healthcare delivery. In the background section a brief introduction about interoperability and its importance in the healthcare environment. The *intelligent agents* in interoperability section present a promising technology for interoperability implementation, namely the multi-agent technology. Combining the issues mentioned in the previous sections, a solution, the AIDA platform, is presented. In its section its architecture as well as its database is described. In order to improve AIDA performance, in the following sections fault forecasting systems are presented either from a database or from machines, which execute AIDA agents. The database, machines and agents' workload are also presented and discussed in these sections. In the last section the strengths, weaknesses, opportunities and threats of AIDA are analysed.

BACKGROUND

HIS around the world are in rapid transition, moving from the traditional, paper-based practices to computerized processes and systems to ensure the delivery of health care and improve the quality of the services (Weber-Jahnke, Peyton, & Topaloglou, 2012). The healthcare domain, specifically HIS have been a very attractive domain for Computer Science researchers and it is facing a growing number of challenges. HIS are at the heart of all these challenges. They can provide a better coordination among medical professionals and facilities, thus reducing the number and incidence of medical errors. At the same time, they can reduce healthcare costs and may provide a means to improve the management of hospitals (Palazzo et al., 2013).

HIS provide a composed environment of complex information systems, heterogeneous, distributed and ubiquitous, speaking different languages, integrating medical equipment and customized by different entities, which in turn were set by different people aiming at different goals. Everyday new applications are developed to assist physicians in their work, but those systems are built in "silos" and they have a little impact on their environment constituting isolated information islands, that limit the flow of information, while lack the ability to interact and communicate with other systems (Miranda et al., 2012; Palazzo et al., 2013; Peixoto et al., 2012; Weber-Jahnke et al., 2012).

The possibility and the need of communication are one of the main characteristics of the human beings. Similarly the HIS need to communicate and cooperate in order to enhance their overall performance and usefulness, to improve HIS, quality of the diagnosis, but mainly, to improve the quality in patient treatment. Cooperation and exchange of data and information is indeed one of the most relevant features, is the essence for the optimisation of existing resources and the improvement of the decision making process through consolidation, verification and dissemination of information (Miranda et al., 2012).

The perception of integration and interoperation must be introduced into this environment. Integration aims to gather and acquire information of distinct systems in order to reinforce or strengthen them, while interoperation concentrates on the continuous communication and exchange of information across cooperative systems. Therefore, the concept of *interoperability* has been presented; there is no definition for this term, however it can be said that interoperability is the ability of independent systems to exchange meaningful information and initiate actions from each other, in order to operate together for mutual benefit (Miranda et al., 2010). The main goal of interoperability in healthcare is to connect applications and data can be shared and exchanged across the healthcare environment and distributed to medical staff or patients whenever and wherever they need it. Interoperability is no longer a technological option, it is a fundamental requirement for delivering effective care and ensuring the health and well-being of million of patients world-wide (Rogers, Peres, & Müller, 2010).

Motivation

In the last decades interoperability and the respective implications for the delivery of healthcare has been a topic of study, and in 2003 it was found that the level of interoperability between systems in most health institutions was extremely low (Carr & Moore, 2003).

However, since 1987 the *Health Level Seven International (HL7)* was founded. It is a non-profit organization, which the main goal is providing a comprehensive framework and related standards for the exchange, integration, sharing, and retrieval of electronic health information that supports clinical practice and the management, delivery and evaluation of health services. HL7 provides standards for interoperability with multiple objectives like the improvement of care delivery, the optimization of the daily workflow, the reduction of ambiguity and the improving of knowledge exchange between all stakeholders (HL7, 2012).

There has been an intensive effort to develop standards adapted and optimized towards improving healthcare delivery. These standards have been able to give a definite structure or shape to low level interoperability in healthcare, in a firmly established and modular manner. Among these patterns HL7 is considered the most adaptable one in healthcare interoperability. HL7 started as a mainly syntactic healthcare oriented communication protocol at the application layer, the seventh layer of the Open Systems Interconnect (OSI) communication model. The initial versions of the protocol defined the message structure by loosely connected healthcare applications, and by classifying the different types of messages involved in this environment with the aggregation of standardized segments. It was uniquely syntactic, and according to the general models of interoperation is one of the lowest levels of this process. In the current version, the HL7 is focused on semantic interoperability, including the appropriate use of exchanging information in the sense of the communicating application's behaviour. This model contains relations and metadata in an abstract level that may enable far higher levels of integration, namely semantic interoperability and validation of exchanged information, using the relational mapping of each artefact (Miranda et al., 2012, 2010).

Interoperability in Electronic Health Record

Nowadays information technologies in medicine and healthcare are experiencing a difficult situation in which each staff person uses in the daily work a set of independent technologies that in-

volve huge sets of information. This independence may be the cause of difficulty in *interoperability* between information systems. The overload of information systems within a healthcare facility may lead to problems in accessing the total information needed.

HIS have gained great importance and have grown in quality and quantity. With this information overload, it is necessary to infer what information is relevant to be registered in the Electronic Health Record (EHR) and Decision Support Systems (DSS) must allow for reasoning with incomplete, ambiguous and uncertain knowledge (Peixoto et al., 2012). The EHR is a core application which covers horizontally the healthcare unit and makes possible a transverse analysis of medical records along the services, units or treated pathologies, bringing to the healthcare area new methodologies for problem solving, computational models, technologies and tools.

Due to the complexity of each HIS, the possibility of a global information system emerges as something complex and incomplete. However, the need to gather significant information to be shared with other services and to communicate all relevant data related to the patient and the executed procedures, is not only of high value to the institutions, but also to the patient. In order to aggregate and consolidate all significant information, a solid and efficient process of interoperation or integration must be developed. This process must take into consideration scalability, flexibility, portability and security when applied to EHR. The complexity and sensitivity of the exchanged information require more than technological efficiency and pragmatic exchange of information. The dissemination of incoherent information and its introduction into the EHR may cause more than inconsistent records, and they may give rise to a wrong diagnose. In order to avoid this moral and ethical drawback a thorough validation of the exchanged and integrated information must be performed. The development of top-level interoperability frameworks is henceforth of an intrinsic nature or indispensable quality of the healthcare environment. The multitude and intricacy of services that must be performed by the EHR and Group Decision Support Systems (GDSS) require such a framework or otherwise would be inefficiently intertwined with other essential solutions (Miranda et al., 2010).

INTELLIGENT AGENTS IN INTEROPERABILITY

There is a variety of methodologies and architectures through which it is possible to implement interoperability between HIS. These methodologies are based on common communication architectures and standards such as HL7. However, there are still some concerns about the distribution, fault tolerance, and communication standards. The multi-agent technology has stood out in the area of *interoperability*, including interoperability in healthcare, addressing the concerns mentioned above.

This technology is closely related to the basic concepts that define a distributed architecture. The agent-based computing has been vaunted for its ability to solve problems and/or as a new revolution in the development and analysis of software. The agent-based systems are not only a promising technology, it is becoming as a new way of thinking, a conceptual paradigm for analysing problems and develop systems in order to solve problems related to the complexity, distribution and interactivity. Although there is no accepted definition for agent, it can be said that agents are understood as computational artifacts that exhibit certain properties such as (Jose Machado, Abelha, Novais, Neves, & Neves, 2010):

- **Autonomy:** The ability to act without direct intervention from peers, more specifically humans;

- **Reactivity:** Capacity for integration into an environment, perceive through sensors and acting to certain stimuli;
- **Pro-Activity:** Ability to solve intelligent problems as planning their own activities in order to achieve their goals;
- **Social, Emotional and Moral Behaviour:** Ability to interact with other agents and even change their behaviour in response to this interaction. They can communicate through constructs and protocols of low or high level, as well as means of addressing and direct communication. They can cooperate to achieve a certain common goal, as well as their individual goals, i.e. they must have the ability to negotiate with other agents.

In view of the above-described property, agents can be defined as autonomous and problem-solving computational entities capable of effective operation in dynamic and open environments. They are often deployed in environments in which they interact, and maybe cooperate with other agents that have possibly conflicting goals (Luck, McBurney, & Preist, 2003).

Agent-based software should be robust, scalable and secure. To achieve this, the architectures must allow compliant agents to discover each other, communicate and offer a service to one another. These architectures go beyond the capabilities of the typical distributed object oriented programming techniques and tools (Contreras, Germán, Chi, & Sheremetov, 2004).

Multi-Agent Systems for Interoperability

Multi-agent systems (MAS) offer a new and often more appropriate way of development of complex systems, especially in open and dynamic environments. Some key features of the agent technology support these capabilities. The autonomy and pro-activeness features of an agent allow it to plan and perform tasks defined to accomplish the design objectives. The social abilities enable an agent to interact in MAS and cooperate or complete fulfilling its goals. The MAS can be considered as a rich and highly adaptable technology with a keen interest in the area of *interoperability* among HIS (Jose Machado et al., 2010).

To develop these systems specification standard methods are required, and it is believed that one of the characteristics for its high acceptability and recommendation is simplicity. In fact, the use of *intelligent agents* to simulate human decision-making in the medical field offers the potential for software suitable for the development and practical analysis and design methodologies that do not distinguish between agents and humans. These systems can provide skill and effectiveness to monitor the behaviour of its own officers, with a significant impact on the process of acquiring and validating knowledge, i.e. MAS is aware of the evolution process of intelligent systems and it is capable of accomplishing actions, which usually are performed by human beings, as replace elements or delegate tasks.

The MAS is able to manage the entire life cycle of the agent, the availability of the modules of the HIS as a whole, keeping all agents freely distributed. New agents with the same characteristics and objectives can be created through the MAS depending on the needs of the system in which they are inserted. The structure of these agents and the MAS can be developed according to the services they provide and the logical functionality of systems that interact with them.

The agents in a healthcare facility configure applications or utilities that collect information in the organization. Once collected, this information can be provided directly to other entities, e.g. a doctor or to a server, stored in a file or sent by e-mail to someone (J Machado et al., 2010).

HL7 Services in the Multi-Agent System

The *HL7* standard plays an essential role in the implementation of interoperability, in the development of exchange of medical information, the standardization of medical documents into eXtensible Markup Language (XML) structures and vocabulary specification for rugged use in messages and documents. Although health informatics standards like HL7 are completely distinct from agent communication standards, HL7 services can be also implemented under the agent paradigm.

These agents based on HL7 services can communicate with services that follow different paradigms and communicate with other agents that use both the HL7 as communication agents. Although the HL7 standard can be implemented using other architectures, agent-based solutions enjoy a wide *interoperability* capability, being able to be integrated with the specific behaviours. These behaviours may become more effective if they use the machine learning paradigm and other artificial intelligence (AI) techniques in order to adapt to the environment and be able to avoid errors and correct the flow of information and knowledge extraction within the institution.

As mentioned previously, the HL7 standard does not limit its use to any technology or architecture; however, it aims to use regular communications between health systems oriented. There are, obviously, architectures and technologies that have become the most used, but the ones that stand out are those that are present by default in the information systems of specific equipment to perform various diagnostic methods.

However, in the process of communication and exchange of information, we cannot only worry about information systems, although information exchange with the devices is increasingly important. These devices usually communicate through loosely associated standards, i.e. directly with the information system (e.g., Medical imaging Information System, Cardiology Information System) or proprietary systems that may or may not be consistent with other information systems. This type of equipment usually follows a client - server architecture in which the equipment is in most cases only a client. So, it is understandable that there is considerable difficulty in establishing a system of uniformly understanding and fully communicating with all services within a hospital. Even with the adoption of standards, specifically HL7, different flavourings usually require distinct handling of the messages and its events. To resolve this situation, the solution is to refer to the use of agents that enable creating specific behaviours or agents that adapt to any situation by keeping all coupled systems (Miranda et al., 2012).

THE AGENCY FOR INTEGRATION, DIFFUSION AND ARCHIVE OF MEDICAL INFORMATION (AIDA)

Medical informatics is an area supported by two basic sciences, the Computer Science and the Health Sciences, which contributes to the improvement of quality in the provision of health services as it aims to better management of information resources and health. As mentioned in the previous sections, the interaction and communication based on specific protocols are fundamental to the successful implementation, execution and / or management of any HIS. Actually the HIS have to be described as a wide variety of distributed and heterogeneous systems that speak different languages, integrate medical equipment, are customized by different companies, which in turn were developed by different people aimed at different goals. This leads us to consider the solution(s) for a particular problem, part of a process of integration of different information sources, using different protocols through an *Agency for Integration, Diffusion and Archive (AIDA)* medical information, bringing

health care methodologies to solve problems in medical education, computational models, tools and technologies (Duarte et al., 2010).

AIDA is a platform developed to allow the dissemination and integration of information generated in a healthcare environment. This platform includes many different integration capabilities; primarily uses Service Oriented Architectures (SOA) and *Multi-Agent Systems* (MAS) to implement interoperability, in accordance with standards, comprising of all service providers within a health institution (Miranda et al., 2010).

This platform, designed to ensure *interoperability* between the HIS, and is characterized by electronic appliances providing intelligent workers, here understood as software agents, which have a pro-active behaviour and are responsible for tasks such as communication between different sub-systems, sending and receiving information (e.g., clinical or medical reports, images, data collections, prescriptions), management and economics of information and responding to requests, with the necessary resources to carry them out correctly and timely. The main objectives are, as the name implies, integrating, disseminating and archiving large data sets from various sources (i.e., departments, services, units, computers, medical equipment, etc.). However this platform also provides tools to implement and facilitate communication with humans through Web-based services, i.e., the construction of AIDA follows the acceptance of simplicity, common objectives and addressing responsibilities (Duarte et al., 2010; Peixoto et al., 2012).

AIDA Architecture

Figure 1 shows the architecture where one can observe that AIDA is the central element in a healthcare environment, which ensures interoperability and communication between the following systems:

Figure 1. AIDA architecture

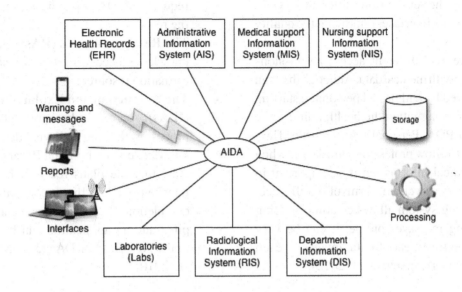

- **The Electronic Medical Record (EHR):** A kind of repository of information on the study of the health of an individual subject of care, in a format that can be processed by computer, stored and transmitted from a secure and accessible by multiple authorized users;

- **The Administrative Information System (AIS):** Seeks to represent, manage and archive the administrative information during the episode. The episode is a collection of all the operations assigned to a patient from start to the end of the treatment;

- **The Medical Information System (MIS):** Seeks to represent, manage and archive clinical information during the episode;

- **The Nursing Information System (NIS):** Seeks to represent and manage archive information on nursing practices during the episode;

- **The Information Systems of all Departments and Services (DIS):** In particular Laboratories (Labs), *Radiology*

Information System (RIS) and Medical Imaging (PACS - Picture Archive and Communication System), which handles images standard DICOM format.

The presented architecture was expected to support medical applications and has the form of intelligent information processing Web systems. Its functional roles and information flowing among them are controlled with adjustable autonomy.

Health professionals gather information and its value is stored and distributed automatically to where it is needed. Every document created within a specialized service honouring certain rules, is kept closer to different departments. The coding tools and ordering are very useful for connecting different data to a particular problem, as the encoded data are very easy to access by AI based decision support systems. The built-in electronic sorting can be used not only for medical equipment or pharmacological prescriptions, but also for the acquisition of laboratory results and study images that are out of service at the origin. Furthermore, it can allow the centralization of exam display, thus allowing the results from different services sharing the same interface, improving the quality of service.

There are also different access permissions when dealing with medical data. Although they can only be viewed by authorized personnel, starting from any terminal within the health unit to even the laptop or PDA. Personal access must be flexible in order to allow professionals to access when needed. Medical information is so important in terms of privacy as well as in terms of significance. The messaging system allows creating, sending and receiving messages online. It can be very useful for the treatment of data, images or even to exchange files (Peixoto et al., 2012).

AIDA as a Multi-Agent System

Considering the previous sections it can be noted that the AIDA platform is a pure communication MAS, i.e., there is no external environment influence and the agents only communicate with each other via messages. However AIDA contains different types of agents:

- **The Proxy Agents (PAs):** Provide the bridges between users and the system in terms of questions that can be explained;, decisions may have to be taken and / or visualization of the results. The system interfaces are based on Web-related front-ends using Hypermedia pages that can be accessed through a standard Web browser;
- **The Decision Agents (DAs):** Provide mediation capacities, acting by accepting a task of PAs. They can break down tasks into sub-tasks, sending them to be processed by the CAs, later integrating the results (returned by CAs);

- **The Computing Agents (CAs):** Accept requests of DAs specific tasks, returning the results;
- **The Resource Agents (RAs):** Have all the knowledge needed to access a specific information resource;
- **The Interaction and Explanation Agents (IEAs):** Act on the basis of argumentative processes that are fed with data and / or knowledge from both the PA and the DAs. Note that the plans received by the DAs may be partial; in that mode, only after the completion of a task, a trace can be compiled and an application can be delivered to the APs and / or DAs (Jose Machado et al., 2010).

AIDA Database

Over the years, organizations have increased use of databases and today they are considered essential for everyday tasks (Godinho, 2011). Particularly in healthcare units, databases have a vital role, since they store very important information about the patients' clinical status, administrative information and other relevant information for the healthcare services. Therefore, it is crucial to ensure the availability, reliability, confidence and safety of databases. As a result, they must have the following characteristics (Bertino & Sandhu, 2005; Drake et al., 2005; A. Rodrigues, 2005):

- **Confidentiality:** The database must have mechanisms to prevent intruders, so that unauthorized persons cannot access and publicize the data stored (Bertino & Sandhu, 2005; Kim et al., 2010; A. Rodrigues, 2005);
- **Integrity:** The database must have mechanisms that prevent modification of data by

unauthorized persons. Thus, it is possible to keep the information from the database incorruptible and inviolable (Bertino & Sandhu, 2005; Kim et al., 2010; A. Rodrigues, 2005);

- **Availability:** The databases must have mechanisms to access the required information in time. In addition, they should have mechanisms for fault prevention and tolerance, so that the system will thereby be able to continue operating despite the failure of any component not affecting the normal operation of the organization (Bertino & Sandhu, 2005; A. Rodrigues, 2005).

In healthcare units, it is important for databases to be available twenty-four hours a day, seven days per week, because the information is vital for solving the patients' problems and for hospital management. For this reason, it is essential to ensure the integrity and permanent availability of data even in the presence of faults (Godinho, 2011).

To achieve these goals, fault tolerance mechanisms based on the data or components redundancy are used. The main databases of CHP – including AIDA - are based on an Oracle Real Application Cluster (RAC) System. This mechanism is provided by Oracle for improving the availability and scalability of databases. A RAC system is composed by a shared database witch can be accessed through the server/computer that contains a database instance and an ASM (Automatic Storage Management) instance. In this way, it is possible access to the database across multiple servers (Ashdown & Kyte, 2011; Drake et al., 2005; Strohm, 2012).

In AIDA database, there is also another fault tolerance mechanism: a data guard solution. This mechanism consists in one or more standby databases (replicas of the original database), which should be in different places. In this way, when the master database is unavailable the replica

can be used in read-only mode. It is essential that the master and the standby databases are synchronized and access is read-only during the recovering (Godinho, 2011). The Figure 2 presents the complete architecture of AIDA database with these two mechanisms.

DATABASE WORKLOAD AND FAULT FORECASTING IN THE AIDA DATABASE

The fault tolerant system adapted to AIDA database mentioned in the Section AIDA Database ensures the availability, reliability and disaster recovery of data. However, these mechanisms do not allow the prediction or prevention of faults. In this context, it emerges the necessity of developing a *fault forecasting* system. To achieve this goal it is essential to monitor database performance, verify the normal workload and then adapt a forecasting model to the database context.

Monitoring Database Performance

The use of monitoring systems by organizations has been growing not only because they are useful to diagnose faults but also because they can help to ensure data security (Nair, 2008). Monitoring is not a simple process, and its complexity increases as it becomes necessary to monitor various components and systems with complex architectures. However, with the Oracle Systems it is possible to take advantage of several tools to help in this process. The performance views are one of these tools that enable to consult useful information for monitoring. The content of these views is refreshed periodically (Chan, 2008; Rich, 2013).

There are several statistics that can be used to characterize the behaviour of the database. According to the objective of preventing faults related to the resource limitation, some of them have been selected to monitor the following statistics (Chan, 2008; Godinho, 2011; Ramos, 2007):

Figure 2. AIDA Database Architecture with RAC and data guard solution systems

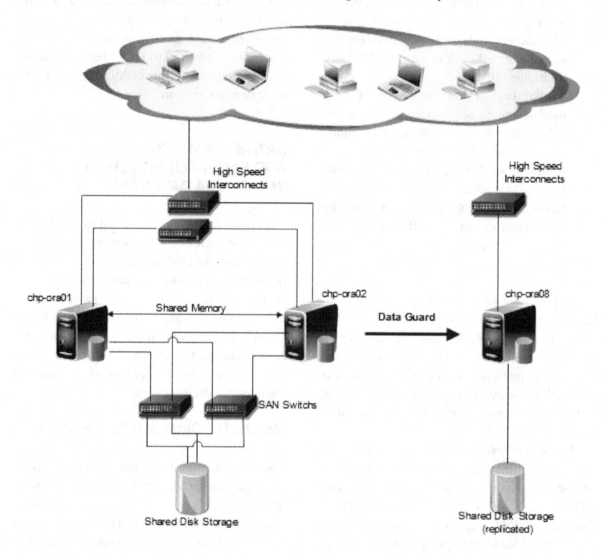

- **DB Time:** Is the time elapsing between the instant of placing of the query by the user to the reception of all results, this time should be the lowest possible. In Oracle systems, this time is a sum of total time (including CPU time, IO time, Wait time) spent on all requests from users. Therefore it is a good indicator of the workload of the system. Typically, this time increases with the number of simultaneous users or applications, but it may also increase due to other system problems (Dias, Ramacher, Shaft, Venkataramani, & Wood, 2005; Godinho, 2011).

- **Numbers of Transactions:** Transactions are indivisible sequences of operations that perform some work on the database. A greater number of transactions can indicate more work. In Oracle databases, the number of transactions can be obtained by adding up the values of statistics "user commits" and "user rollbacks" since each transaction always ends with a "commit" command and any undo operation as a "rollback" command (Godinho, 2011; Schumacher, 2003; Shallahamer, 2007).

- **Number of Executions:** One transaction consists of set of operations in the database depending one the query. It is important to collect information about the number of operations because it may be the case that there are few transactions but many operations. In Oracle databases this information can be obtained by collecting, the "execute count" statistic (Shallahamer, 2007).

- **Calls Ratio (RC):** Ratio between recursive calls and total calls. A recursive call occurs when a user request needs one query SQL that needs another SQL query. The total of calls is the sum of recursive calls and user calls (when a user request can be resolved through a single SQL query). Ideally this ratio should be as low as possible, since the high number of recursive calls can indicate problems with the design of tables or an excessive amount of triggers running at the same time. This ratio can be calculated by the equation (Rich, 2013):

$$RC = \frac{recursive\,Calls}{\left(recursive\,Calls + user\,Calls\right)}$$

- **Number of Current Logons:** Each logon, i.e., session is associated with a piece of memory, so many simultaneous sessions can cause problems. Note that the number of logons does not represent the number of users because each user may have multiple sessions. In Oracle systems, the number of sessions can be obtained by statistic "logons current" (Chan, 2008).

- **Processor Utilization:** It is necessary to constantly monitor its utilization because it is one of the most important database components. Low values of processor utiliza-

tion may indicate problems at the level of I/O. If the values are too high, it can compromise the functioning of the database. The percentage of utilization can be obtained thought a command of the operating system (Chan, 2008).

- **Memory Utilization:** The memory is a key component to the speed of the database systems. Depending on the data location the access speed changes. If the data is in memory, speed is greater. However, if the data is on disk, the access velocity is lower. This statistic is also accessible through the operating system commands (Schumacher, 2003).

- **Size of Redo File:** Represents the amount of redo entries (Kbytes). The redo files are used to store information about changes made to the database. An increase in the size of these files, indicates a higher number of operations and therefore a higher database load (Rich, 2013).

- **Buffer Cache Ratio (BC):** This ratio shows the percentage of data that is in memory cache, rather than in the disk. Normally, the BC is very high, so it is necessary to pay attention if BC decreases, this may indicate a lack of memory problems. BC can be calculated:

$$BC = \frac{\left(1 - physical\,Reads\right)}{\left(consistent\,Gets + block\,Gets\right) \times 100}$$

- **Amount of I/O Requests:** The I/O operations need a long time to process. A large number of these operations can indicate memory problems and frequent access to disc (Chan, 2008).

- **Amount of Redo Space Requests:** Indicates the lack of space to write in the buffer. Some delays may occur because it is necessary to write some data to disk to release memory. This can happen due to a poorly sized buffer, or excess entries generated simultaneously.

- **Volume of Network Traffic:** The network that interconnects all the components of the database. Therefore, the network is very important for database performance. If a volume of the network is increasing greatly, the database can be slow and compromise users' requests (Chan, 2008).

Modified Early Warning Score

In medicine, a model called the Modified Early Warning Score (MEWS), has been used for the prediction, in advance, of serious health problems. This model uses a decision table, like the Table 1, to evaluate the clinical status of the patient according to the monitoring of patients' vital signs. The set of these values represents the clinical status of the patient. (Albino & Jacinto, 2009; Gardner-Thorpe, Love, Wrightson, Walsh, & Keeling, 2006; Subbe, Kruger, Rutherford, & Gemmel, 2001).

Normally, if any of the parameters have a score equal to two, the patient must be in observation. In case, the sum of scores is equal to four, or an increase of two values, the patient requires urgent medical attention. In a more extreme situation, if a patient has a score higher than four, he is at risk of life (Devaney & Lead, 2011; Subbe et al., 2001).

Score Table

To evaluate the behaviour of the database it is essential to study its normal workload. So, after collecting the values of the statistics mentioned in the previous subsection during a month, it was possible to evaluate the state of the database based on percentiles and classifying the state through a decision table (Table 2). The statistics collected about the database (as mentioned in a previous section) are evaluated individually through the score table. Depending on the value of the deviation, abnormal situations are assigned granted scores such as in MEWS.

According to the scores, two situations can happen: less serious situations wherein the sum of all parameters' score is equal or less than four and serious situations wherein the sum is more than four. The value four was elected because in MEWS the value four also means the limit between less and more serious situations. Furthermore, the system's administrators agreed that this should be the limit. They also agreed that this value may not be e permanent and could be changed. In the first situation a visual warning will be issued on the dashboard responsible for monitoring the system

Table 1. MEWS scores

MEWS Score	3	2	1	0	1	2	3
Temperature (C)		< 35.0	35.1-36.0	36.1-38.0	38.1-38.5	> 38.6	
Heart rate (min⁻¹)		< 40	41-50	51-100	101-110	111-130	> 131
Systolic BP (mmHg)	< 70	71-80	81-100	101-199		> 200	
Respiratory rate (min⁻¹)		< 8		8-14	15-20	21-29	> 30
SPO$_2$	< 85	85-89	90-93	> 94			
Urine output (ml/kg/h)	Nil	< 0.5					
Neurological		New confusion		Alert	Reacting to voice	Reacting to pain	Unresponsive

Table 2. Database severity scores

SCORE	0	1	2	3
Value	< p75	p75-p80	p80-p90	> p90
Severity	Normal	Low Severity	Grave	Critical

and in the second warnings will be sent (via email) to the database administrator, allowing him to take speedy action to prevent the occurrence of a fault in the database.

New limits are calculated at the end of each day, based on new measurements that are periodically collected.

AIDA Database Workload

The most critical period detected in the AIDA's *database workload* during a normal day in CHP was between 10:00 to 12:00. Three peaks were detected: DB time (6.9 seconds), percentage of processor utilization (32.63%) and number of sessions (941).

Verifying the following points it is possible to verify the average values of several statistics related to AIDA database:

- Transactions per second – 214;
- Percentage of processor utilization – 18;
- Percentage of the memory utilization – 98;
- DB time per second – 6;
- Number of sessions – 681;
- Number of I/O requests per second – 632;
- Number of operations per second – 742;
- Buffer cache ratio – 0.998;
- Number of redo size (KB/s) – 152;
- Recursive calls ratio – 0.14;
- Network traffic volume (bytes/s) – 686 135;
- Redo log space requests per second – 0.55.

It is possible to conclude that AIDA database has a high utilization. The average number of sessions is 681. Furthermore, one can observe that on average about 214 transactions per second are processed, resulting on about 742 operations per second in the database.

Figure 3 presents six graphs for the following metrics: number of sessions, percentage of memory, volume of network traffic, number of transactions, operations and requests for I/O per second. In all these graphs there are four lines, the green corresponds to the 75th percentile, the yellow to the 80th percentile, the red to the 90th percentile and the blue is the value measured every minute. This excerpt was taken from one of the critical periods of the day, verifying that the blue line with some frequency exceeds the limits established by the percentiles indicating the presence of an abnormal situation.

If only considering the last measurement, it shows that the number of sessions and the volume of network traffic are above the 90th percentile, the number of operations per second is above the 80th percentile, and the number of requests for I / O operations is between percentile 75 and 80. The other metrics are in a normal situation, below the 75th percentile. In this case, the sum of the overall score would be 9, which would provide a warning email of abnormality. However, this situation does not cause database fault and for this reason it is necessary to update limits. Limits are updated at the end of the day taking account of all measured values that do not cause a fault, in this way the model improves its ability to represent reality.

It is important to note, that emails are sent only 15 to 15 minutes in order mean values be used to compare; thus avoiding the impact of small variations during the interval.

Figure 3. Extracting results from the monitor dashboard of AIDA

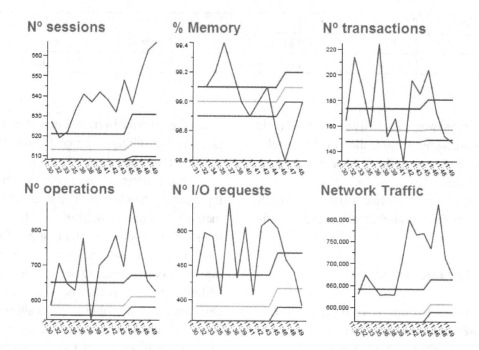

AGENTS WORKLOAD AND FORECASTING AND DETECTION OF FAULTS IN THE AIDA

Besides monitoring and preventing faults of the database, it is also important to monitor the behaviour of the agents individually as well as the computers they execute their tasks. It is also essential to monitor the agents and computers performance.

Monitoring Agents and Computer Performance

In order to collect information about the performance of the agents and computers the Windows Management Instrumentation (WMI) technology was used. WMI is the Microsoft approach for Web-Based Enterprise Management (WBEM), which is an industry initiative to develop a standard technology for accessing management. WMI uses the Common Information Model (CIM) standard to represent managed components such as systems, applications, networks, devices or even files. CIM is a standard, unified, object-oriented framework for describing physical and logical objects in a managed environment. To provide a common framework, CIM defines a series of objects taking into account a basic set of classes, classifications and associations. WMI objects can be accessed from scripts running either on a local machine or, security permitting, across a network. Besides that, it offers a powerful set of services including the retrieval of information and the event notification system. Furthermore, its utilization is easy because WMI uses a query-based language named Windows Query Language (WQL), which is a subset of the standard SQL (Structured Query Language) (Boshier, 2000; Costa & Silva, 2010; Lavy & Meggitt, 2001).

To characterize the agent performance, three metrics are collected (Microsoft, 2013a, 2013b):

- **Percent Processor Time:** Percentage of elapsed time that all of threads of the agent's process used the processor to execute instructions.
- **Working Set:** Maximum number, in megabytes, in the working set of the agent's process at any point in time. The working set is the set of memory pages touched recently by the threads in the process.
- **I/O Data Kbytes per Second:** Rate at which the agent's process is issuing read and write input/output (I/O) operations. This property counts all I/O activity generated by the process, including file, network, and device I/O operations.

On the other hand, to analyse the computer performance, information about RAM memory and CPU and further about the disk free space is collected. These three metrics are collected in the available percentage of CPU, RAM memory and disk space. Being aware of these three parameters, it is possible to characterize the computer performance, as well as identify situations where the machine is at a crash state (Microsoft, 2013c, 2013d, 2013e).

Agents and Computer Workload

During a month, the workload of the AIDA computers and agents was collected. As Figure 4 shows, among the five machines that execute AIDA agents, the hsa-aida08 computer is the one that consumes more CPU (an average of 14.09%) and the hsa-aida01 is the one that consumes more memory RAM (an average of 42,38%). On the other hand, hsa-aida01 is the one that consumes less CPU (an average of 5.5%), and hsa-aida08 and hsa-aida04 are the ones that consume less memory RAM (an average of 14.23% and 12.93%, respectively). It was also possible to confirm that the CPU's consumption was constant only varying from 5 to 10 percent in maximum. The consumption of RAM memory was very constant.

In Figure 5, the activity of the agent 101 during a day is presented. This agent is executed continu-

Figure 4. Extracting results from the monitor dashboard of AIDA machines

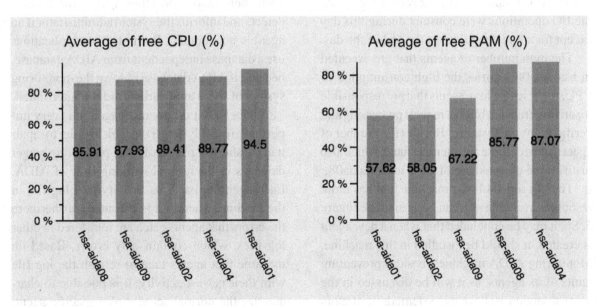

Figure 5. Extracting results from the monitor dashboard of AIDA agents. Activity of the agent 101 during a day (from 00:00 to 23:59) in hsa-aida01. Number of processes, average of CPU usage (%), RAM memory consumption (Mbytes) and I/O operations per second (Kbytes). On the right the number of processes and CPU consumption is highlighted

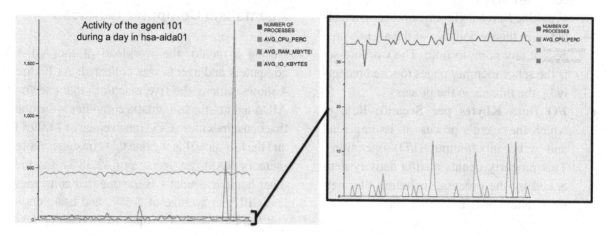

ously in hsa-aida01. As it can be seen on the left side of Figure 5, the average of RAM memory consumption is constant and it rounds the 400-450 Mbytes. On the right side of Figure 5, it can be observed that the number of processes produced by agent 101 is about 35. These are the reasons for the high consumption of RAM in hsa-aida01. In Figure 5 it also can be observed that the average of CPU consumption badly exceeds the 10% and the I/O operations were constant during this day except for some operations at the end of the day.

The high number of agents that are executed in hsa-aida08 justifies the high consumption of CPU. In these machine agents that are responsible for archive transfer, billing, request processing and verifications are installed. Besides the number of agents, most of these are often executed, which also justifies the elevated use of CPU in hsa-aida08.

The hsa-aida04 is the machine that has more resources available as it can be seen in the Figure 5. So, it may be concluded that when a new agent is created, it should be installed in this machine. Monitoring AIDA machines, besides preventing faults of its agents, as it will be discussed in the next subsection, it allows the system administrators

to manage the resources of AIDA computers in order to take advantage of them in the best way.

Forecasting and Detection of Faults

In this subsection two applications will be presented. One that prevents faults in AIDA computers (where agents are executed) and inherence prevents agent faults too. The other application quickly detects and informs the system administrator if an agent is not running. Both of these applications use a database independent from AIDA database, because if AIDA database is down the monitoring system of these applications are not interrupted.

When a fault occurs in an agent it is very important to quickly detect the fault in order to repair it in the shortest period of time, preventing bigger damages in the normal working flow of AIDA. Each agent registers its activity in a log file in the machine wherein it is executed, furthermore the errors that agents catch are registered in other log files, which contain only errors. Based on the time that agents take to refresh the log file with their newest activity, it is possible to characterize the normal activity of a specific agent, so it is possible to know how often an agent is executed. A minimum period of time (about two weeks) is useful to collect the intervals of time that characterize the agent activity. With a set of data collected about the intervals of time that an agent is executed and using a score table based on percentiles (similar with the score table presented in the previous section) it is possible to classify the state of agents activity, assigning a score such as it is done in MEWS.

Once the only variable used to calculate the score is the interval of time, the table for this situation has five states (from zero to four), moreover after doing tests the intervals between the percentiles 85, 90, 95 and 97.5 were assigned to this score table (instead of going from the percentile 75 until 90 such as the score table mentioned in the previous section). As for the model used on the database for *fault forecasting*, if the score obtained was less than four then a visual warning was issued on the monitoring dashboard, if the score was equal to four an email was sent to the system administrator in order to take speedy action to restore the normal working flow and prevent future damages. New limits are constantly calculated for each agent improving the application's efficacy. In relation to the errors recorded in the respective log file, the application detects when a new error appears and informs (by email) the administrator. To finish, this application is endowed with persistence in relation to the database state. If the database is down, all SQL statements are recorded in a file and the administrator is warned. When the database returns back to normal state, records are committed and the limits are refreshed. During the database down time, scores do not stop being

calculated and abnormal situations are detected. However the limits are not refreshed and the limits used in the score table are the last ones.

The application related to the computer monitoring also uses a score table to identify critical situations. This application prevents faults in the AIDA machines and by inherence prevents agent faults too. Initially, there was an attempt to create a score table based on percentiles as the tables previously presented, but it did not succeed. The application sent several false positive warnings per day. The computer performance limits for a good operation is an issue that varies a lot. Those limits depend of the objectives that the system administrator wants for a specific machine. For example, the hsa-aida01 machine has agents that are running continuously and they are responsible for archiving transfers and provide Web services. This behaviour provokes, as it is possible to see in the previous section, a high consumption of RAM memory. In this case, the system administrator should increase the RAM limits in order to avoid being warned in regular situations. So, the score table was created with default fixed limits that also were discussed among the system administrators for the available percentage of CPU, memory and disk space and through a management page, the system administrator can change these limits for each metric either generally or specifically for one machine. The default score table for all computers, based on MEWS, are presented in Table 3.

Once again, if the sum of all parameter scores is more than four, serious situations are detected and a warning (email) is sent to the administrator. For example, if a machine has 12% of CPU available, 6% of RAM memory and 14% of disk's free

Table 3. Default scores table for fault forecasting in the AIDA computers

Scores	0	1	2	3
Available CPU (%)	> 50	50-25	25-10	< 10
Available RAM memory (%)	> 15	15-10	10-5	< 5
Disk's Free Space (%)	> 15	15-10	10-5	< 5

space, the score is five, this situation is considered critical and the administrator will be informed to take preventive actions.

AIDA - SWOT ANALYSIS

Once the AIDA is a vital element of the normal operation of the HIS, it is very important to ensure that it offers the best functionalities and that users are satisfied. This analysis is intended to gather information about AIDA, in order to improve it. The *SWOT analysis* can reveal what are the great strengths of AIDA as well as its weaknesses. Furthermore, the opportunities are highlighted and the key threats to AIDA are alerted. The acronym SWOT means: strengths, weaknesses, opportunities and threats. Strengths represent the internal power that an organization owns to fight against the rivalry. Weaknesses represent aspects that reduce the quality of the product and/or of the service taking into account the customers opinion and/or competitive environment. Opportunities are defined as a set of conditions suitable for achieving certain objectives at the right moment, and threats are any inappropriate event or force in the external environment that causes damage to the organization's strategy. When this analysis is complete it is possible to use the strengths to develop new strategies; once weaknesses detected, these may be eliminated and some strategies may be reinforced; the opportunities should be explored; the threats should be countered. Strengths and weaknesses may be detected by an internal evaluation, on the other hand opportunities and threats by an external one. The organizational environment wherein the SWOT analysis is performed involves a huge number of elements and complex relationships of cause-and-effect, and is split in the internal and external environment. The first one can be controlled by the organization since it is very sensitive to the strategies implemented. There are internal factors such as

management, culture at work, finance, research and development, staff, operational efficiency and capacity, technical frameworks and organizational structure. Nonetheless, external factors such as political, economic, cultural, social, technological and ambient, define the external environment, which is not controlled by the organization and acts homogeneously in all organizations included in the same market and the same area. It may be concluded that opportunities and threats affect all organizations, however the probability of their impacts may be reduced by each organization (Dyson, 2004; Pereira et al., 2013).

In the following subsections the items of AIDA SWOT analysis in the CHP are presented.

AIDA Strengths

- Power management of change in the system;
- Ability to personalize objects like interface;
- High availability and full-time support;
- High accessibility;
- Security;
- Technologically modern system (R. Rodrigues et al., 2012; Santos, Portela, & Vilas-Boas, 2011) ;
- Ease of maintenance;
- Ease of use (Pereira et al., 2012);
- Credibility of the management team;
- Immediate access to detailed clinical information;
- Reports customized to meet the needs required;
- High computing power;
- Interoperability (Miranda et al., 2010);
- Ability to remotely access the system in a safe way;
- Failures prediction of databases (Silva et al., 2012);
- Fast detection of agents' abnormal activity;
- Failures prediction of machines wherein agents are executed.

AIDA Weaknesses

- System documentation non-existent;
- Graphical interface slightly confusing;
- Necessity of paper documentation in some services of the CHP;
- Insufficient education and training of health professionals;
- Computers are old and consequently slow.

Opportunities to AIDA

- Ability to integrate other applications;
- Ability to provide information via Internet;
- Ability to expand and sustain new services;
- Increasing importance of digital files;
- Government incentives;
- Extinction of paper use in the CHP;
- Modernization and organizational development;
- Projection of more efficient and usable interfaces;
- Developing better and more effective security protocols;
- Increasing expectation of citizens to obtain answers of clinical services faster and, at the same time, reliably;
- Use of mobile devices to access the system;
- Use of new technologies in order to enrich the system.

Threats to AIDA

- High degree of competition from other systems;
- Expansion of software companies for the health market;
- Competition/market pressure;
- Competition for scarce talented IT resources;
- Economic-financial crisis and subsequent financial constraints;
- Readiness to recover from disasters;
- Cyber attacks (hackers);

- System is based on Internet Explorer.

It may be concluded that AIDA in the CHP is a system of high relevance, endowed with many positive points such as interoperability, good usability, faults forecasting and high availability. On the other hand, a small number of weaknesses were detected such as the inexistent system documentation. This weakness is overcome by the full-time presence of technicians, who are always available to assist any healthcare professional.

The computerization of the entire clinical process in all services of the CHP is not an easy task. Nonetheless, all the efforts are being made for concretizing this main goal.

Relatively to interface, the Portuguese legislation forces the healthcare units to save all information about every patient, consequently when a professional accesses the clinical process of a specific patient, every clinical information about him has to be displayed, which can make the reading process a bit confusing.

The current Portuguese financial situation and the high cost of new technology acquisition made difficult replacing old computers. So it is very important to look at opportunities that may improve the AIDA. For example, the increasing importance of digital files creates a good opportunity to extinct the use of paper in the CHP. The other opportunities such as integrating new applications and services, improving security protocols and using mobile devices should be well exploited in order to fight against the competition.

The *SWOT analysis* shows few threats that the administration should realize. The biggest threat is the competition from other systems, despite the economic and financial crisis represents a big threat as well.

Security is an issue that the administrators should be always aware of, in spite of AIDA providing a high level of security. It is very important to ensure the security and confidentiality of its information and prevent cyber attacks. It is also very important to ensure the availability of the system. That means the system should have alternatives to disaster situations; if the system crashes, the CHP must not paralyze its activities.

CONCLUSION

This chapter demonstrates the importance and the impact that the interoperability causes in healthcare information systems. The usage of the HL7 standard embedded in a multi-agent system (endowed of autonomy, reactivity, pro-activity and social, emotional and moral behaviour) is fundamental to improve communication among heterogeneous systems, i.e., to achieve the interoperability among the healthcare information systems.

The intelligent and dynamic framework called AIDA is presented in this chapter. It constitutes a solution to accomplish the interoperability in healthcare units surpassing functional needs as well as financial and technical restrictions among clinical, medical and administrative systems.

The main core of AIDA platform is its database. The AIDA database must guarantee its confidentiality and integrity as well as its availability, which are ensured by fault tolerance mechanisms.

In order to prevent fault in AIDA database, a fault forecasting system based on MEWS model was adapted to the database context. Besides this system prevents database faults, it was possible to study the normal workload of AIDA database. In the Centro Hospitalar do Porto, a high utilization and workload of AIDA database (an average of 681 sessions, 214 transactions per second and 742 operations per second) was verified. It was also identified that the critical workload of AIDA is the period between 10:00 and 12:00.

A similar fault forecasting system for the computers wherein agents are executed was implemented. Detection of the faults system was also implemented. It enables detecting the agent fault in order to repair in the shortest period of time possible, preventing bigger damages in the normal working flow of AIDA. Furthermore, it was possible to study the computer and agents workload for the purpose of allowing the system administrators to manage the resources of AIDA machines and agents.

The SWOT analysis demonstrates that the system has a lot of strong points, as well as fewer weak ones. Through the identification of the system weaknesses, the system administrators can make up their minds. The evaluation proved to be a powerful tool, which has provided useful information to improve the quality of AIDA.

ACKNOWLEDGMENT

This work is funded by National Funds through the FCT - Fundação para a Ciência e a Tecnologia (Portuguese Foundation for Science and Technology) within project PEst-OE/EEI/UI0752/2014.

REFERENCES

Albino, A., & Jacinto, V. (2009). *Implementação da escala de alerta precoce - EWS*. Portimão.

Ashdown, L., & Kyte, T. (2011). *Oracle Database Concepts, 11g Release 2 (11.2)*. Oracle.

Bertino, E., & Sandhu, R. (2005). Database security - Concepts, approaches, and challenges. *IEEE Transactions on Dependable and Secure Computing, 2*(1), 2–19. doi:10.1109/TDSC.2005.9

Boshier, A. (2000). Windows Management Instrumentation: A Simple, Powerful Tool for Scripting Windows Management. *MSDN Magazine, 4*.

Carr, C. D., & Moore, S. M. (2003). IHE: A model for driving adoption of standards. *Computerized Medical Imaging and Graphics, 27*(2-3), 137–146. doi:10.1016/S0895-6111(02)00087-3 PMID:12620304

Chan, I. (2008). *Oracle Database Performance Tuning Guide, 10g Release 2 (10.2)*. Oracle.

Contreras, M., Germán, E., Chi, M., & Sheremetov, L. (2004). Design and implementation of a FIPA compliant Agent Platform in.NET. *Journal of Object Technology*, *3*(9), 5–28. doi:10.5381/jot.2004.3.9.a1

Costa, L., & Silva, F. (2010). Um Software de gerenciamento baseado no padrão WBEM-WMI. *Sistemas de Informação & Gestão de Tecnologia*, *5*.

Devaney, G., & Lead, W. (2011). *Guideline for the use of the modified early warning score (MEWS)*. Academic Press.

Dias, K., Ramacher, M., Shaft, U., Venkataramani, V., & Wood, G. (2005). Automatic performance diagnosis and tuning in Oracle. In *Proceedings of the 2005 CIDR Conf*. CIDR.

Drake, S., Hu, W., McInnis, D., Sköld, M., Srivastava, A., & Thalmann, L. … Wolski, A. (2005). Architecture of Highly Available Databases. In M. Malek, M. Reitenspieß, & J. Kaiser (Eds.), Service Availability (Vol. 3335, pp. 1–16). Springer.

Duarte, J., Salazar, M., Quintas, C., Santos, M., Neves, J., Abelha, A., & Machado, J. (2010). Data Quality Evaluation of Electronic Health Records in the Hospital Admission Process. In *Proceedings of International Conference on Computer and Information Science*, (pp. 201–206). Academic Press.

Dyson, R. G. (2004). Strategic development and SWOT analysis at the University of Warwick. *European Journal of Operational Research*, *152*(3), 631–640. doi:10.1016/S0377-2217(03)00062-6

Gardner-Thorpe, J., Love, N., Wrightson, J., Walsh, S., & Keeling, N. (2006). The value of Modified Early Warning Score (MEWS) in surgical in-patients: a prospective observational study. *Annals of the Royal College of Surgeons of England*, *88*(6), 571–575. doi:10.1308/003588406X130615 PMID:17059720

Godinho, R. (2011). *Availability, Reliability and Scalability in Database Architecture*. Universidade do Minho.

HL7. (2012). *HL7 Website*. Retrieved from http://www.hl7.org/

Kim, S., Cho, N., Lee, Y., Kang, S.-H., Kim, T., Hwang, H., & Mun, D. (2010). Application of density-based outlier detection to database activity monitoring. *Information Systems Frontiers*, 1–11.

Lavy, M. M., & Meggitt, A. J. (2001). *Windows Management Instrumentation (WMI)*. New Riders. Retrieved from http://www.google.pt/books?id=DD1jA3RgFEMC

Luck, M., McBurney, P., & Preist, C. (2003). *Agent technology: Enabling next generation computing (a roadmap for agent based computing)*. AgentLink/University of Southampton.

Machado, J., Abelha, A., Novais, P., Neves, J., & Neves, J. (2010). Quality of service in healthcare units. *International Journal of Computer Aided Engineering and Technology*, *2*(4), 436–449. doi:10.1504/IJCAET.2010.035396

Machado, J., Miranda, M., Gonçalves, P., Abelha, A., Neves, J., & Marques, J. A. (2010). *AIDATrace: Interoperation platform for active monitoring in healthcare environments*. Academic Press.

Microsoft. (2013a). *WMI Overview*. Retrieved August 16, 2013, from http://technet.microsoft.com/en-us/library/cc753534.aspx

Microsoft. (2013b). *Win32_PerfFormattedData_PerfProc_Process class*. Retrieved August 16, 2013, from http://msdn.microsoft.com/en-us/library/windows/desktop/aa394277(v=vs.85).aspx

Microsoft. (2013c). *Win32_PerfFormattedData_PerfOS_Processor class*. Retrieved August 16, 2013, from http://msdn.microsoft.com/en-us/library/windows/desktop/aa394271(v=vs.85).aspx

Microsoft. (2013d). *Win32_PerfFormattedData_PerfOS_Memory class*. Retrieved August 16, 2013, from http://msdn.microsoft.com/en-us/library/windows/desktop/aa394268(v=vs.85).aspx

Microsoft. (2013e). *Win32_PerfFormattedData_PerfDisk_LogicalDisk class*. Retrieved August 16, 2013, from http://msdn.microsoft.com/en-us/library/windows/desktop/aa394261(v=vs.85).aspx

Miranda, M., Duarte, J., Abelha, A., Machado, J., & Neves, J. (2010). Interoperability in healthcare. In *Proceedings of European Simulation and Modelling Conference*. ESM.

Miranda, M., Machado, J., Abelha, A., & Neves, J. (2013). In G. Fortino, C. Badica, M. Malgeri, & R. Unland (Eds.), *Healthcare Interoperability through a JADE Based Multi-Agent Platform* (Vol. 446, pp. 83–88). Intelligent Distributed Computing, VI: Springer. doi:10.1007/978-3-642-32524-3_11

Miranda, M., Salazar, M., Portela, F., Santos, M., Abelha, A., Neves, J., & Machado, J. (2012). Multi-agent Systems for HL7 Interoperability Services. In Procedia Technology (Vol. 5, pp. 725–733). Elsevier.

Nair, S. (2008). The Art of Database Monitoring. *Information Systems Control Journal*, (Ccm), 1–4.

Palazzo, L., Sernani, P., Claudi, A., Dolcini, G., Biancucci, G., & Dragoni, A. F. (2013). *A Multi-Agent Architecture for Health Information Systems*. Retrieved from http://netmed2013.dii.univpm.it/sites/netmed2013.dii.univpm.it/files/papers/paper5.pdf

Peixoto, H., Santos, M., Abelha, A., & Machado, J. (2012). Intelligence in Interoperability with AIDA. In *Proceedings of 20th International Symposium on Methodologies for Intelligent Systems* (LNCS), (Vol. 7661). Berlin: Springer.

Pereira, R., Duarte, J., Salazar, M., Santos, M., Abelha, A., & Machado, J. (2012). Usability of an Electronic Health Record. *IEEM, 5*.

Pereira, R., Salazar, M., Abelha, A., & Machado, J. (2013). SWOT Analysis of a Portuguese Electronic Health Record. In Collaborative, Trusted and Privacy-Aware e/m-Services (Vol. 399, pp. 169–177). Springer.

Ramos, L. (2007). *Performance Analysis of a Database Caching System In a Grid Environment*. FEUP.

Rich, B. (2013). *Oracle Database Reference, 11g Release 2 (11.2)*. Oracle.

Rodrigues, A. (2005). *Oracle 10g e 9i: Fundamentos Para Profissionais*. Lisboa: FCA.

Rodrigues, R., Gonçalves, P., Miranda, M., Portela, F., Santos, M., & Neves, J. … Machado, J. (2012). Monitoring Intelligent System for the Intensive Care Unit using RFID and Multi-Agent Systems. In *Proceedings of IEEE International Conference on Industrial Engineering and Engineering Management (IEEM2012)*. IEEE.

Rogers, R., Peres, Y., & Müller, W. (2010). Living longer independently - A healthcare interoperability perspective. *E&I Elektrotechnik und Informationstechnik, 127*(7-8), 206–211. doi:10.1007/s00502-010-0748-8

Santos, M. F., Portela, F., & Vilas-Boas, M. (2011). *INTCARE: Multi-agent approach for real-time intelligent decision support in intensive medicine*. Academic Press.

Schumacher, R. (2003). *Oracle Performance Troubleshooting With Dictionary Internals SQL & Tuning Scripts*. Kittrell: Rampant TechPress.

Shallahamer, C. (2007). *Forecasting Oracle Performance*. Berkeley, CA: Apress.

Silva, P., Quintas, C., Duarte, J., Santos, M., Neves, J., Abelha, A., & Machado, J. (2012). Hospital database workload and fault forecasting. In *Step Towards Fault Forecasting in Hospital Information Systems*. Academic Press.

Strohm, R. (2012). *Oracle Real Application Clusters Administration and Deployment Guide, 11g Release 2 (11.2)*. Oracle.

Subbe, C. P., Kruger, M., Rutherford, P., & Gemmel, L. (2001). Validation of a Modified Early Warning Score in medical admissions. *QJM*, *94*(10), 521–526. doi:10.1093/qjmed/94.10.521 PMID:11588210

Weber-Jahnke, J., Peyton, L., & Topaloglou, T. (2012). eHealth system interoperability. *Information Systems Frontiers*, *14*(1), 1–3. doi:10.1007/s10796-011-9319-8

KEY TERMS AND DEFINITIONS

AIDA: Platform developed to ensure interoperability between healthcare information systems.

Database Workload: Database performance based on its main statistics.

Fault Forecasting: Prevention of failures through the monitoring of the performance of the object intended.

HL7: Standard for interoperability in healthcare.

Intelligent Agent: Autonomous programs that operate in an environment in order to achieve a goal.

Interoperability: Autonomous ability to interact and communicate.

Multi Agent System: System with multiple agents working together in order to achieve a global goal.

SWOT Analysis: Picking and discussion of strengths, weaknesses, opportunities and threats with the purpose of know better and improve a system.

Chapter 6
Efficient Healthcare Integrity Assurance in the Cloud with Incremental Cryptography and Trusted Computing

Wassim Itani
Beirut Arab University, Lebanon

Ayman Kayssi
American University of Beirut, Lebanon

Ali Chehab
American University of Beirut, Lebanon

ABSTRACT

In this chapter, the authors propose the design and implementation of an integrity-enforcement protocol for detecting malicious modification on Electronic Healthcare Records (EHRs) stored and processed in the cloud. The proposed protocol leverages incremental cryptography premises and trusted computing building blocks to support secure integrity data structures that protect the medical records while: (1) complying with the specifications of regulatory policies and recommendations, (2) highly reducing the mobile client energy consumption, (3) considerably enhancing the performance of the applied cryptographic mechanisms on the mobile client as well as on the cloud servers, and (4) efficiently supporting dynamic data operations on the EHRs.

INTRODUCTION

The healthcare industry is considered one of the main sectors that can take advantage of the services offered by the cloud computing model. By outsourcing the storage and processing of EHRs to remote cloud providers, healthcare institutions are guaranteed unlimited opportunities summarized in the following points:

1. On-demand abundance in fault-tolerant storage capacities.

DOI: 10.4018/978-1-4666-6118-9.ch006

2. Powerful processing on clusters of commodity computing machinery. This contributes to reducing the physicians' practice times as well as the patient's waiting times.

3. Better compliance with regulatory policies such as HIPAA (Annas, 2003) by migrating the EHRs to HIPAA-compliant cloud providers.

4. Mobile universal access that enhances the seamless sharing of medical information among physicians, patients, and insurance companies. This results in better dissemination of medical expertise among physicians and in major time and cost savings.

5. Adaptable pay-as-you-go pricing schemes that ensure the cost-effective management of the ever-growing patient data.

Despite the manifold advantages inherently provided by cloud computing in the healthcare field, several challenges are hindering its widespread adoption and impeding the process of medical data and software migration to the cloud. A chief concern is represented in safeguarding the integrity of the patient medical information as it is stored and processed in the cloud. The integrity assurance of patients' data should be given exceptional attention since any malicious modification on EHRs may result in fallacious medical decisions and hence life-threatening consequences. The patients concern about the integrity of their medical records is highly justified and has its roots in the intrinsic structure of the cloud computing model where everything is under the jurisdiction of the cloud provider. In cloud computing, EHRs are stored and processed on top of, possibly, untrusted servers that are not owned, controlled, or even managed by the respective healthcare institution. If the cloud service provider happens to have malicious intentions, it may undetectably jeopardize the integrity of the patients' medical records.

In addition to the integrity threats posed by malicious and "misbehaving" cloud providers, other sources of risk on healthcare cloud data include traditional internal and external attacks on the cloud network.

EHRs are characterized by a set of security, regulatory, and operational constraints that distinguish them from generic cloud data as far as integrity assurance is concerned:

1. EHRs are governed by strict regulatory policies, such as HIPAA, that all medical institutions must comply with by law. HIPAA specifies the administrative, technical, and physical protection mechanisms that need to be applied to safeguard the privacy and integrity of medical records.

2. Individual EHRs consist of relatively large data sets represented in medical imagery (X-Rays, CT scans, MRIs, radiology scans), lab test reports, physician diagnosis and transcripts, etc. that increase continuously over the life span of the respective patient subject. The healthcare integrity enforcement system should be designed to operate efficiently on large data records.

3. Individual EHRs may be modified and updated frequently depending on the respective patient case. The healthcare integrity enforcement system should be able to securely support dynamic operations on cloud data as it is stored and processed in the cloud.

4. A considerable portion of EHRs is, currently, generated, analyzed, and updated using battery-powered mobile and portable devices on the client side. The healthcare integrity enforcement system should be designed with energy-awareness in mind to preserve the battery resources of energy-limited devices operated by physicians and medical personnel.

5. EHRs should be preserved in storage and kept accessible for relatively long periods of time (minimum EHR retention periods can reach up to thirty years in the majority of medical institutions in the US.). This fact stresses

on the need for having high-performance and energy-efficient security mechanisms to assure the integrity of the ever-growing EHRs during these long retention periods.

The above-mentioned constraints render the design of the integrity enforcement mechanisms on EHRs quite intricate and challenging. Any healthcare integrity protocol should target the EHR security, regulatory, and operational requirements to stipulate the migration of medical records to the cloud. Relying on traditional integrity mechanisms such as message authentication codes and digital signatures in their classical forms would not suit the constraints of healthcare services in the evolving cloud computing infrastructure.

In this chapter, we propose the design and implementation of an integrity-enforcement protocol for detecting malicious modification on EHRs stored and processed in the cloud. The proposed protocol leverages incremental cryptography premises and trusted computing building blocks to support secure integrity data structures that protect the medical records while: (1) complying with the specifications of regulatory policies and recommendations, (2) highly reducing the mobile client energy consumption, (3) considerably enhancing the performance of the applied cryptographic mechanisms on the mobile client as well as on the cloud servers, and (4) efficiently supporting dynamic data operations on the EHRs. The trusted computing components prevent any undetectable modification on the EHRs by unauthorized internal or external entities, including the cloud provider itself. The incremental cryptography mechanisms contribute to reduce the energy consumption of the cryptographic operations on the mobile client side and enhancing the performance of the overall integrity enforcement protocol. The central property that gives incremental cryptography algorithms their merits in the healthcare domain is the following: if we apply the incremental cryptography algorithm on a medical record and afterwards this record gets

modified, it is feasible to update the result of the algorithm by merely using the modified record blocks instead of re-computing the algorithm on the whole document. This property contributes to major performance and energy efficiencies in a healthcare setting due to the large size of medical documents and the frequent update mechanisms that are performed on them.

The proposed system design will be analytically analyzed and experimentally implemented in a real cloud computing environment to demonstrate the performance and energy savings it provides in a healthcare setting.

BACKGROUND

Incremental cryptography has its basis in the work by Bellare, Goldreich, and Goldwasser (1994). The main property aimed in their work is to devise a set of encryption and hashing algorithms that can be efficiently and rapidly applied on the modified chunks of updated input documents instead of re-operating on the whole documents from scratch. As stated previously, this property contributes to major performance and energy savings in the medical domain due to the intrinsic nature of EHRs and the computational patterns applied on them. In other words, the relatively large size of medical documents and the frequency of update mechanisms that are performed on them renders incremental cryptography algorithms a very efficient choice for ensuring the integrity of EHRs stored and processed in the cloud. Bellare, Guerin, and Rogaway (1995) introduced the XOR MAC authentication structure. XOR MAC is a message authentication code algorithm characterized by being parallelizable, incremental, and provably secure. The incremental property of the XOR MAC algorithm is graphically demonstrated in Figure 1.

Trusted computing-based systems and protocols are believed to be a natural trend that the cloud computing market will follow in the coming years to resolve the different data privacy and integrity

Figure 1. A graphical demonstration of the XOR MAC incremental property

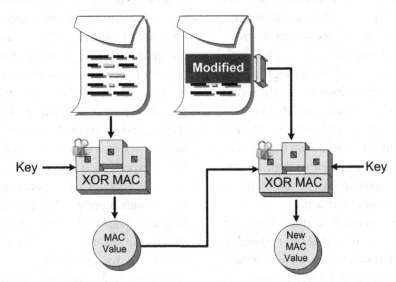

challenges hampering the wide adoption of cloud computing, particularly in healthcare and financial applications. This fact is corroborated by a set of signals received from the IT industry itself:

1. The considerable advancement in physical security mechanisms and packaging technology and the assortment of secure applications that can be implemented on top of physically-secure cryptographic coprocessors.

2. The availability of a set of successful cryptographic coprocessor implementations meeting the strictest FIPS 140 security standards (Dyer et al., 2001).

3. The emergence of general-purpose open-source cryptographic coprocessor designs that provide competitive performance and higher functionality as compared to commercial products with one to two orders of magnitude reduction in cost.

4. The proposed work of the Trusted Computing Group (Berger, 2005) for developing a set of cloud security services and protocols based on their Trusted Platform Module (TPM) (Bajikar, 2002).

Cryptographic coprocessors (Best, 1980; Tygar & Yee, 1991) represent a prominent trusted computing building block that is believed to play a major role in building secure cloud protocols. Cryptographic coprocessors aid in providing secure and isolated processing containers in the computing cloud that are physically and logically protected against unauthorized access (even from the cloud service provider itself). A cryptographic coprocessor is a hardware card that interfaces with the main computer or server, mainly through a PCI-based interface. It is a complete computing system that is supported with a processor, RAM, ROM, backup battery, non-volatile persistent storage (mainly used to securely store cryptographic data structures and keying material) and an Ethernet network card. For economical reasons, a crypto coprocessor is generally less capable in terms of processing and memory resources than the main server system it interfaces to. The main property that gives a crypto coprocessor its secure capabilities is the tamper-proof casing that encloses it and makes it resistant to physical attacks. A secure coprocessor tamper-resistance or tamper-responding mechanisms should reset the internal state of the coprocessor (RAM, persistent storage, processor registers) upon detecting any suspicious physical activity on the coprocessor hardware.

The only logical interface to the functionality of the coprocessor is done through a *root* highly-privileged process burned at manufacturing into the ROM of the coprocessor. This process represents a minimal operating system for the coprocessor. The input/output access to the cryptographic coprocessor can be either done locally via the main server system bus, or remotely via the coprocessor network interface.

It is worth mentioning here that substantial research efforts had been carried out to develop tamper resistant hardware technologies for supporting data and platform integrity assurance protocols. The Trusted Computing Group led the way in this field by developing tamper-resistant TPM modules. Moreover, virtualization support has been lately developed for TPMs (Perez, Sailer, & van Doorn, 2006; Sadeghi, Stüble, & Winandy, 2008) allowing operating systems and applications running in virtual machines to utilize the trusted computing capabilities of these modules. Nevertheless, TPM modules are typically equipped with limited processing and memory resources which makes them suitable for mere personal integrity enforcement on single user devices. This fact renders TPMs infeasible for supporting virtualized multiuser processing in enterprise service environments as is the case in cloud computing.

Many cloud computing research works have dealt with the security and confidentiality of customer data at the storage level within the boundaries of the cloud IT infrastructure. The proposed approaches mainly focused on encrypting the storage facility contents at rest in its physical location, typically, in relational and object database systems. The main drawback of such approaches resides in the necessity to decrypt the encrypted data before being processed by the cloud computing units which can

impose a considerable performance impact and can induce several limitations on certain native database operations such as comparison queries and updates on encrypted data. For this reason, the notion of partial data encryption was introduced to decrease the performance impact of encryption/decryption operations and to relax some of the restrictions on the basic database operations. In spite of this, a significant performance decline is still experienced when accessing and updating encrypted data or when performing comparison searches and queries on an encrypted partition in large cloud storage facilities. An extensive discussion on the different confidentiality and integrity approaches for securing data at rest is presented in Bowers, Juels, and Oprea (2009); Kamara and Lauter (2010); Wang et al., (2010).

The work in Li and Jha (2010) aims at providing a secure execution environment for virtual machines running on top of untrusted management operating systems. This work targets type-I virtualization architectures such as the Xen virtualization system (Barham et al.,, 2003). The main concept behind this work is to reduce the Trusted Computing Base (TCB) of the virtualization system by excluding the management OS out of this TCB. This exclusion reduces the size of the trusted code and thus aids in limiting the number of attacks that can jeopardize the security of the entire execution environment. Unlike the scheme that we present in this chapter, the security model presented in Li and Jha (2010) is susceptible to hardware, side-channel, and direct memory access attacks.

Wang et al., (2010) propose a cloud storage integrity verification mechanism that is based on erasure codes to ensure the correctness and availability of clients' data. This is done by providing redundancies that localize the misbehaving servers responsible of data corruption. Their scheme supports dynamic operations on stored data including block modification, deletion, and insertion.

We believe that Wang et al., (2010) suffers from a set of limitations that are addressed in the following points:

- The threat model presented by the authors is not realistic in cloud computing environments since most of the analysis is based on the number of misbehaving or corrupt servers. In cloud computing, all the storage servers, facilities, and resources are under the full control of the cloud service provider. In this respect, all the servers can be assumed to be effectively compromised if the cloud provider is a misbehaving one. We believe that the presented threat model better suits a traditionally distributed system with replicated storage resources rather than a cloud computing environment. Only in a traditionally distributed system the security analysis based on the number of compromised servers makes sense. In cloud computing environments, all remote cloud resources should be assumed compromised from the early stages of application or service deployment.

- The authors do not mention the system model regarding the dynamic operations on cloud stored data. In other words, we believe that there should be a discussion on the entities that can carry out this kind of dynamic operations and in what domain. This property is very important in cloud computing since if the operations are to be locally carried out on the client device then this is fine from a security point of view. However, if these dynamic operations are to be executed in the cloud, i.e. in the cloud provider's address space (this is the usual scenario in cloud computing), then all the security properties and guarantees will be violated since, in this case, the provider

needs to posses the secret keying material to be able to execute the processing operations.

The work in Ateniese et al. (2007); Schwarz and Miller (2006); Shacham and Waters (2008); Curtmola et al. (2008) follow analogous concepts.

SYSTEM MODEL

The system model assumed in this work consists of three main entities: a mobile client that consumes the medical cloud storage services, a cloud service provider that manages and operates the cloud storage facility, and a trusted third party (TTP) that configures and distributes tamperproof cryptographic coprocessors for installation in the remote cloud. The TTP is the organizational unit trusted by both, the cloud provider and customer. In a cloud computing infrastructure, a crypto coprocessor should be installed on every physical server running virtual machine for customers registered in the medical cloud service. To make the solution economically feasible, the system allows the resources of the crypto coprocessor to be shared among more than one cloud customer. In fact, it is this sharing mechanism that necessitates the presence of a TTP to load the cryptographic data structures and keying material of more than one cloud customer on the crypto coprocessor. Technically, the main responsibility of the *TTP* is to load a set of public/private key pairs into the persistent storage of the crypto coprocessor. Every public/private key pair (PU_{ID}/PR_{ID}) is to be allocated to a single healthcare customer when the latter registers with the cloud integrity service. Upon registration, the healthcare customer will securely receive a copy of her public/private key pair. This can be achieved through a face-to-face transaction or a secure electronic session.

The PU_{ID}/PR_{ID} key pair set can be remotely updated by the *TTP* even after the crypto coprocessor is installed in the computing cloud. This remote key update mechanism is very important to support the registration of new customers and the service revocation of existing customers.

In addition to loading the customer's PU_{ID}/PR_{ID} key pair, the *TTP* also loads its own private master key, K_M, into the persistent storage of the crypto coprocessor. This key is needed by the *TTP* to remotely authenticate to the crypto coprocessor and to securely execute commands against it. Due to the security sensitive responsibilities of the *TTP*, serious measures should be employed to fortify the *TTP* site against the different forms of system and network penetration attacks.

After the mobile client registers with the service, it executes an authenticated version of the Diffie-Hellman key management protocol (Diffie, Van Oorschot, & Wiener, 1992) to exchange and share a secret Key K_s with the crypto coprocessor in the cloud.

Threat Model

The attacker in the system threat model can jeopardize the integrity and authenticity of the EHRs in two main forms: (1) by executing weak man-in-the-middle attacks on network traffic or by (2) compromising the cloud site itself. The attack on the cloud site could either be executed by an outsider or the cloud provider itself. In other words, the attacker is assumed to have the necessary expertise and tools to conduct any type of modification and fabrication attack on the EHR data marshaling on the network links or that stored and processed in the cloud infrastructure.

The main axiom we consider in this work is that a secure coprocessor is capable of ensuring the privacy and integrity of the data it possesses in its address space. In fact, every security protocol depends on a set of assumptions, which if respected, supports the proper fulfillment of the promised security properties and mechanisms. For instance, when designing cryptographic protocols, it is usually assumed that encryption algorithms are computationally-secure in resisting cryptanalysis and that a successful brute force attack on the key space is highly expensive considering current technological and computational capabilities. Thus, analogously, we believe that it may be possible to violate the physical security protections of a crypto coprocessor but this would require enormous effort and resources that are not currently possessed by attackers. Based on this, we do not associate the protocol designs we present in this work with any available crypto coprocessor design technology, but rather present their using a generic crypto coprocessor model that serves the physical security axiom we initially assumed. In other words, we believe that just as cryptographic algorithms can be evolved and modified to increase, beyond feasibility, the cost required to break them; tamper-proof security packaging technology can be enhanced to increase the cost and effort required to breach the crypto coprocessor physical security mechanisms.

System Design

The system design is divided into three phases: the initialization phase, the data update phase, and the integrity verification phase. The protocol steps in each phase are presented and followed by a mathematical analysis of the energy savings realized. A schematic diagram detailing the interaction among the cloud entities in each protocol phase is presented in Figure 2.

The Initialization Phase

In this phase, the mobile data is prepared with the incremental authentication codes before migration to the cloud. For every client EHR EHR_x marked for cloud migration, an incremental MAC MAC_x

Figure 2. Protocol interaction among the mobile client, cloud provider, and the crypto coprocessor

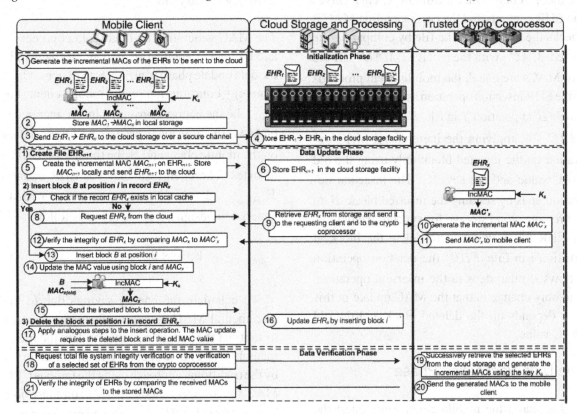

is created using the shared key K_s. The generated incremental MACs are stored locally on the mobile client side and the corresponding files are transferred to the cloud storage.

The Data Update Phase

This phase demonstrates how the incremental cryptographic concepts can be utilized for securely and efficiently supporting dynamic operations on the cloud data. Three main dynamic operations are adopted: EHR creation, EHR block insertion, and EHR block deletion. Note that the insertion and deletion operations form the building block for other file operations such as block replacement, block swapping, and block move.

EHR creation: the EHR creation steps are analogous to those followed in the initialization phase. To secure the integrity of a newly created

EHR EHR_{n+1}, the mobile client generates an incremental MAC on this file using the shared secret K_s. MAC_{n+1} is stored locally while EHR_{n+1} is transferred to the cloud for remote storage.

EHR block insertion: to insert a block B at position i in file EHR_x, the mobile client checks the availability of the EHR in local storage before applying the integrity operations. If EHR_x is not available, the mobile client requests it from the remote cloud storage. The cloud service provider processes the EHR request by retrieving the record from storage and sending a copy to the mobile client as well as to the trusted crypto coprocessor. Upon receiving EHR_x the trusted coprocessor generates the incremental MAC MAC'_x using the shared key K_s and sends this MAC value to the mobile client. Once the mobile client receives the EHR contents and the corresponding MAC it checks the integrity of the file by comparing the stored MAC_x with the received MAC'_x. If the two MACs are equal, the mobile client proceeds to the EHR insertion operation as follows: it inserts block B at position i in file EHR_x and updates MAC_x by applying the incremental MAC operation on the inserted block only using the old MAC value and the key K_s. The insertion operation ends by sending the inserted block B to the remote cloud storage for synchronization.

EHR block deletion: to delete the block at position i in File EHR_x the deletion operation follows similar steps to the insertion operation. The only change is that the MAC update in this case depends on the deleted block and the old MAC value.

The Data Verification Phase

In this phase, the mobile client can request the integrity verification of an EHR, collection of EHRs, or the whole medical record system stored in the remote cloud. To avoid expensive data transfer operations to retrieve the EHRs to be verified from the remote cloud storage and to reduce the processing overhead resulting from client-side integrity verification, the core integrity checking mechanism is offloaded to the crypto coprocessor. This phase starts by the mobile client requesting the integrity verification of a set of EHRs or the whole medical record system from the trusted crypto coprocessor. The trusted coprocessor successively retrieves the selected EHRs from the cloud storage, generates their incremental MACs using the shared secret K_s, and sends the generated values to the mobile client. The mobile client can verify the integrity of files by applying cheap comparison operations between the stored and received MAC values.

Energy Analysis

The MAC generation by the crypto coprocessor and the incremental MAC update mechanism in the data update phase contributes to major savings in energy consumption on the mobile client. Let E_{IMac} be the energy consumed by the incremental MAC function when processing 1 byte of data on the mobile client and S_x be the size of EHR_x in bytes. The energy savings per EHR update, $E_{MAC-Gen}$, due to the crypto coprocessor MAC generation design choice is given as follows:

$$E_{MAC-Gen} = E_{IMac} \times S_x \qquad (1)$$

To calculate the energy savings due to the incremental MAC update mechanism, we need to subtract the energy cost incurred by the incremental MAC update operation from that incurred by the traditional approach using the famous CBC MAC function to generate a MAC on the whole file contents. Let E_{CBC} be the energy consumed by the CBC MAC algorithm when processing 1 byte of data and M_x be the percent data modification applied on EHR_x due to block insertion or deletion. Since

$$E_{IMac} = 1.05 \times E_{CBC}$$

(Bellare, Goldreich, & Goldwasser, 1995) then the energy savings per EHR update E_{update} is given as follows:

$$E_{update} = \\ S_x \times E_{IMac} \times \left(1 / 1.05 - M_x\right) \qquad (2) \\ \approx S_x \times E_{IMac} \times \left(1 - M_x\right)$$

The energy savings increase as M_x decreases since the incremental function is processing fewer bytes compared to the total EHR size. The energy savings in the verification phase has two main components: a processing component and network reception component. Let $S_{1 \to r}$ be the combined size of the EHRs to be verified by the crypto coprocessor in bytes and $E_{Net-recv}$ be the energy consumed by the mobile client transceiver upon receiving 1 byte of data. The total application-layer energy savings in the verification phase on the mobile client due to delegating the MAC generation to the crypto coprocessor is given as follows:

$$E_{verify} = S_{1 \to r} \times (E_{IMac} + E_{Net-recv}) \quad (3)$$

Economic Feasibility Analysis

The cryptographic coprocessor represents the main cost factor in the realization of the security system. A brief economic study shows that commercial cryptographic coprocessors range in price from hundreds to thousands U.S. Dollars. The cost of the coprocessor mainly depends on the processing and memory capabilities of the coprocessor, the degree of physical security and tamper-resistance supported, the compliance of the coprocessor with FIPS standards, and the crypto functionality (hardware acceleration and cryptographic implementations) provided. We believe that the cost of the incremental integrity solution presented can be greatly reduced based on a set of external economic factors, as well as internal design choices related to the protocol architecture itself. These factors are summarized in the following points:

1. The increase in demand on cryptographically secure facilities to provide practical security solutions, particularly to computing clouds, will increase the competitiveness in the crypto coprocessor commercial market and will gradually result in a higher functionality/cost ratio.

2. The technological advancements in computing and memory hardware, as well as in physical packaging mechanisms, will result in delivering cost-effective cryptographic coprocessors.

3. The emergence of open-source cryptographic processor designs will support the elimination of monopoly in the coprocessor market, and hence will lead to considerable price reductions.

4. The coprocessor sharing mechanism employed (where more than one healthcare customer shares the resources of a particular crypto coprocessor) participates in mitigating the cost of the incremental integrity services provided and reducing the payback period of the cloud provider investment (the payback period is the length of time required for investment to recover its cost). This sharing mechanism plays a major role in the cost-effectiveness of the security solution. To illustrate this, we will derive a general equation to calculate the payback period of the cloud provider investment in the incremental integrity service. Without loss of generality, we calculate the payback period of a single crypto coprocessor as follows: Let C_{sp} denote the capital cost of the cryptographic coprocessor unit. C_{sp} consists of the following cost components: (1) The cost of the crypto coprocessor hardware, (2) the coprocessor configuration and distribution, (3) the coprocessor installation in the computing cloud, and (4) the operational and maintenance costs including power consumption and network bandwidth usage for carrying out remote configuration. Let R and R_{sp} represent the cost of computation

per hour on the main server processor and crypto coprocessor respectively. Let M be the ratio of R_{sp} to R ($M = R_{sp}/R$). Let L represent the average number of customers sharing the resources of the crypto coprocessor per hour. The payback period in months, PB_m, is calculated as follows:

$$PB_m = \frac{C_{sp}}{L \times M \times R \times 24 \times 30} \qquad (4)$$

Assume that C_{sp} is \$ 10,000, L is 3 users, M is 2 (the cost of 1 computing hour on the crypto coprocessor is double that on the main server processor) and R is \$ 0.48 per hour (based on the Amazon EC2 Windows standard on-demand instance rate using the Large AMI profile). Therefore, based on Equation 4, PB_m is equal to 4.82 months. This payback period is very reasonable in return of the incremental integrity service provided. From the cloud provider's perspective, we believe that the payback period will be even shorter as the number of security-demanding customers increase and as the cost of the crypto coprocessor decrease with the technological advancements in packaging technology.

5. The light-weighted nature of the incremental cryptography protocol supports a better utilization of the crypto coprocessor and avoids any unnecessary loads on its resources. This aids in reducing the resource requirements, and hence the price, of the coprocessor.

6. The functional requirements of the protocol design do not rely on any form of hardware cryptographic implementation or acceleration. All the cryptographic mechanisms can be implemented in software at the expense of a slight decrease in performance.

7. Cloud computing security research is giving more attention to trusted hardware security approaches to provide technical solutions for solving several data privacy and integrity issues in the computing cloud. This fact is supported by the proposed work of the Trusted Computing Group for developing a set of cloud security services and protocols based on their TPM modules.

System Implementation

The system design is experimentally tested by a proof of concept implementation using an emulated cloud computing unit. The virtualization layer is provided using VMware Workstation 7.1 (VMware, 2013). The mobile client is a Nokia N 97 smart phone running the Symbian OS v 9.4. The protocol implementation on the mobile phone was carried out on the Nokia QT 4.7.2 mobile platform (QT software, 2013) using the C++ programming language. The network connectivity of the Nokia N97 phone is provided via an 802.11g wireless DSL router. We evaluated the energy savings by executing a set of fifty typical insertion and deletion commands (add/delete a line of text, add/delete a paragraph, cut/paste lines and paragraphs, add/remove an image, etc.) on thirty MS Office Word documents. The file sizes range from 100 KB to 2 MB. The power measurements are carried out using the Nokia Energy Profiler tool v 1.2 (Nokia Energy Profiler, 2013).

The average execution time of the incremental MAC generation on the mobile device was found to be 41 ms compared to 403 ms of the traditional integrity approach that generates the file CBC MAC from scratch. This is over 95% reduction in processing requirements. The average energy consumption of the incremental MAC generation on the mobile phone was found to be 9.6×10^{-8} J/Bytes compared to 93×10^{-8} J/Bytes for the CBC MAC approach. It is worth noting that the processing and energy savings are relatively proportional in this case, since the incremental MAC and the CBC MAC functions employ analogous system operations.

Security Discussion

The security assumptions in the system revolve around the cryptographic integrity enforcement mechanisms provided by the incremental MAC structures and the tamperproof capabilities of the cryptographic coprocessor. The security properties of the incremental MAC structures are comprehensively discussed and analyzed with rigorous proofs in Bellare, Guerin, and Rogaway (1995). The main purpose behind using the MACs is to prevent any undetectable malicious tampering on the EHRs stored in the cloud storage facilities. The computational logic responsible of generating the incremental MACs on the cloud side is executed in the cryptographic coprocessor. This entity represents a safe and isolated processing container that is physically and logically protected against any unauthorized access. This fact allows the cloud-side MAC generation on the EHRs to be executed safely in the address space of the cryptographic coprocessor and protects it from any external or internal attacks (refer to the "*System Design*" section).

FUTURE RESEARCH DIRECTIONS

As far as future directions are concerned, we strongly believe that as the cloud computing platform expands further and further, the need will be highly compelling towards protecting the integrity of the massive amounts of cloud data, specifically that of a sensitive and critical nature such as healthcare records and financial documents. Intelligent and efficient cryptographic data structures and mechanisms such as the incremental cryptography building blocks presented in this chapter should be employed to enhance the security, performance, and energy consumption of the cloud business logic and computing units.

We are currently researching several probabilistic and randomized algorithms and data structures for achieving this purpose and promising results are expected on this front.

CONCLUSION

In this chapter we presented a security system for enforcing the integrity of EHRs in the cloud. The protocols presented rely on incremental cryptography mechanisms and trusted computing technologies to protect the integrity of medical documents during their different processing and storage lifecycle stages in the cloud. The main contribution is to design and implement a set of protocol building blocks that (1) comply with the specifications of regulatory policies and recommendations, (2) operate in a performance- and energy-efficient manner on the mobile client devices and cloud servers, and (3) efficiently supports dynamic data operations (insertions, deletions, and modifications) on the EHRs.

REFERENCES

Annas, G. J. (2003). HIPAA regulations-a new era of medical-record privacy? *The New England Journal of Medicine*, *348*(15), 1486–1490. doi:10.1056/NEJMlim035027 PMID:12686707

Bajikar, S. (2002, June 20). *Trusted platform module (tpm) based security on notebook pcs-white paper*. Mobile Platforms Group, Intel Corporation.

Barham, P., Dragovic, B., Fraser, K., Hand, S., Harris, T., & Ho, A. et al. (2003). Xen and the art of virtualization. *ACM SIGOPS Operating Systems Review*, *37*(5), 164–177. doi:10.1145/1165389.945462

Bellare, M., Goldreich, O., & Goldwasser, S. (1994). Incremental cryptography: The case of hashing and signing. In Advances in Cryptology—CRYPTO'94 (pp. 216-233). Springer.

Bellare, M., Goldreich, O., & Goldwasser, S. (1995). Incremental cryptography and application to virus protection. In *Proceedings of the Twenty-Seventh Annual ACM Symposium on Theory of Computing* (pp. 45-56). ACM.

Bellare, M., Guérin, R., & Rogaway, P. (1995). *XOR MACs: New methods for message authentication using finite pseudorandom functions.* Springer.

Berger, B. (2005). Trusted computing group history. *Information Security Technical Report, 10*(2), 59–62. doi:10.1016/j.istr.2005.05.007

Best, R. M. (1980). Preventing software piracy with crypto-microprocessors. [). IEEE.]. *Proceedings of IEEE Spring COMPCON, 80*, 466–469.

Bowers, K. D., Juels, A., & Oprea, A. (2009). HAIL: A high-availability and integrity layer for cloud storage. In *Proceedings of the 16th ACM Conference on Computer and Communications Security* (pp. 187-198). ACM.

Diffie, W., Van Oorschot, P. C., & Wiener, M. J. (1992). Authentication and authenticated key exchanges. *Designs, Codes and Cryptography, 2*(2), 107–125. doi:10.1007/BF00124891

Dyer, J. G., Lindemann, M., Perez, R., Sailer, R., Van Doorn, L., & Smith, S. W. (2001). Building the IBM 4758 secure coprocessor. *Computer, 34*(10), 57–66. doi:10.1109/2.955100

Li, C., Raghunathan, A., & Jha, N. K. (2010). Secure virtual machine execution under an untrusted management OS. In Proceedings of Cloud Computing (CLOUD), (pp. 172-179). IEEE.

Nokia Energy Profiler Tool Home Page. (n.d.). Retrieved from http://www.forum.nokia.com/Library/Tools_and_downloads/Other/Nokia_Energy_Profiler/

Perez, R., Sailer, R., & van Doorn, L. (2006). vTPM: Virtualizing the trusted platform module. In *Proceedings of the 15th Conference on USENIX Security Symposium* (pp. 305-320). USENIX.

QT Software Homepage. (n.d.). Retrieved from http://qt.digia.com/

Sadeghi, A. R., Stüble, C., & Winandy, M. (2008). Property-based TPM virtualization. In *Information Security* (pp. 1–16). Springer.

Tygar, J. D., & Yee, B. S. (1991). *Dyad: A system for using physically secure coprocessors.* Academic Press.

VMware Workstation Homepage. (n.d.). Retrieved from http://www.vmware.com/workstation

Wang, Q., Wang, C., Li, J., Ren, K., & Lou, W. (2009). Enabling public verifiability and data dynamics for storage security in cloud computing. [Springer.]. *Proceedings of Computer Security–ESORICS, 2009*, 355–370.

KEY TERMS AND DEFINITIONS

Cloud Computing: Is a computing model that supports outsourcing execution and storage services for end customers to remote virtualized data centers.

Confidentiality: Is a security service that ensures that only authorized parties can understand the contents of a message.

Cryptographic Coprocessor: A cryptographic coprocessors is a tamper-proof supporting processor that aids in providing secure and isolated processing containers that are physically and logically protected against unauthorized access.

Electronic Healthcare Record (EHR): An EHR is a document that contains sensitive medical information referring to one or more patient.

Incremental Integrity: Is ensuring the integrity of a document by, merely, applying the security algorithms on modified chunks of this document without the need to apply it on the whole document from scratch.

Integrity: Is a security service that ensures the detection of any unauthorized modification on data when processed, stored, or exchanged over the network links.

Message Authentication Code (MAC): Is a security mechanism that enforces the integrity verification of data.

Chapter 7
Auditing Privacy for Cloud-Based EHR Systems

Jonathan Sinclair
RepKnight Ltd., UK

Benoit Hudzia
Stratoscale Ltd., UK

Alan Stewart
Queen's University Belfast, UK

ABSTRACT

An EHR is a modern specialisation of a Customer Relationship Management that specifically focuses on the collection and exchange of electronic health information about individual patients between healthcare organisations. Electronic Heath Records systems hold personally identifiable information, especially that which falls under the category of sensitive personal data. As with all industries, the eHealth industry sees potential in cloud-based service offerings and the reduced infrastructure cost they imply, whilst realising the issues regarding security and privacy that may be encountered from outsourcing processing and storage to untrustworthy Cloud Service Providers (CSPs). In this chapter, the authors propose an approach to handle and audit data privacy requirements by leveraging a carefully designed architecture deployed for auditing data privacy in cloud ecosystems.

INTRODUCTION

Most organisations manage their customer data through a Customer Relationship Management (CRM) system. CRM is a widely adopted strategy for enhancing and maintaining customer relationships and the information that pertains to the customer through the phases of administration, marketing, sales and support. Most commercial CRM offerings didn't provide the support and services required for the health industry and, therefore, a specialised form of CRM, the Electronic Health Record (EHR) system was developed. An EHR is a modern specialisation of a CRM which specifically focuses on the collection and exchange of electronic health information about individual patients between healthcare organisations. EHR systems hold personally identifiable

DOI: 10.4018/978-1-4666-6118-9.ch007

information especially that which falls under the category of sensitive personal data. As with all industries the eHealth industry sees potential in cloud-based service offerings and the reduced infrastructure cost they imply, whilst realising the issues regarding security and privacy that may be encountered from outsourcing processing and storage to untrustworthy CSPs. The loss of control has been highlighted as a concern in regards to the compliance of privacy laws and is required in order to control and enforce the access to records by third parties.

In this chapter, we first propose an approach to defining data privacy requirements. Second, we present an architecture deployed for auditing data privacy. Third we present the validation and verification of a data locality results and finally propose a pragmatic approach to breach of compliance prediction in the light of analysis.

BACKGROUND

E-Health

E-Health refers to the utilisation of information systems within the healthcare industry (I.T. Union 2008). Two goals of e-Health as mentioned by Edworthy (2001) are:

1. To provide greater efficiency; and
2. To scale patient services.

Moreover, the World Health Organisation (WHO) defined e-Health in 2005 as:

Use of information and communications technologies (ICT) in support of health and health-related fields, including health-care services, health surveillance, health literature, health education, knowledge and research.

The E-Health domain is heavily regulated, and Figure 1 shows important healthcare laws taken from the EU, UK and US. Current laws highlighted in red; superseded laws are displayed in black. These laws typically address electronic healthcare considerations but do not extend to issues arising from the use of cloud and virtualisation technologies. Revisions of current laws to address issues arising from technological advances are pending.

E-Health Technologies

Various E-Health related technologies have been developed. They aim to provide a unified platform for processing health records, which delivers services to a variety of types of user. But also, enable access to health records from a range of platforms and devices while providing integration of health records across different health-care domains and deliver an efficient health management and administration process.

The recent development and evolution of e-Health systems needs address the economies of

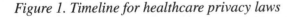

Figure 1. Timeline for healthcare privacy laws

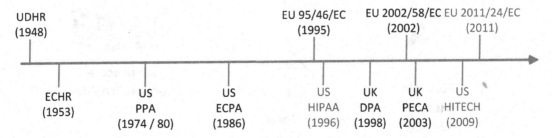

scale while providing efficient data management processes which operate across cross-jurisdictional boundaries without compromising patients' data privacy rights. It has been identified that, despite the development of laws in some jurisdictions to deal with privacy in EHR's, many in the field argue that regulation is providing an insufficient level of granularity regarding the use of EHR's in the context of the technology stack (WHO, 2005).

Electronic Medical Record (EMR), Electronic Health Record (EHR)

Often the terms electronic medical record (EMR), electronic health record (EHR) and personal health record (PHR) are used interchangeably. However, there is a clear difference between the three kinds of record in both their content and in the underlying technology. EMRs were the first mainstream system that medical professionals used to record the diagnosis and treatment of medical conditions for patients. EHRs were derived from EMRs and record information about all aspects of patient health, not just medical conditions. Figure 2 shows how the technology supporting EHRs allows different departments, sites and organisations to share patient information. Finally, PHRs are derived from an EHR and allow patients to view and administer aspects of their healthcare records.

Many implementations of EMR, EHR and PHR systems exist with different architectures, communication standards and deployment methods. Here we consider the OpenVistA project in a virtualised context. OpenVistA is an open source

Figure 2. Source composition for EHRs

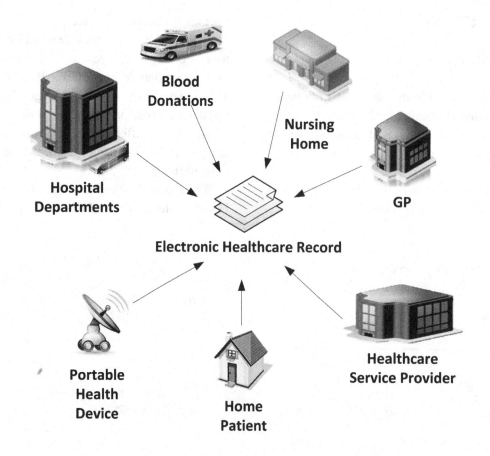

implementation of an EHR system, VistA. An existing deployment of VistA in the US supports 8 million patients, 180,000 health professionals in 163 hospitals, 800 clinics and 135 nursing homes.

Cloud Supply Chains

Cloud supply chains are a new field of research driven by an evolution of supply chains through the adoption of cloud computing as described by Lindner et al., (2010) and Zhou et al., (2012). The concept of the cloud supply chain is a convergence of existing of different business models as depicted by Kijl (2005), Bouwman (2006), and Porter (1980). These models cover all aspects of the supply chain and business lifecycle acknowledging regulations as an influencing factor of dynamic business models such as that involving cloud computing. Lindner et al., (2010) describe how Cloud supply chains are defined as two or more parties linked by the provision of Cloud services, related information and funds.

eHealth Cloud Supply Chain

The e-Health Cloud supply chain shown in Figure 3 is a concept used to describe the different actors and parts involved throughout the end-to-end life cycle of health care related Cloud services. As a result, the eHealth Cloud supply chain is a system of business processes that are executed in order to satisfy the demands of Cloud consumers as described by Lindner et al., (2010,2011), in this case health care providers. This concept is similar to a typical supply chain where a product/service exists at the beginning of the chain and a customer at the end. However, within the context of Cloud computing, the product/service would be a Cloud offering in the form of Software as a Service (SaaS), Platform as a Service (PaaS), Infrastructure as a Service (IaaS) or a combination of these. Lindner et al., (2011a) present how these can be combined to offer an aggregated service to consumers providing them with value-adding services. There can be a number of actors and

Figure 3. Audit supply chain

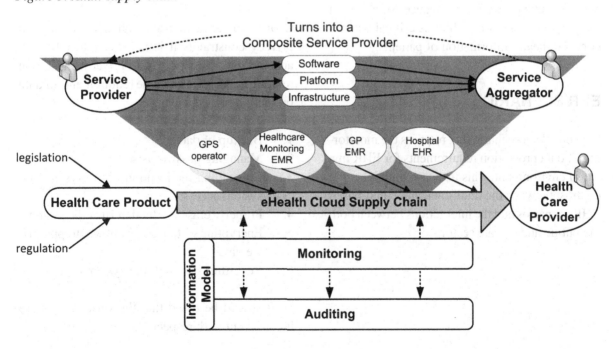

components involved in the Cloud supply chain such as the Cloud service provider, the Cloud consumer and possibly a Cloud broker. The Cloud broker's role is to establish a relationship with various Cloud providers to find the best offering to suit the consumer's needs. As well as a number of components existing within a Cloud, consumers can utilise more than one type of cloud, however this causes complexities throughout the supply chain, because of the various clouds and the different components in each of these (Lindner et al., 2011a). Other components that are passed through the Cloud supply chain include information and funds. Cloud services are traditionally consumed through a pay-per-use model, where the consumer only pays for how much they use. However, other methods of payment include pay monthly (subscription-based method) or fixed price. E.g., if a Cloud consumer uses more than one cloud to fulfil a service, each cloud may have its own payment model and the cloud consumer may pay monthly for one cloud and pay-per-use for another cloud. As a result, this can increase significantly the complexity of the EHR supply chain. Stewart (2009) present how this make it more difficult to ensure compliance and carry out the process of auditing which is critical when it comes to health information of patients.

EHR SCENARIO

We consider a scenario that requires the monitoring of data protection requirements for EHR in a cloud environment. This use case highlights the contrast between the traditional and cloud-based EHR scenarios and the interactions between both the public and private sector.

Data Protection Compliance for EHR Systems

The challenges of assessing the data privacy compliance of cloud-based EHR systems are complex. Interactions between multiple parties and devices occur in real-time. Individuals have the ability to access their medical records; held by third-party healthcare service providers, using a range of wireless devices. Services that utilise stored information about a patient's diet, medication and location access sensitive personal information (subject to privacy legislation). An individual should be provided with guarantees about how their personal data is managed. Health institutions store details in addition to an individual's medical history. A patient should be able to monitor who has access to their personal information. Figure 4 shows an EHR system composed of an EHR Database, EHR Client, Patient WebPortal and EHR Imaging services.

DEFINING EHR DATA PRIVACY REQUIREMENT

In order to define international, national or local privacy constraints it is necessary to take into account the diversity of data privacy legislation relating to healthcare. Some requirements of data protection laws involve:

1. Backup of data;
2. Managing passwords;
3. Controlling the location of the system and system access;
4. Properly erase media that runs the system;
5. Encrypting system processes when appropriate; and
6. Recording and auditing system usage.

It should be noted that the various laws are inconsistent with respect to:

Figure 4. EHR system as a service

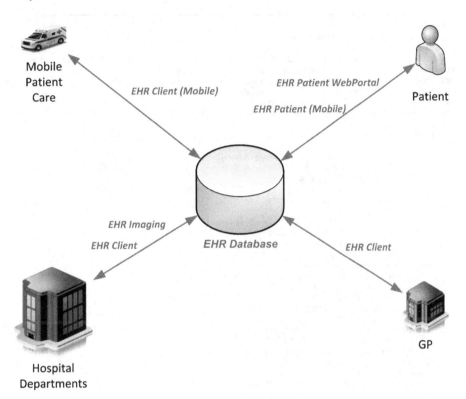

1. Retention duration;
2. Encryption standards;
3. Locality restrictions; and
4. Audit frequencies.

One way to represent variations in privacy laws is to parameterise requirements (see Figure 5).

EHR Service Level Agreements

In the remainder of this chapter, we will focus attention on location constraints that arise from data privacy laws (e.g. running services within a specific geographic region, or preventing access and data transfer to/from different geographies). An SLA template for geolocation constraints for an OpenVistA EHR service is shown in Listing 1. In line 2 the name of the agreement, EHRAgreement, is defined. Following this lines 3 through 10

Figure 5. Compliance WS-agreement structure

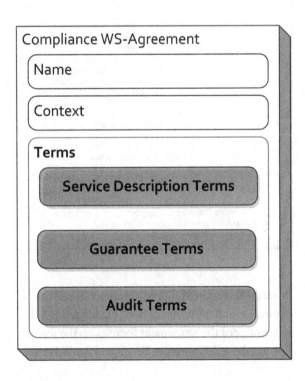

Listing1. Example EHR SLA,frame

```
 1   <wsag:Agreement AgreementId=``AGSV2032">
 2       <wsag:Name> EHRAgreement </wsag:Name>
 3       <wsag:AgreementContext>
 4           <wsag:AgreementInitiator>uuid:d9769f3d-0ab0-4fb8-803b-0d1120ffcf54</wsag:AgreementInitiator>
 5           <wsag:AgreementResponder>medsphere.com</wsag:AgreementResponder>
 6           <wsag:ServiceProvider>AgreementResponder</wsag:ServiceProvider>
 7           <wsag:ExpirationTime>1396674000</wsag:ExpirationTime>
 8           <wsag:TemplateId>3287</wsag:TemplateId>
 9           <wsag:TemplateName>EHRTemplate</wsag:TemplateName>
10       </wsag:AgreementContext>
11       <wsag:Terms>
12           <wsag:All>
13               <wsag:ServiceDescriptionTerm wsag:Name=``geoLocation"
14                       wsag:ServiceName="openVistA EHR">
15               </wsag:ServiceDescriptionTerm>
16               <wsag:ServiceProperties wsag:Name=``locationProp"
17                       wsag:ServiceName="EHR">
18                   <wsag:VariableSet>
19                       <wsag:Variable wsag:Name=``ipLocation"
20                           wsag:Metric="country">
21                       </wsag:Variable>
22                   </wsag:VariableSet>
23               </wsag:ServiceProperties>
24               <wsag:ServiceReference wsag:Name=``locationRef"
25                   wsag:ServiceName="EHR">
26               </wsag:ServiceReference>
27               <wsag:GuaranteeTerm wsag:Name=``validLocations"
28                   Monitored="True">
29                   <wsag:ServiceLevelObjective>
30                       ipLocation IS_WITHIN EU
31                   </wsag:ServiceLevelObjective>
32               </wsag:GuaranteeTerm>
33               <wsag:AuditTerm wsag:Name=``geoLocation"
34                       ComplianceName=``UK DPA"
35                       Continuous=``True">
36                   <wsag:AuditScope>
37                       <wsag:Audit>...</wsag:Audit>*
38                       <wsag:AccessControl>...</wsag:AccessControl>*
39                       <wsag:DataSource>...</wsag:DataSource>*
40                       <wsag:DataPersistence>...</wsag:DataPersistence>*
41                       <wsag:DataTransport>...</wsag:DataTransport>*
42                       <wsag:DataConsumer>...</wsag:DataConsumer>*
43                       <wsag:RiskManagement>...</wsag:RiskManagement>*
44                   </wsag:AuditScope>
45                   <wsag:AuditCondition>
46                       <wsag:GuaranteeName>...</wsag:GuaranteeName>
47                       <wsag:RequiredValue>...</wsag:RequiredValue>
48                       <wsag:PreferredValue>...</wsag:PreferredValue>
49                       <wsag:Restrictions>...</wsag:Restrictions>
50                   </wsag:AuditCondition>*
51                   <wsag:ServiceLevelObjective Type=``xs:string">
52                       ...
53                   </wsag:ServiceLevelObjective>*
54                   <wsag:BusinessValueList>
55                       ...
56                   </wsag:BusinessValueList>
57               </wsag:AuditTerm>
58           </wsag:All>
59       </wsag:Terms>
60   </wsag:Agreement>
61
```

describe the context for the agreement in terms of expiration and the template used for definition. The remainder of the agreement focuses on the terms; Service-based, GuaranteeTerms and AuditTerms.

The ServiceDescriptionTerms, ServiceProperties and ServiceReferences describe different aspects of a service referring to the service name, openVistA EHR. The ServiceProperties defines a location property, locationProp in line 16 which has a variable set, lines 18-21, used to measure the location in terms of IP with a metric range of countries. The GuaranteeTerms section provides the monitoring conditions for the ipLocation variable of the service property, locationProp.

The condition on line 30 states the ipLocation variable should be a country within the predefined set of countries which represent the EU. Finally lines 33-57 describe the extended audit terms section. It refers to the ServiceDescriptionTerm, named geoLocation in line 13 and associates it with a compliance law, UK DPA, indicating that it should be continuously monitored. Lines 36-44 defined the scope for the audit in terms of the proposed novel framework. Finally lines 45-50 define the conditions of the compliance audit.

CONTINUOUS COMPLIANCE AUDITING SERVICE (CCAS) SYSTEM LANDSCAPE FOR EHR

The CCAS system has been customised for the OpenVistA EHR example. The OpenVistA services have been deployed on an OpenNebula Cloud Infrastructure (see Figure 6). The Cloud architecture consists of a management machine which hosts the OpenNebula Cloud Manager, a Service Broker and a Service Hoster which execute the service lifecycle and five cloud machines which are used to host OpenVistA services and the service auditor.

Specification of System Architecture

The specifications of the machines used in the cloud ecosystem are detailed below in Table 1

EHR CLOUD ECOSYSTEM

An EHR Cloud ecosystem is the evolution of an EHR system which incorporates distributed and mobile sources (see Figure 7). The cloud supply chain, for the OpenVistA EHR cloud system is shown in Figure 3. EHR cloud supply chains utilise a number of virtualised services (deployed within the cloud environment). In Figure 6 we show how the CCAS is deployed alongside an EHR system (as described in Figure 7) in the cloud. Each EHR service has an audit probe that interacts with it and provides auditing data.

Figure 6. CCAS system landscape

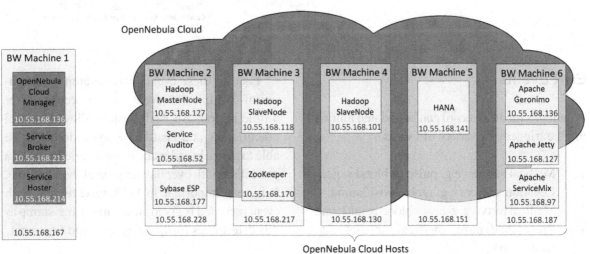

Table 1. System specification

	BW 1	BW 2	BW 3	BW 4	BW 5	BW 6
CPU (Cores/Threads)	8/16	4/8	4/8	4/8	12/24	4/8
Memory	8 Gb	16 Gb	16 Gb	16 Gb	128 Gb	6 Gb
Hard Disk	300 Gb	500 Gb	500 Gb	500 Gb	1 Tb	300 Gb
Network Interfaces	3	2	2	2	2	2

Figure 7. EHR use case architecture

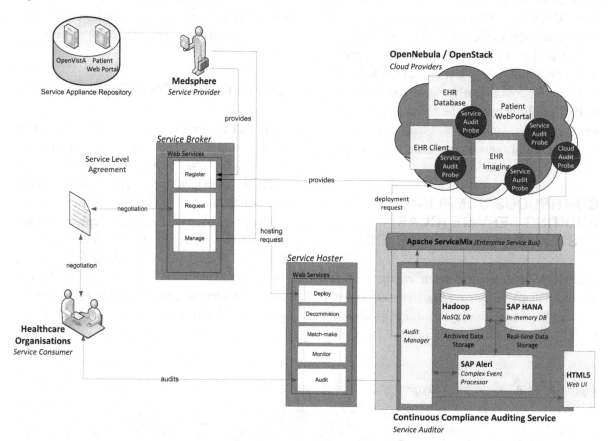

EHR Events

A patient's medical record can be updated following the trigger of a variety of events:

1. Medical sensors e.g. pulse or blood sugar;
2. Location sensors e.g. global positioning;
3. Medical tests e.g. x-ray or blood results; and
4. Prescribed care, medical or diet e.g. medication.

Each of these events may be atomic or consist of multiple sub-events which occurred over a time period. An EHR system allows medical practitioners and healthcare professionals to be able to gain a broader and more detailed view of a patient's health over the duration of their lifetime. It is very important in EHR systems that each event recorded is given an accurate time-stamp as this determines further diagnosis and treatment.

EHR Logs

There are two common types of log / messaging formats used within EHR systems; HL7 used to store details of a patient's diagnosis, care and treatment to include medical history such as known allergies (shown in Figure 8 and CCR used to store detailed information regarding prescribed care, medication or diet over a continuous period (as per example in Listing 2). The HL7 example in Figure 8 shows that an event took place at 11.23 18/08/1988 for a patient PATID1234, William Jones; who has an allergy to penicillin which brings him out in hives, the event had a diagnosis of primary malignant neoplasm of liver. The CCR example in Listing 2 details the prescription of medication to patient 001 of 90 doses of 0.125mg of Digoxin. Each of these formats is normalised using adapters in the messaging bus defining standard parsing methods to conform to the CCAS logging format in Figure 9.

EHR Complex Event Processing

In order to assess the overall compliance of business processes against a given principle (i.e.

locality) an event processing network (EPN) is generated from the relevant input sources, requirements and measurement databases in order to determine an output, this approach was previously used by Rozsnyai et al., (2007) to cope with the deluge of data.

The Event Processing Network for locality (Figure 10) consists of input windows for HANA, Hadoop and SQL Anywhere (SQA) databases. The information for location of relevant services is then aggregated from both the HANA and Hadoop databases into a `ServiceLocations' input stream whilst the confidence values for relevant services are mapped to a `ServiceConfidence' input stream. Each of these streams along with the locality requirements from a `ServiceRequirements' input stream (determined at service deployment) and Locations input stream (sourced from an IP database) are all fed into an output window `CurrentLocation'. This output window is the trigger to run an assessment of each service by the `NonCompliant' output stream, which in turn is initiated by the `Location10' flex stream.

In the Figure you can see the event processing agent (EPA) query for the flex stream written in Continuous Computation Language (CCL).

Figure 8. HL7 log format

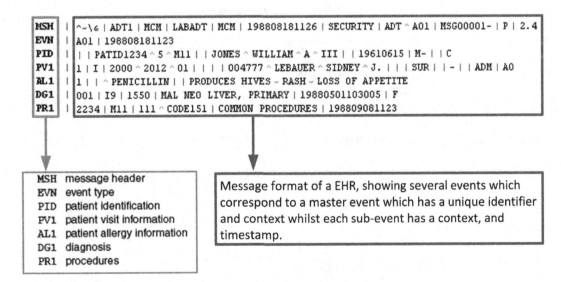

```
MSH | |^~\& | ADT1 | MCM | LABADT | MCM | 198808181126 | SECURITY | ADT ^ A01 | MSG00001- | P | 2.4
EVN | |A01 | 198808181123
PID | | | PATID1234 ^ 5 ^ M11 | | JONES ^ WILLIAM ^ A ^ III | | 19610615 | M- | | C
PV1 | |1 | I | 2000 ^ 2012 ^ 01 | | | | 004777 ^ LEBAUER ^ SIDNEY ^ J. | | | SUR | | - | | ADM | A0
AL1 | |1 | | ^ PENICILLIN | | PRODUCES HIVES ~ RASH ~ LOSS OF APPETITE
DG1 | |001 | I9 | 1550 | MAL NEO LIVER, PRIMARY | 19880501103005 | F
PR1 | |2234 | M11 | 111 ^ CODE151 | COMMON PROCEDURES | 198809081123
```

MSH message header
EVN event type
PID patient identification
PV1 patient visit information
AL1 patient allergy information
DG1 diagnosis
PR1 procedures

Message format of a EHR, showing several events which correspond to a master event which has a unique identifier and context whilst each sub-event has a context, and timestamp.

Listing 2. An example Continuity Care Record (CCR)

```
1  <?xml version=``1.0" encoding=``utf-8"?>
2  <ContinuityOfCareRecord xmlns='urn:astm-org:CCR'>
3      <CCRDocumentObjectID>MedDoc</CCRDocumentObjectID>
4      <Language>
5          <Text>English</Text>
6      </Language>
7      <Version>1.0</Version>
8      <DateTime>
9          <ExactDateTime>1374598308</ExactDateTime>
10     </DateTime>
11     <Patient>
12         <ID>001</ID>
13     </Patient>
14     <Medications>
15         <Medication>
16             <Description>
17                 <Text>Digoxin 0.125mg, 1 qDay, #90</Text>
18             </Description>
19             <Product>
20                 <ProductName>Digoxin</ProductName>
21                 <Strength>
22                     <Value>0.125</Value>
23                     <Units>mg</Units>
24                 </Strength>
25             </Product>
26             <Quantity>
27                 <Value>90</Value>
28             </Quantity>
29             <Directions>
30                 <Direction>
31                     <Dose>
32                         <Value>1</Value>
33                     </Dose>
34                     <Frequency>
35                         <Value>qd</Value>
36                     </Frequency>
37                 </Direction>
38             </Directions>
39         </Medication>
40 </ContinuityOfCareRecord>
41
```

Figure 9. Event log format

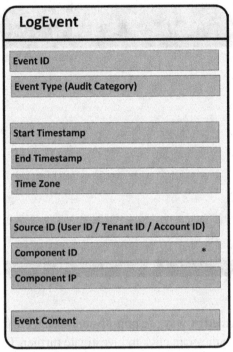

* not required for physical device logs

This EPA query calculates the time window for checking non-compliance every 10s. The resultant output of the non-compliance check is fed back to a HANA database.

Once triggered the output window compares the IP of a service with the IP database in order to determine a location and furthermore compares this location with the given ipLocation requirement to produce a compliance result which is stored in the Hadoop database. If non-compliant an alert is produced and sent to the HANA database to be visualised on the dashboard in real-time.

EHR Audit

CCAS provides the audit results by means of a Web portal. This allows data to be visualised and presented to the consumer in different forms depending on the context of the data.

Initially the consumer would be presented with a services tab (Figure 11) listing all their services, active or inactive, that have been registered with

Figure 10. EHR locality complex event process

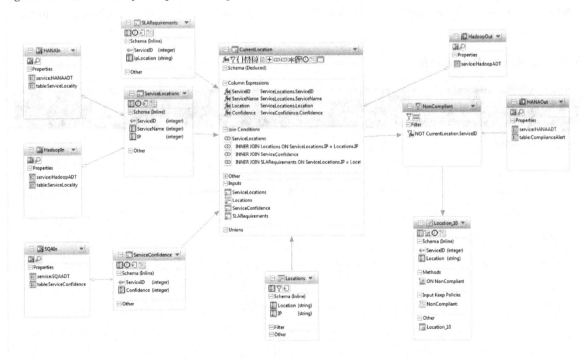

Figure 11. Audit portal - EHR consumer

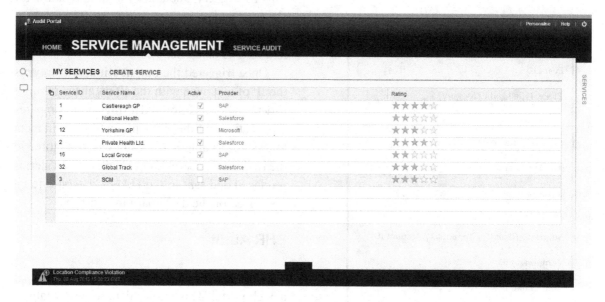

the CCAS system to be audit assessed. Information such as ID, name and active status are provided by the service broker, whilst provider and rating are from the service registry. From this screen the auditor provides integration with the service marketplace allowing easy access to create services. Whilst on this screen if a compliance breach is detected for an active service the consumer is

informed by way of a pop-up announcement upon which they can click to investigate further. These alerts are also able to be navigated in audit alerts tab of the service audit section (Figure 12). This page presents the user with an inbox of alerts, giving a title of each compliance breach, its occurrence data, other information such as status and priority may supplement this. On clicking an audit alert,

Figure 12. Audit alerts dashboard

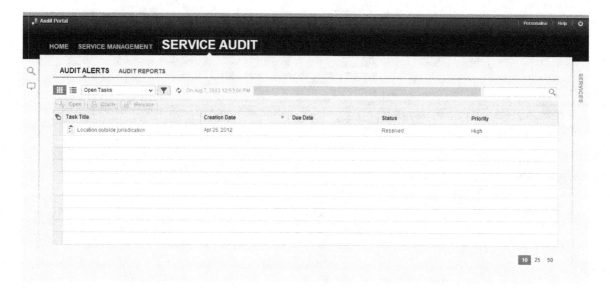

Figure 13. Location audit alert map

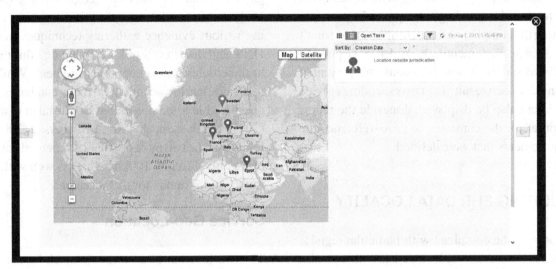

either on the services pop-up or the audit alert page, a window will be presented describing the detail of the compliance breach. In the case of a geo-location breach the window presented (Figure 13) shows a map of the service components and their location indicating compliance using the traffic light system (green for compliant, orange for compliant risk, red for non-compliant). This window also shows a summarised view of the audit alerts table which allows the user quickly to scroll through and change the content of the window to show details of a different alert.

Most importantly the audit portal allows the consumer to select a service and open an audit report. This report (Figure 14) shows a breakdown of the laws and their corresponding principles

Figure 14. Audit report - EHR service

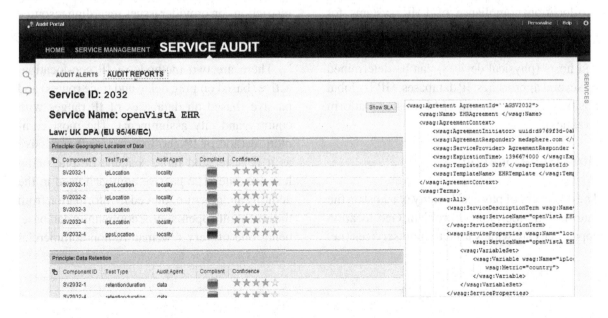

presenting a table of the service components and the test they have undergone to prove the principle stating the compliance for each, although we don't go as far as implementing confidence we provide a visualisation of how this could be presented alongside each result. The corresponding service SLA can also be displayed alongside the report in order for the consumer to cross-reference the requirements that were defined.

AUDITING EHR DATA LOCALITY

In order to be compliant with particular legislation, consumers may only store data within certain geographical locations as described by Peterson (2011) Whilst it was possible for the consumer to enforce their own security measures for on-premise solutions, the cloud computing model makes them reliant upon the service providers to implement the required measures. Therefore a degree of trust is necessary between the consumer and service providers in the context of managing the geographic deployment and storage of services and data.

The SLA extensions implemented and the CCAS and corresponding distributed architecture implemented are utilised to provide an audit of geo-location compliance of EHR systems for privacy legislation.

The locality of services (virtual instances), and hosts (physical devices) can be determined by several approaches; IP databases, GPS (global positioning systems) and TPM (trusted platform modules).

Host Geo-Location

The discovery of physical locality of a host on the Internet is a widely known problem. Geo-location approaches are widely used to limit services (i.e.

gambling and television) to geographic regions. IP databases used for geo-location are setup using various evidence gathering techniques from DNS and Internet topology mapping, through to traceroutes and latency measurement. Whilst it is said that the accuracy of these databases is questionable as demonstrated by Huffaker et al., (2011) and Poese et al., (2011), Siwpersad (2008) found that the two most popular commercial databases only differ by 100km, which is well within satisfactory bounds for this research.

Service Geo-Location

The geo-location of a service is much harder to determine and can only be relied upon when it is cross-referenced with the location of the physical host upon which the service resides. IP proxies, service composition and service migration are some of the reasons why cross-referencing is necessary.

IP Geo-Location

Mapping IP addresses to a geographic location has become of key importance for the adoption of enterprise cloud computing and the Internet of services. Service locality is key to enforcing restrictions on provider issues regarding resource allocation and service migration for legal requirements of consumers.

There are two methods of IP geo-location; active (based on ping delay and trace routes) and passive (based on databases of IP ranges with country and city assignment). The most common method of IP geo-location used is passive as it is faster and more scalable despite being less accurate. The passive approach used in the auditing architecture sourced IP information from the hostip.info open-source community database, being one of very few mature non-commercial

Listing 3.

```
# Probe configuration
geoProbe.id=location
geoProbe.sleep=30
geoProbe.proxy.host=proxy.lon.sap.corp
geoProbe.proxy.port=8080
...
public void init(IProperties properties)
{
        this.properties = properties;
        logger.debug(``GeoProbe.properties \n {}," properties);
        // Initialise XML Parser
        parser = new ParseGeoJSON();
        // Load AMQP Automatic reconnect properties
        {
        reconnect = properties.getBoolean(``amqp.reconnect.enabled," true);
        reconnectSleepBase = properties.getInt(``amqp.reconnect.sleep," 1 *
1000);
        reconnectExponentialBackoff = properties.getBoolean(``amqp.reconnect.
exponential-backoff," true);
        reconnectMaxSleep = properties.getInt(``amqp.reconnect.max-wait," 10 *
60 * 1000);
                if (!run)
                {
                        reconnectSleepActual = reconnectSleepBase;
                }
        }
        // Load probe configuration
        {
                id = properties.getString(``geoProbe.id");
                sleepDuration = properties.getInt(``geoProbe.sleep," 30);
        }
        // Connect to AMQP Broker
        {
                String host = properties.getString(``amqp.broker.host");
                int port = properties.getInt(``amqp.broker.port," 5672);
                int timeout = properties.getInt(``amqp.timeout," 10);
                connection = new Manager(host, port, timeout);
                key = properties.getString(``amqp.publish.key," ``monitor.up-
date.geo");
                exchange = properties.getString(``amqp.publish.exchange,"
``amq.topic");
        }
```

continued on following page

Listing 3. Continued

```
        // Add manager listener
        {
                connection.addListener(new ManagerListener()
                {
                        @Override
                        public void closed()
                        {
                                logger.warn(``Connection lost");
                                restart = true;
                                runThread.interrupt();
                        }
                });
        }
}
private GeoData getData() throws IOException
{
        return parser.parse();
}
private MetricCollection buildProtobuf(String id, GeoData data)
{
        MetricCollection.Builder metrics = MetricCollection.newBuilder();
        metrics.addMetrics(buildMetric(id, ``location.country," data.coun-
try));
        metrics.addMetrics(buildMetric(id, ``location.city," data.city));
        metrics.addMetrics(buildMetric(id, ``location.longitude," data.longi-
tude));
        metrics.addMetrics(buildMetric(id, ``location.latitude," data.lati-
tude));
        return metrics.build();
}
private Metric buildMetric(String id, String name, String value)
{
        Metric.Builder metric = Metric.newBuilder();
        metric.setId(id);
        metric.setName(name);
        metric.setValueType(Type.STRING);
        metric.setStringValue(value);
        metric.setTimestamp(now);
        return metric.build();
}
```

continued on following page

Listing 3. Continued

```
private Metric buildMetric(String id, String name, float value)
{
        Metric.Builder metric = Metric.newBuilder();
        metric.setId(id);
        metric.setName(name);
        metric.setValueType(Type.FLOAT);
        metric.setFloatValue(value);
        metric.setTimestamp(now);
        return metric.build();
}
```

Figure 15. Example HostIP.info query result

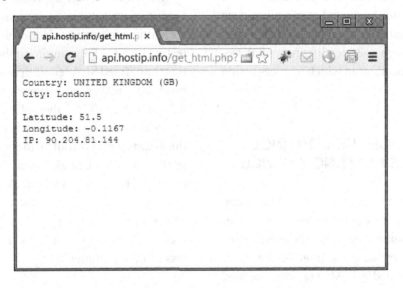

offerings. In Listing 3 an extract of the properties file and java code used by the locality agent of the audit probe to determine the geo-locality of a service is given. Figure 15 shows an example of the output returned from querying the database.

Intel Trusted Execution Technology (Intel TXT)

Intel Trusted Execution Technology (TXT) provides enhanced hardware components enabling the protection of sensitive information from software-based attacks. Features such as micro-processor or I/O subsystem integration enable this technology, allowing the operating system or hypervisors to access these capabilities.

The utilisation of a prototype feature on the trusted platform module (TPM) of the Intel TXT chipset for geo-tagging provides a foundation for future cryptographic hardware methods of attestation.

Geo-Location Migration

Geo-location migration is assessed based on the service location throughout it's lifetime or over a given time period. A service may be singular or be a composite being made up of multiple services. Each deployed entity of a service not only needs to be assessed based upon the location it has been deployed to, but also any location to which an entity of the service resides through the audit period. This is necessary due to virtualisation and the use of migration by the cloud provider for resource utilisation and disaster recovery / backup mitigation. Although a compliance audit can be done as a 'point in time' action (as shown in Figure 14, audits conducted over a given time period (i.e. annually, or bi-annually) may assess compliance through a service lifetime and therefore require all locations in which services reside to be compliant.

EVALUATION OF THE CONTINOUS COMPLIANCE AUDITING SERVICE

An evaluation of the CCAS approach has been determined through a comparative assessment against existing audit processes. These processes were illustrated by simplification of the audit work-flows as defined by ISACA (as implemented by companies such as PwC). The knowledge for the evaluation was verified by an experienced IT systems auditor.

The existing approach by auditors to assess the compliance of IT controls within a system is divided into two work-flows; planning and testing. The planning work-flow (Figure 16) assesses the effect that IT complexity has on the auditor's ability to study and evaluate the controls implemented within the system. This approach allows the auditors to determine whether or not it is both possible and worthwhile to conduct the required audit tests. The testing work-flow (Figure 17) is only conducted if a positive outcome is produced from the planning work-flow. This work-flow assesses the complexity of the IT environment in order to determine how and what tests to perform on the system, these results are evaluated and compliance breach risk is determined as being of high or low value. If high, tests are re-run, otherwise any deficiencies are documented, identified, remediation attempted and penalties issued.

Each step of the existing process requires manual interaction by the auditor. Under most circumstances, distributed cloud-based systems are regarded as being too complex and therefore more audits are unable to be conducted using current auditing methods.

The CCAS Audit approach (Figure 18) provides a more automated approach to auditing in which the auditor is aided in both planning and testing. In CCAS the auditor only needs to assess that the defined SLA requirements match the necessary compliance requirements in order to prepare an audit plan. CCAS then allows the auditor to utilise compliance tests already conducted by the third-party auditing tool, or to conduct substantive testing on historical electronic logs. Evaluation of this existing material enables the auditor to quickly determine the compliance breach risk and any further actions. CCAS has the advantage of enabling the auditor to assess all systems regardless of their complexity.

CONCLUSION

Auditing for e-Health compliance conformance in a cloud context is a topic that tackles relatively new research questions discussing the problems that hinder the adoption of cloud computing for Health Care. As systems become more dynamic, virtualised and distributed it becomes impractical for auditors to undertake a manual approach to assess the compliance of IT systems. In order to provide a tool which bridges the gaps between both the legal and technical domains and provides an auditor with a more automated approach to help

Figure 16. Manual audit plan

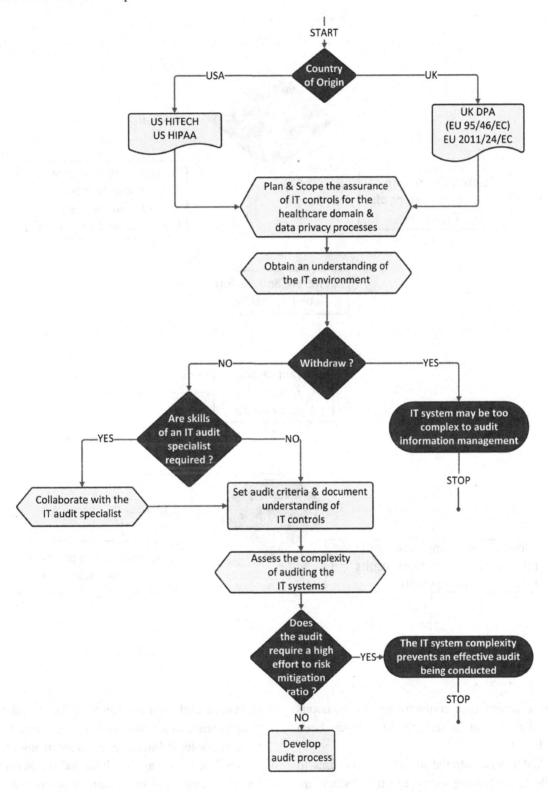

Figure 17. Manual audit test

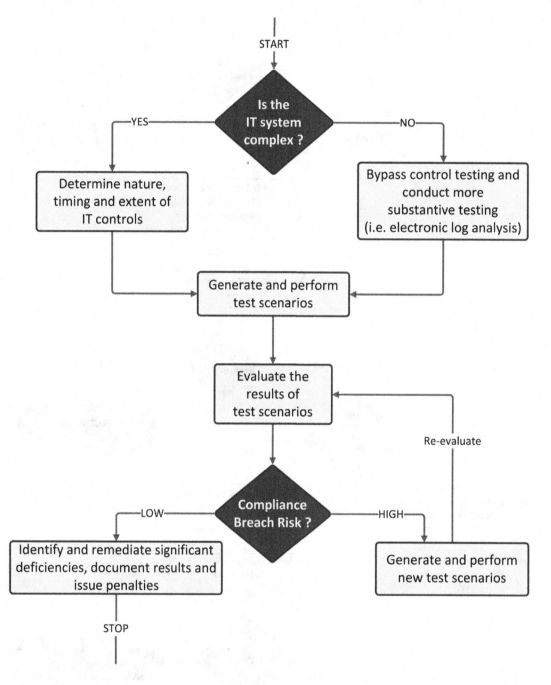

achieve compliance conformance a continuous compliance auditing service (CCAS) has been developed.

CCAS demonstrated in this chapter aims to tackle the following three objectives which are

fundamental challenges of auditing for compliance conformance in a cloud context: legal specification, scalable architecture and visualising audit results. The CCAS approach for auditing services for compliance was implemented in a real world

Figure 18. CCAS audit process

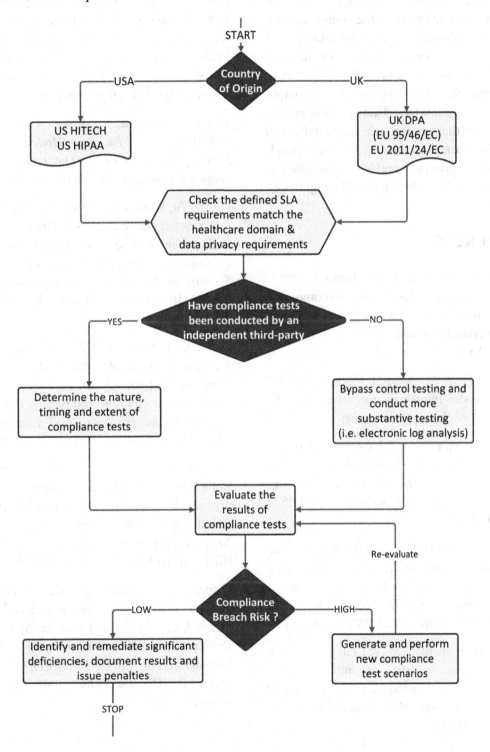

scenario for EHR systems providing an overview of its function and output in the context of geo-location compliance. An in-depth example of SLA definition, a complex event processing and audit visualisation where provided. To finish an evaluation of the CCAS approach and its output was provided against the existing process and has demonstrated that it can provide audit capabilities to IT environments (such as distributed and cloud-based) which have been previously classified as too complex to be audited for legal compliance.

REFERENCES

Abbadi, I. M., Namiluko, C., & Martin, A. (2011, December). Insiders analysis in cloud computing focusing on home healthcare system. In Proceedings of Internet Technology and Secured Transactions (ICITST), (pp. 350-357). IEEE.

Bouwman, H., & MacInnes, I. (2006). Dynamic business model framework for value webs. []. IEEE.]. *Proceedings of System Sciences, 2*, 43–43.

Edworthy, S. M. (2001). Telemedicine in developing countries: May have more impact than in developed countries. *British Medical Journal, 323*(7312), 524. doi:10.1136/bmj.323.7312.524 PMID:11546681

Gunter, T. D., & Terry, N. P. (2005). The emergence of national electronic health record architectures in the United States and Australia: models, costs, and questions. *Journal of Medical Internet Research, 7*(1). doi:10.2196/jmir.7.1.e3 PMID:15829475

Huffaker, B., Fomenkov, M., & Claffy, K. (2011). Geocompare: a comparison of public and commercial geolocation databases. In *Proceedings of Network Mapping and Measurement Conference (NMMC)*. NMMC.

Kifor, T., Varga, L., Álvarez, S., Vázquez-Salceda, J., & Willmott, S. (2006). Privacy issues of provenance in electronic healthcare record systems. In *Proceedings of the 1st Int. Workshop on Privacy and Security in Agent-Based Collaborative Environments (PSACE 2006)*. PSACE.

Kijl, B., Bouwman, H., Haaker, T., & Faber, E. (2005). *Dynamic Business Models in Mobile Service Value Networks: A Theoretical and Conceptual Framework*. FRUX Deliverable.

Li, M., Yu, S., Ren, K., & Lou, W. (2010). Securing personal health records in cloud computing: Patient-centric and fine-grained data access control in multi-owner settings. In *Proceedings of Security and Privacy in Communication Networks* (pp. 89–106). Springer. doi:10.1007/978-3-642-16161-2_6

Lindner, M., Galán, F., Chapman, C., Clayman, S., Henriksson, D., & Elmroth, E. (2010). The cloud supply chain: A framework for information, monitoring, accounting and billing. In *Proceedings of 2nd International ICST Conference on Cloud Computing (CloudComp 2010)*. ICST.

Lindner, M., McDonald, F., McLarnon, B., & Robinson, P. (2011). Towards automated business-driven indication and mitigation of VM sprawl in Cloud supply chains. In *Proceedings of Integrated Network Management (IM)* (pp. 1062–1065). IEEE. doi:10.1109/INM.2011.5990505

Lindner, M. A., McDonald, F., Conway, G., & Curry, E. (2011). Understanding Cloud Requirements-A Supply Chain Lifecycle Approach. In *Proceedings of Cloud Computing 2011, The Second International Conference on Cloud Computing, GRIDs, and Virtualization* (pp. 20-25). Academic Press.

Milojicic, D., Llorente, I. M., & Montero, R. S. (2011). Opennebula: A cloud management tool. *IEEE Internet Computing, 15*(2), 11–14. doi:10.1109/MIC.2011.44

Peterson, Z. N., Gondree, M., & Beverly, R. (2011). A position paper on data sovereignty: The importance of geolocating data in the cloud. In *Proceedings of the 8th USENIX confErence on Networked Systems Design and Implementation.* USENIX.

Poese, I., Uhlig, S., Kaafar, M. A., Donnet, B., & Gueye, B. (2011). IP geolocation databases: Unreliable? *ACM SIGCOMM Computer Communication Review, 41*(2), 53–56. doi:10.1145/1971162.1971171

Rozsnyai, S., Vecera, R., Schiefer, J., & Schatten, A. (2007). Event cloud-searching for correlated business events. In *Proceedings of E-Commerce Technology and the 4th IEEE International Conference on Enterprise Computing, E-Commerce, and E-Services,* (pp. 409-420). IEEE.

Siwpersad, S. S., Gueye, B., & Uhlig, S. (2008). Assessing the geographic resolution of exhaustive tabulation for geolocating Internet hosts. In *Proceedings of Passive and Active Network Measurement* (pp. 11–20). Springer. doi:10.1007/978-3-540-79232-1_2

Stewart, J. A., Day, M., Print, C., & Favato, G. (2009). Compliance in the supply chain: implications of Sarbanes-Oxley for UK businesses. *ICFAI Journal of Supply Chain Management, 6*(1), 8–19.

IT Union. (2008). *Implementing e-health in developing countries.* ITU Tech Report.

World Health Organisation. (2005). *58th World Health Assembly Report.* WHO Tech Report.

Zhou, L., Zhu, Y., Lin, Y., & Bentley, Y. (2012). Cloud Supply Chain: A Conceptual Model. In *Proceedings of European, International Working Seminar on Production Economics.* Innsbruck, Austria: Academic Press.

KEY TERMS AND DEFINITIONS

Auditing: Collecting and evaluating evidence to determine whether a computer system (information system) safeguards assets, maintains data integrity, achieves organizational goals and consumes resources efficiently.

Cloud Supply Chain (CSC): Two or more parties linked by the provision of Cloud services, related information and funds.

Cloud: A model for enabling ubiquitous, convenient, on-demand network access to a shared pool of configurable computing resources (e.g., networks, servers, storage, applications, and services) that can be rapidly provisioned and released with minimal management effort or service provider interaction.

Compliance: The assurance that processes, defined by both government and regulators, which require that businesses manage data safely, are being adhered to.

Customer Relationship Management (CRM) System: Maintains customer information for the purposes of administration, marketing, sales and support.

Electronic Health Record (EHR) Systems: Special forms of CRM systems customised for the health-care domain used to collect and store patient health information.

Service Lvel Agreement (SLA): Is a contract between a service provider and a consumer that specifies, usually in measurable terms, the conditions upon the service has been provisioned.

Chapter 8
Sharing Medical Information by Means of Using Intelligent Agents and Cloud Computing

Mauricio Paletta
Universidad Nacional Experimental de Guayana (UNEG), Venezuela

ABSTRACT

From birth to death, every human being leaves a long medical history consisting of laboratory exams, records of medical consultations, records, and hospitalizations, as well as any other important information that affects the patient's health. These are known today as Electronic Health Records (EHR) or Electronic Medical Records (EMR). However, because a person's lifestyle and health are continuously changing, most of this medical information is distributed among different institutions, cities, and even countries where the specific processes were undertaken, in possession of health insurance providers or even hidden inside a drawer of the patient's home. Therefore, aiming to enhance the availability of improved medical services at reduced costs, modern information technology is being increasingly used in the healthcare sector. Researchers, developers, and companies have made efforts to develop mobile, Web, desktop, and enterprise e-health applications raising the importance of interoperability and data exchange between e-health applications and Health Information Systems (HIS). In this regard, Cloud Computing (CC) promises low cost, high scalability, availability, and disaster recoverability, which can be a natural solution for some of the problems faced in storing and analyzing EMRs. However, CC, which is mainly defined to address the use of scalable and often virtualized resources, is still evolving. New, specific collaboration models among service providers are needed for enabling effective service collaboration, allowing the process of serving consumers to be more efficient. In this chapter, the current state and trends of CC in healthcare are presented as well as a detailed collaboration model based on intelligent agents focusing on the EHR sharing subject. This model for enabling effective service in cloud systems is based on a recent research proposal related to defining a collaboration mechanism by means of Scout Movement. The chapter also includes details on the way in which services and service providers are clearly defined in this particular system.

DOI: 10.4018/978-1-4666-6118-9.ch008

INTRODUCTION

Imagine a situation in which a patient's complete medical history is available online. If so, then for example every time a person takes a laboratory exam the institution would register the results online, making them available for every physician or hospital that examines the patient so they would upgrade the patient's medical information, and so on. If this could be possible, then a patient's medical information could be accessible anytime and anywhere it might be needed, either by doctors or health care facilities as well as by the patient him/herself. In this scenario then, if a patient needs to visit a new doctor, for example, or a specialist, then the first thing the doctor could do is to take a look to the patient's medical information online instead of asking routine questions like: Have you ever had any major surgeries? Can you tell me anything about your family history? Do they take any medication? Are you on any medication? And so on. Also notice that a patient can be better helped if the patient's relative medical information is easily accessible online. In the event of a fatality, moreover, the information would continue to be stored online to help relatives.

Furthermore, it is interesting to consider what happens to a patient's laboratory results taken during his or her lifetime. What happens to these results? Could these results be stored somewhere where they might be accessible at any time by both the patient and the physician or healthcare provider? Could these results be organized into graphics or charts that could, for example, show how the patient's cholesterol levels have evolved over time?

According to Wilson (2012), "The healthcare industry has traditionally underutilized technology as a means of improving the delivery of patient care. Even today, organizations still rely on paper medical records and handwritten notes to inform and make decisions. Digital information is siloed between departments and applications, making access to a patient's longitudinal record difficult,

if not impossible. This lack of access costs the healthcare industry millions of dollars each year in duplication and waste" (p. 4). In the same order of ideas, Kuo (2011) states that "Health care, as with any other service operation, requires continuous and systematic innovation in order to remain cost effective, efficient, and timely, and to provide high-quality services" (p. e67). Moreover, "One of the areas with greatest needs having available information at the right moment and with high accuracy is healthcare. Right information at the right time saves lives" (Lupşe et al., 2012, p. 81).

Because the healthcare industry specifically is under significant pressures to lower the costs associated with providing their services, this idea of sharing Electronic Health Records (EHR) or Electronic Medical Records (EMR) is not new. However, "the ability of healthcare providers to adopt new technologies that drive better patient care has always been a challenge, born out of the cost and complexity of rolling out new technologies" (Wilson, 2012, p. 10).

An EMR is a computerized legal medical record (patient record) created in an organization that delivers care. It has three parts (Li et al., 2010):

1. **The Patient's Data:** Basic information of a patient: name, address, date of birth, insurance information, and so on.
2. **The Patient's Profile:** Summary of a patient's family history as well as details of the patient's life style.
3. **The Clinical Data:** Information related to symptoms, diagnosis, and treatment of each of a patient's medical cases.

Due to the fact that a patient' EMR can be distributed between hospitals, research clinics, private health care institutions, doctors/physician, insurance companies, pharmacies, laboratories, imaging centers, and even the same patient, it sounds reasonable then to maintain the information in a distributed environment. Another possible option to consider could be centralization but it is difficult overall if considered for worldwide distribution. Nevertheless, distribution means that all these institutions could share the information with each other and so a set of specific rules must be defined. Moreover, obtaining and upgrading the information in a distributed system can be better as it can be associated with the concept of service in the Web i.e. a Service Oriented Architecture (SOA).

In this regard, Cloud Computing (CC) is emerging as a solution for this area related to a distributed system that works toward providing reliable, customized, and "quality of service" guaranteed dynamic computing environments for end-users (Weiss, 2007). It is primarily based on service-level agreements that provide external users with services under request. However, the success of achieving this goal in proper time (efficiency) and/or to obtain higher quality results (effectiveness) in these dynamic and distributed environments depends on implementing an appropriate collaboration model between service providers in the cloud.

It must be noticed, related specifically to this healthcare related subject of sharing a patient's EMR information, that the relevance of obtaining and upgrading a patient's EMR information both efficiently and effectively in such a complex distributed system consisting of all those entities that can form any part of the patient's EMR has been noticed. Moreover, it is important to understand that the amount of digital information available is directly proportional to the ability to manage this data. Because a patient is a living subject his or her information is continuously growing, which makes healthcare a good example of large data continuously increasing and managing it becomes a growing problem.

This chapter focuses on explaining the way in which services and service providers are clearly defined in this particular CC distributed system. Originated from previous work (Paletta, 2012c), the chapter also includes an explanation of why Intelligent Agents (IAs) organized in a Multi-Agent

System (MAS), is a good option to implement a cloud computing system in general. Moreover and because Scout Movement or Scouting has been a very successful youth movement in which the collaboration of its members can be observed, a previous work aiming to design a framework that defines MASs based on the principles of Scouting and adapted for CC environments is used in this chapter to design the cloud computing system by sharing the EMR information.

Aiming to address the aforementioned content this chapter is structured in the following sections. Besides this introductory section, the next section below contains a detailed explanation of why I believe CC is the best way to reach a solution to the problem addressed in this chapter including some previous related work. The third section discusses the details of why I believe IAs and MAS are good options for implementing CC systems. A particular experience combining MAS and CC by using Scouting principles and called CCS-Scout is presented in the fourth section. The fifth section presents the details of sharing EMR information by using CCS-Scout. Finally, the last sections are concerned about the direction of future research and the corresponding conclusions of this chapter.

Why Cloud Computing?

This section features some explanation as to why CC should be considered the appropriate technology for sharing EMR information. It begins with some definitions related to CC given by different authors and it also includes a brief state of art related to the subject of sharing EMR information by means of CC.

According to Buyya et al., (2009) "Cloud is a parallel and distributed computing system consisting of a collection of inter-connected and virtualized computers that are dynamically provisioned and presented as one or more unified computing resources based on service-level agreements (SLA) established through negotiation between the service provider and consumers."

Vaquero et al., (2008) state "Clouds are a large pool of easily usable and accessible virtualized resources (such as hardware, development platforms and/or services). These resources can be dynamically reconfigured to adjust to a variable load (scale), allowing also for optimum resource utilization. This pool of resources is typically exploited by a pay-per-use model in which guarantees are offered by the Infrastructure Provider by means of customized Service Level Agreements."

In the same order of ideas, "Cloud Computing is the evolution of a variety of technologies that have come together to alter an organization's approach to building out an information technology infrastructure. Like the Web a little over a decade ago, there is nothing fundamentally new in any of the technologies that make up cloud computing" (Reese, 2009, p. 1). "At its simplest, cloud computing is the dynamic delivery of information technology resources and capabilities as a service over the Internet. Cloud computing is a style of computing in which dynamically scalable and often virtualized resources are provided as a service over the Internet. It generally incorporates infrastructure as a service (IaaS), platform as a service (PaaS), and software as a service (SaaS)" (Sarna, 2011, p. 2).

Finally, a definition given by the National Institute of Standards and Technology (NIST) states that "Cloud computing is a model for enabling convenient, on-demand network access to a shared pool of configurable computing resources (e.g., networks, servers, storage, applications, and services) that can be rapidly provisioned and released with minimal management effort or service provider interaction. This cloud model promotes availability and is composed of five essential characteristics: on-demand self-service, broad network access, resource pooling, rapid elasticity, and measured service; three service models: infrastructure as a service, platform as a service, and software as a service; and four deployment models: private, community, public, and hybrid" (Mell & Grance, 2009, p. 50).

Distributed computing system, computing resource, service, negotiation, and infrastructure provider are keywords extracted from these previous definitions and are related with CC technology. As we will see in the next section of this chapter these keywords are relevant for discovering the relationship between CC systems and multi-agent based collaboration distributed systems. Moreover, this relationship can also be analyzed by identifying the key characteristics of CC (Armbrust et al., 2009):

1. The illusion of infinite computing resources.
2. The elimination of an up-front commitment by cloud users.
3. The ability to pay for usage as needed.

Additionally, Voorsluys et al., (2011) present the following features desired for a cloud:

1. **Self-Service:** Consumers of CC services expect on-demand, nearly instant access to resources. For that reason clouds must allow the use of services without human intervention (Mell & Grance, 2009).
2. **Per-Usage Metering and Billing:** CC eliminates up-front commitment by users. Services must be priced on a short-term basis and released as soon as they are not needed (Armbrust et al., 2009). This means that users will only pay for what is used.
3. **Elasticity:** CC gives the illusion of infinite computing resources available on demand (Armbrust et al., 2009), so that users expect clouds to provide a quantity of resources at any time efficiently (rapidly) and effectively (with quality).
4. **Customization:** A great disparity between user needs is common in a multi-tenant cloud. So then, resources must be highly customizable.

Moreover, Rochwerger et al., (2011) enumerate the basic principles of CC by highlighting the fundamental requirement from the providers of CC that allows virtual applications to freely migrate, grow, and shrink:

1. **Federation:** Service providers in a CC environment have a finite capacity. In order to grow beyond this capacity, "Cloud Computing providers should be able to form federations of providers such that they can collaborate and share their resources."
2. **Independence:** Service providers in a CC environment should be able to manage their infrastructure without exposing internal details to their customers or partners so that users should be able to utilize the services of the cloud without relying on any specific tool. Therefore, "services need to be encapsulated and generalized such that users will be able to acquire equivalent virtual resources at different providers."
3. **Isolation:** Users in a CC environment need warranties from services providers so that their personal computer items are completely isolated from others. "Users must be ensured that their resources cannot be accessed by others sharing the same cloud and that adequate performance isolation is in place to ensure that no other user may possess the power to directly affect the service granted to their application."
4. **Elasticity:** It is the CC ability to provide or release resources on-demand. In order to meet demand variations, CC providers should enact this ability automatically.
5. **Business Orientation:** CC providers should develop mechanisms to ensure quality of service and proper support for service-level agreements.
6. **Trust:** Establishing trust is one of the most critical issues to be addressed before CC can become the preferred computing paradigm. Therefore, the mechanisms allow building and maintaining trust between consumers and providers, as well as between providers are essential for the success of CC systems.

To complete this brief review about CC, a brief explanation of the three service models that compose CC established by NIST are presented below (Jha et al., 2011): Software as a Service (SaaS), Platform as a Service (PaaS), and Infrastructure-as-a-Service (IaaS). In this regard, Mohan (2011) states "From a technology viewpoint, as of today, the IaaS type of cloud offerings have been the most successful and widespread in usage. However, the potential of PaaS has been high. All new cloud-oriented application development initiatives are based on the PaaS model. The significant impact of enterprises leveraging IaaS and PaaS has been in the form of services whose usage is representative of SaaS on the cloud."

1. **SaaS:** Provides ready-to-run services that are deployed and configured for the user.
2. **PaaS:** Provides the ability to deploy custom applications on the infrastructure of the CC providers. These applications are developed using the programming languages and the application programming interfaces defined by the provider.
3. **IaaS:** Provides low-level virtualized resources such as storage, networks, and other fundamental computing resources via self-services to the user. In general, the user can deploy and run arbitrary software, which usually includes operating systems as well as applications.

After this brief review of the CC's conceptual aspects, I should now highlight why CC is the most appropriate technology to address the specific issues related to sharing medical information in particular and healthcare related information in general. I believe that the best way to proceed is both to mention some previous work belonging to the state of the art of this subject and to enumerate what other authors or institutions think about this. From the vast amount of research that exists in this area, the following is a list of some of the corresponding previous work:

- Botts et al., (2010) detail the architectural design for a personal health record system called "HealthATM" that utilizes and integrates services from Google's cloud computing environment. Services are integrated into an unobtrusive and easy way to use an ATM-style interface for health consumers and care providers to manage and track their health.

- Deng et al., (2011) focus on a home healthcare system based on cloud computing. It introduces several use cases and draws architecture based on the cloud. Security and privacy challenges are identified in the proposed cloud-based home healthcare system. A functional infrastructure plan is provided to demonstrate the integration between the proposed application architecture with the cloud infrastructure.

- Dimitrova et al., (2012) present a framework for design of novel interfaces for Cloud compatible medical services called User Interface as a Service (UIaaS) aiming to support seamless and ubiquitous health monitoring based on flexible and useful Cloud services for healthcare. The work describes the methods and new interfaces for health monitoring that have recently been developed for the proposed framework.

- Ekonomou et al., (2011) present a cloud-based healthcare system that integrates a formal care system (DACAR) with an informal care system (Microsoft Health Vault). The proposal provides high levels of security and privacy within a cloud environment, enabling sharing of both health records and access rights, along with the patient's pathway.

- Guo et al., (2012) discuss an important research tool related to health information sharing and integration in Healthcare Cloud (HC) and investigate the arising challenges and issues. Authors also describe many potential solutions to provide more opportunities to implement EHR cloud as well as to introducing the development of a HC related collaborative healthcare research example.

- He et al., (2013) proposal of a private cloud platform architecture, which includes six layers according to the specific requirements. It utilizes message queue as a cloud engine, and each layer thereby achieves relative independence by these loosely coupled means of communications with publish/subscribe mechanism. A plug-in algorithm framework is also presented, and massive semi-structured or unstructured medical data are accessed adaptively by this cloud architecture.

- Hu et al., (2012) propose a cloud computing solution for sharing healthcare information based on Google App Engine (GAE). The authors claim that they achieve interoperability among different healthcare centers and between healthcare providers and receivers with high stability and availability.

- Khansa et al., (2012) propose an intelligent cloud-based electronic health record (ICEHR) system which has the potential to reduce medical errors and improve patients' quality of life, in addition to reducing costs and increasing the productivity of healthcare organizations. The authors developed a set of best practices that encompass end-user policies and regulations, identity and access management, network resilience and service level agreements, advanced computational power, "Big Data" mining abilities, and other operational/managerial controls that are meant to improve the privacy and security of the

ICEHR and make it inherently compliant to healthcare regulations. These best practices serve as a framework that offers a single interconnection agreement between the cloud host and healthcare entities, as well as streamline access to private patient information based on a unified set of access principles.

- Kuo et al., (2012) propose a cloud-based data-mining platform for sharing research data/results through the Internet while remaining cost effective, flexible, secure, and where privacy is preserved. The work also evaluates the implementation challenges of the cloud based platform and provides potential solutions to handle the identified issues so that other similar research can use this study as a reference to determine whether to migrate from traditional to cloud-based services.

- Lupşe et al., (2012) propose a solution based on cloud computing implemented for hospital systems having as a result a better management, high speed for medical processes, and increased quality of medical services. The paper suggests a model for the architecture of the information systems in two key departments of a hospital, Pediatrics and Obstetrics, and Gynecology (OB GYN) by using interoperability for better access to information and preparing the system for future connectivity.

- Ming et al., (2013) propose a novel patient-centric framework and a suite of mechanisms for data access control to PHRs stored in semi-trusted servers aiming to assure the patients' control over access to their own PHRs. Authors leverage attribute-based encryption (ABE) techniques to encrypt each patient's PHR file. They focus on the multiple data owner scenario, and divide the users in the PHR system into multiple security domains that greatly reduces the key management com-

plexity for owners and users. The authors claim that a high degree of patient privacy is guaranteed simultaneously by exploiting multiauthority ABE.

- Papakonstantinou et al., (2011) introduce a scenario to implement a cloud-based service for ePrescribing. The physician that uses the application is connected to the PHR (Personal Healthcare Record) system. He / she reads a summary of the medical history of each patient's records and selects a list of drugs. The application validates the selection of drugs based on their interaction with other drugs, patient allergies, and medication history of the patient.

- Pardamean and Rumanda (2011) present a model as an integrated EMR (Electronic Medical Record) sharing medical data between medical units. The application is developed on a cloud platform that keeps the EMR system on the form of SaaS and can be used by Government, Hospitals, Doctors, Patients, Pharmacies and Health Insurance Organizations, through the Internet.

- Rao et al., (2010) use the concept entitled "Pervasive Cloud" which means "Accessing the Power of a Cloud through Pervasive Access of Mobile Communications," to present "Dhatri," a Pervasive Cloud Based Healthcare Application targeted towards Healthcare needs specifically for Rural and Deep Rural Areas. It inherits the powerful features of a typical Cloud Computing and enables the Pervasive Healthcare Access.

- Radwan et al., (2012) present a data exchange mechanism and interoperability between Health Information Systems (HIS) and e-health applications across a cloud-based service. The proposed service provides a single point of entry for retrieving Electronic Medical Records (EMR) among the various HISs that a patient record is stored in and for any e-health application seeking such information. The work also proposes a unified secure platform that provides developers, health care providers, and organizations access to a framework to retrieve and manage medical records and Personal Health Records (PHR) among various subscribers.

- Sobhy et al., (2012) present details of an architectural design for a personal health record system called "MedCloud" that utilizes and integrates services from Hadoop's ecosystem in conjunction with HIPAA privacy and security rules. The work also examines the impact of cloud computing on improving healthcare services.
- Wang and Tan (2010) provide the proposal of a medical and health information system infrastructure based on CC. The authors applied in this architecture the three kinds of application mode: SaaS, PaaS, and IaaS.
- Yu et al., (2011) provide a service-modeling approach to model the requirement and design of different Service Oriented Architecture (SOA) based services by using Service Oriented Modeling and Architecture (SOMA) and employing Service Oriented Modeling Framework (SOMF) modeling styles and assets. It also includes the development of a u-Healthcare Web based software system, which uses the service model as a foundation to ensure secure provisioning of health services to its prospective clients.
- Zhang and Liu (2010) present important concepts related to EHR sharing and integration in healthcare clouds and analyze the arising security and privacy issues in access and management of EHRs. The authors describe an EHR security reference model for managing security issues in healthcare clouds, which highlights three

important core components in securing an EHR cloud. They also illustrate the development of the EHR security reference model through a use-case scenario and describe the corresponding security countermeasures and state of the art security techniques that can be applied as basic security guards.

The following are several issues extracted from both related work and previous documentation I found during while researching:

- According to the Microsoft Official Blog, "Cloud computing promises enormous benefits for the healthcare world. These could include improved patient care, better health for the overall populations providers serve, and new delivery models that will make healthcare more efficient and effective. And cloud computing can help do all of this in a cost-effective way" (Aylward, 2010).
- Hitachi Data Systems claims that "Enter cloud computing. A panacea? Probably not; however, it is perhaps the biggest potential change to the healthcare industry since the computer. Embracing cloud technology in healthcare may be the answer to enabling healthcare organizations to focus their efforts on clinically relevant services and improved patient outcomes" (Wilson, 2012).
- "Cloud computing introduces a new business model and way of delivering service and value to the medical community, as medical-related trading partners, business associates and customers. There are a number of benefits—point-of-care service delivery, cost-savings, the leveraging of new applications and support for an increas-

ingly mobile workforce—that are enabled through adoption of cloud technologies." (Rabi et al., 2012).

- "Cloud computing paradigm is one of the popular health IT infrastructure for facilitating EHR sharing and EHR integration" (Zhang & Liu, 2010).

- "Cloud computing is one of the long dreamed visions of Healthcare Cloud (HC), which matches the need of healthcare information sharing directly to various health providers over the Internet, regardless of their location and the amount of data" (Guo et al., 2012).

- "Cloud computing promises low cost, high scalability, availability, and disaster recoverability which can be a natural solution for some of the problems faced in storing and analyzing patients' medical records" (Sobhy et al., 2012)

- "Cloud computing owns the pervasive and on-demand service-oriented natures, which can fit the characteristics of healthcare services very well" (He et al., 2013).

- "Most healthcare organizations are in the right place to reap significant benefits from cloud computing, because they have aging technology infrastructure that has not seen significant investments in some time, and they are being asked to implement major new technology-based initiatives such as EMR. Instead of buying their own servers and software for providing general office productivity functions, managing patient records, handling patient billing, or tracking patient care, healthcare organizations can purchase applications from an external provider with experience in the healthcare industry. They can take the opportunity to migrate away from older servers and applications that are outside of their support contracts, and identify and implement solutions that will facilitate better flexibility, faster provisioning of services, and better

interoperability with their partners. This approach will give them access to the newest technologies impacting their industry, and can help them remain in compliance with the ever-changing government regulations for healthcare services." (Alley et al., 2012) Moreover, "In the same way that doctors used telephone call centers to extend their office hours and give their patients access to them round the clock, they can now use cloud computing services to expand their technology reach, and compete on a more even footing with larger organizations." (Alley et al., 2012).. Additionally, having Health Information Exchange (HIE), Physician Collaboration Solutions (PCS) and Clinical Information Systems (CIS) in the cloud "can facilitate better operability between healthcare providers" (Alley et al., 2012). Finally, as claimed by the same authors, the primary benefits of EMR in the cloud are: 1) Reduced implementation time; 2) Much lower initial costs, especially for smaller organizations; 3) Partnership of compliance; and 4) Better scalability, without initial over-provisioning of equipment.

- "Cloud computing can play a critical role in containing healthcare integration costs, optimizing resources and ushering in a new era of innovations. Current trends aim towards accessing information anytime, anywhere, which can be achieved when moving healthcare information to the cloud" (Ahuja et al., 2012). "One of the key benefits will be the ability to exchange data between disparate systems" (Ahuja et al., 2012). "Cloud computing has given opportunities for clinics, hospitals, insurance companies, pharmacies, and other healthcare companies to agree in collaborating between them and share healthcare information to offer better quality of service and reduce costs. Looking over the changes occurring in the market, it appears that cloud-based systems will likely become the norm in healthcare once all the challenges it brings are overcome" (Ahuja et al., 2012). "By adopting the cloud in medical services both patients and healthcare organizations would obtain a huge benefit in patient's quality of service, collaboration between healthcare organizations as well as reductions in IT cost in healthcare companies. ... Therefore, hospitals, clinics, imaging centers, pharmacies and insurance companies can efficiently share patient's medical records, prescription information, X rays, test results, physician's references, physicians availability, etc. that can be accessed anywhere and everywhere by authorized entities. All this information would be used for making decisions, obtaining better diagnosis and treatments to yield better results, scheduling physician's appointments, speeding insurance approval, etc. which highly improves patient's quality of service" (Ahuja et al., 2012).

- "Cloud computing technologies, if implemented and used appropriately, have a response to all these requirements. Thus, cloud computing provides to the health care environment the opportunity to improve services for patients, to easily share information, to improve operational efficiency, and to streamline costs" (Blaisdell, 2013).

- More about positive reasons to use CC for sharing medical healthcare information can be found in both Kuo (2011) and Bollineni and Neupane (2011).

In addition to all the above information, the following are five advantages that cloud computing offers for the health care industry according to Blaisdell (2013):

1. **Collaboration:** Through cloud technologies, the information is synchronized and shared in real time, aiming to allow specific information to be accessed by different health services providers at the same time.

2. **Speed:** Cloud-based tools can not only upgrade and improve their features faster, less expensively and with minimal or no service interruption, but they also enable faster access to important information for health services providers and their patients.

3. **Mobility:** By storing data and computing power in the cloud, health care services providers enable their staff to have access to information anywhere and anytime.

4. **Security and Privacy:** Cloud services providers are required in order to comply with privacy standards such as HIPAA (Health Insurance Portability and Accountability Act) and today there exist several cloud providers designed to offer HIPAA compliance.

5. **Decreased Costs:** There is no need for the health care institution and doctors to invest in hardware infrastructure and maintenance because these concerns are already taken care of by cloud computing providers.

The information presented above shows that CC has recently become important in the healthcare industry. However, although CC offers significant advantages to this industry, it presents some disadvantages that must be taken into account. According to Blaisdell (2013), the most common concerns are those that make any business, from any industry, be reluctant to adopting cloud technologies: security and confidentiality of patient information, interoperability and compliance with government regulations. Rabi et al., (2012) claim that this model has the following disadvantages: 1) No fail-over system in case of communication failure; 2) Smaller hospitals and physician practices do not have the IT staff required to support new technologies (although the cloud removes the burden of hiring internal IT staff to maintain it); and 3) It is necessary to maintain a secure, safe, and authorized environment for the prevention of information leakage.

In my opinion, finding an adequate way to deal with the CC concept and taking into account key aspects like "collaboration" can help reduce or perhaps even eliminate the possible disadvantages mentioned above. This is precisely one of the reasons why a third concept related to MAS is included to this couple CC-healthcare. This is the goal of the next section.

WHY MULTI-AGENT SYSTEMS?

This section presents the motivational aspects involved in the implementation of CC by means of MAS-based frameworks. In this regard, Service-Oriented Architecture (SOA) is extensively used at present for the design of development models of Internet systems, being the Web Services (WS) technology[1] one of the most relatively important technologies. In a SOA, software resources are packaged as "services," which are well-defined, self-contained modules that provide standard business functionality and are independent of the state or context of other services. Services are described in a standard definition language and

have a published interface (Papazoglou & Van den Heuvel, 2007). In reference Weerawarana et al., (2005) the following three items of the SOA triangle are indicated (see *Figure 1*) in order to: 1) provide an abstract definition of the service; 2) publish details about the services so that those who want to use them can understand what they do and can obtain the information necessary for connecting and utilizing them; 3) find a way to discover which services that meet the required needs are available.

The emergence of WS open standards has significantly contributed to improving advances in the domain of software integration (Papazoglou & Van den Heuvel, 2007). "Web services can glue together applications running on different messaging product platforms, enabling information from one application to be made available to others" (Voorsluys et al., 2011). While some WSs are published with the intent of serving end-user applications, their true power resides in WS's interface being accessible to other services. An enterprise application that follows the SOA paradigm is a collection of services that together perform complex business logic (Papazoglou & Van den Heuvel, 2007).

It can be clearly seen that there is a relationship between CC and SOA. It is natural then to use WS as the base for an implementation of a CC system. On the other hand, WS-based systems and MAS

Figure 1. The SOA triangle (Weerawarana et al., 2005)

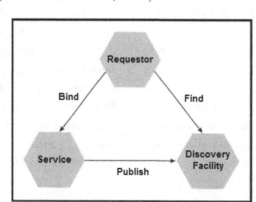

share a motivation in trying to find information systems that are flexible and adaptable. That is why it is natural to consider a conceptual relation among these technologies in the following common themes (Dickinson & Wooldridge, 2005):

- **No Conceptual Distinction:** There is no conceptual difference between a WS and an Intelligent Agent (IA) because both are active building blocks in a loosely-coupled architecture.
- **Bi-Directional Integration:** IAs and WSs can interoperate with each other by initiating communications.
- **IA Invokes WS:** Agents invoke WSs as component behaviors, while the IA level is represented by autonomy and intent.

Besides the relationship between CC and WS together with the relationship between WS and MAS, there exist a number of other factors influencing the implementation of CC by using a MAS:

- In order to meet the principle of "federation" there exist collaboration models utilized in MASs that can be used to form federations of services providers.
- To meet the principle of "independence" that CC should have, the autonomy that IAs have is an important factor.
- The principle of "isolation" can be met by managing the characteristics of delegation that IAs can have.
- To make "elasticity" of the CC system possible, any combination of the following characteristics can be used: autonomy, personality, communication, degradation in style, cooperation, and expectations.
- "Business orientation" can be focused through the IA's task-resolution strategies because the domain of an agent is flexible.

- "Trust" in CC can be achieved as there is trust with IAs. Trust in IAs is derived from the characteristics of autonomy and delegation of the agents.

On the other hand, by considering the cloud of a CC as the environment of a MAS, the following can be said about the cloud:

- It is accessible because all services are available.
- It is deterministic because agents know which services the other agents provide.
- It is episodic because the task an agent has to perform depends on a discrete number of services.
- It is dynamic because the environment changes while agents are collaborating.
- It is discrete because the number of possible services is finite and fixed.

In order to implement a CC based on IAs a MAS-based collaboration model is needed. Any node in the cloud environment (both service requestor and provider) is endowed with an IA of the MAS. A corresponding agent autonomously manages the needs of a particular requestor. The collaboration and negotiation between service providers made to meet all the requesting services are also autonomously managed by the corresponding agent of each provider. The following observations should be noted about the processes that MAS platforms should allow:

- Adding or removing nodes in a CC system implies the creation and termination of agents respectively.
- The unique identification address of any node in the cloud environment is the unique identification address any agent in a MAS needs.

- WS technology provides a registration system where agents can publish their capabilities.
- The necessary communication channel that nodes in a CC system has been the only channel for communication that the agents in a MAS need.

Aiming to define appropriate collaboration mechanisms for enabling effective service collaboration in CC systems, a MAS-based model with emphasis in agent collaboration may be an interesting suggestion to consider (Paletta & Herrero, 2010). Moreover, an important question to be considered is this: what is the right MAS framework that can be used to implement a CC system, taking into account all or most of the subjects identified above?

Services providers, collaboration, negotiation, and task distribution encouraged me to focus on the principles of the Scout Movement or Scouting in order to define a MAS framework for implementing CC. Scouting is a globally known connotation for a youth movement in which organization, cooperation, trust, leadership, learning, communication, roles, rules, obligations, prohibitions, and history among others are present. As a result of the above and by using MAS-Scout (Paletta, 2012a & 2012b), a MAS framework designed for the organization of IAs in MASs by means of the worldwide known Scout Movement, "Intelligent Cloud" was defined in a previous work (Paletta, 2012c) derived from the fact that it is a CC system managed by IAs. The main goal of using MAS-Scout is to have a strategy that can be used for designing a CC system and for defining the way in which tasks can be resolved by distribution. Due to the fact that this strategy is based on Scouting, the cooperation between agents is the key to achieving the desired goals. The next section presents further details.

CLOUD COMPUTING BY MEANS OF SCOUT MOVEMENT

Details of CCS-Scout i.e. CC by means of MAS-Scout are presented in this section. Because the importance of the concept, the section starts with a brief explanation of Scouting.

Scout Movement

Scout movement or Scouting is a global connotation that refers to a youth movement which stated goal is to support young people in their physical, mental, and spiritual states so that they can play a constructive role in society. Scouting dates back to 1907, when Robert Baden-Powell, Lieutenant General of the British Army, held the first Scout camp on Brownsea Island in England. After that, Baden-Powell wrote the principles of Scouting in *Scouting for Young People* (Baden-Powell, 1908). During the first half of the 20th-century, the movement grew to encompass three major groups for boys: Cub Scout (Pack), Boy Scout (Troop), and Rover Scout (Clan). In 1910, a new organization, Girl Guides, was created for girls.

In the words of its founder: "Scouting is a game of boys, led by them, and for which older brothers can give to younger ones a healthy environment, and encourage them to indulge in those activities that are conducive to healthily awaken the virtues of citizenship." This method makes use of motion scout, a non-formal education program with emphasis on practical outdoor activities such as camping, woodcraft, aquatics, hiking, walking, and sports. Another feature of this method is the movement that recognized the mandatory use of the Scout uniform. This movement intends to hide all social differences and strives for equality.

Scouting principles remain unchanged throughout the world, where all Scouting associations are joined together to respect the same values and laws. The emphasis on "learning by doing" provides members with experiences that serve them as a practical method of learning and building confidence. These experiences, coupled with an emphasis on honesty and personal honor, help members develop responsibility, character, confidence, reliability, and willingness leading to collaboration and leadership. Various activities and games carried out outdoors provide not only a fun way to develop skills such as dexterity, but also provide interaction with the natural environment.

In the same order of ideas, principles and laws of the scouts are the same worldwide. Many of such principles and laws derived from the code followed by medieval knights of the Middle Ages. Therefore, the organization ensures the homogeneity of global processes. The precepts to be observed by scouts are: 1) a Scout puts his honor aside in order to be trustworthy; 2) a Scout is loyal; 3) a Scout is useful and helpful to others without thought of reward; 4) a Scout is everyone's friend, and brother to all other Scouts without distinction of creed, race, nationality or social class; 5) a Scout is courteous and gentlemanly; 6) a Scout sees in nature the work of God, he protects animals and plants; 7) a Scout obeys without question and does nothing by halves; 8) a Scout smiles and sings through difficulties; 9) a Scout is economical, hard-worker, and concerned for the good of others; 10) a Scout is clean and healthy, pure in thoughts, words, and actions.

A Scout group consists of different members grouped in organized units that still maintain the original hierarchical structure. Groups are made up of three divisions. A fourth division exists in order to support new activities to society. The first three divisions (pack, troop, and clan) are designed to train young people and consist of young people between ages 6-11, 11-16 and 16-21 years old respectively.

Because of the age differences between the boys, each subgroup/division is organized somewhat differently. However, they always have a guide or leader to guide them. All guides must submit a plan in advance that the young Scouts must meet in order to obtain medals as well as for personal growth. The number and name of each medal is defined by each National organization.

Likewise, the effort made among the leaders of each subgroup and the young members is not the same. In a pack, 100% of the initiative and responsibility lies in the leader. In a troop, responsibility is divided by 50% between the leaders and the members, as the boys are more grown-up and should be given some responsibility as well as discipline, always under adult supervision. Somewhat similarly, Scouts in a clan are older and therefore have more freedom and because of that they are expected to propose activities and to be oriented by their leader.

A troop is a unit of Scouts that brings together Scout patrols. A Scoutmaster and his assistants run a troop (Baden-Powell, 1908). The troops are formed by patrols and every Scout belongs to a patrol. A patrol is made up of a maximum of eight members and each patrol must have a name in order to be distinguished within the troop. Every Scout in the patrol is properly identified with a number. The leader (guide) of the patrol is identified with the number 1, the sub-guide or second in command is identified by the number 2, and so on. These guides and sub-guides are elected by the entire patrol and they are responsible for the performance of the patrol at the same time as they are responsible for reporting to the Scoutmaster. On the other hand, Scouts can only accomplish assigned goals in pairs or groups. According to Baden-Powell, a Scout Patrol is the basic unit of Scouting because it is the base needed for members to learn how to work in teams toward the satisfaction of common goals.

All the members of the patrol elect number 1 or the Patrol Leader. Number 1 is the leader and, therefore, the link between the patrol members and the Scoutmaster (troop's leader). In addition, within each troop a court of honor is defined. A court of honor deals with all matters related with any patrol (work programs, rewards, punishments, etc.). It consists of the Scoutmaster and the patrol leaders. Decisions are made by secret ballot and the Scoutmaster does not vote. Moreover, without the Scoutmaster the patrol leaders are responsible for making decisions for the troop.

In summary, organization, communication, cooperation, trust, learning, and leadership are features related to Scouting that can be used to organize a MAS.

Basic Definitions

To help understand the MAS-based framework CCS-Scout, relevant terms are defined below.

Definition 1: *Activity*: Is any action A_i that is necessary to perform in order to achieve a task.

Definition 2: *Level of complexity*: Is denoted by $\rho(A_i)$ and measured by a number between 1 and 3 that indicates whether A_i is easy, average, or difficult respectively.

Definition 3: *Skill*: Is denoted by $\Pi(A_i) = \{s_1, \ldots, s_k\}$ and it represents the set of skills/abilities s_i needed to accomplish the activity A_i. It is worth noting that there is a finite set of possible pre-defined skills s_i allowed in the set $\Pi(A_i)$. It is also worth noting that, as there is a set of skills $\Pi(A_i)$ related with any activity A_i, there is also a set of skills $\Pi(a)$ associated to an IA-Scout agent a. Initially, agents in the systems do not have to or have not learned any skill ($\Pi(a) = \varnothing$). Skills will be acquired by each agent a through a learning process (see details bellow in this section).

Definition 4: *Completion time*: Is the amount of time, expressed in milliseconds, necessary to complete the activity A_i; it is denoted by $\tau(A_i)$.

Definition 5: *Task*: Is the representation of a main goal and it consists of a set of activities A_i i.e. $T = (A_1, \ldots, A_n)$. In CCS-Scout a CC service is represented as a task. Therefore, a service consists of a set of activities each of which has a level of complexity and requires a set of skills to be completed. Notice that the level of complexity and/or the required skills any activity has can be used to determine a value to this specific activity. This value could be an amount that may be charged for the completion of the activity. Therefore, a cost estimation of one service may be calculated by totalizing the cost of all the corresponding activities. Related to this, expression (1) as depicted in Box 1 calculates the cost $\varsigma(T)$ of achieving service/task $T = (A_1, \ldots, A_n)$ based on the costs of achieving activities A_i, $\varsigma(A_i)$ that are calculated based on the corresponding skills $\Pi(A_i)$. It is worth noting that since $\Pi(A_i)$ is a set of specific skills s_j, $\varsigma(A_i)$ may be calculated by using a weighted average expression aiming to express the importance of each skill $s_j \in \Pi(A_i)$. Therefore, the more specialized the skill, the greater its influence on the calculation of $\varsigma(A_i)$.

Definition 6: *IA-Scout*: Is any of the IA that is part of the MAS defined by means of the CCS-Scout framework.

Definition 7: *IA-Scout Age*: Related with the IA-Scout a, it is the agent execution time $\Gamma(a)$.

Definition 8: *Organization*: Is the way in which IA-Scout agents in a CCS-Scout system are arranged. This is done in the same way as Scouts are organized in Scouting. This means that there are three kinds of groups: clan, troops, and patrols. There are also

Box 1.

$$\varsigma(T) = \sum_{i=1}^{n} \varsigma(A_i); \quad \varsigma(A_i) = p_1\varsigma(s_1) + p_2\varsigma(s_2) + \ldots + p_k\varsigma(s_k); \quad s_j \in \Pi(A_i) \tag{1}$$

Table 1. Summary of the messages exchanged between IA-Scout agents in a CCS-Scout environment

Between	Message Type	Description	Data
Members of the same group	Broadcast	Look for cooperation	Task information
	P2P	Confirm cooperation	Activity
	P2P	Inform that cooperation is no longer required	No
	P2P	Send a task that must be accomplished	Task information
	P2P	Send the response to the tasks that were given to be solved	Response information
An IA-Scout and its leader	P2P	Request activities to perform	No
	P2P	Send the response to the tasks that were given to be solved	Response information
IA-Scout leader and the members of the group	P2P	Assign tasks or activities to be performed	Task information
Between patrol leaders	Broadcast	To convoke a court of honor	No
	Broadcast	To inform about the best candidate of the troop	IA-Scout information
Between a patrol leader and its troop leader	P2P	To inform about the candidate selected to be promoted	IA-Scout information
	P2P	To ask the balance account	No
Between the troop leader and the corresponding patrol leaders	P2P	To inform which IA-Scout should be promoted	IA-Scout information
	P2P	To send the balance account	How much the patrol leader has to pay to the troop leader or get as reimbursement from it
Between troop leaders	Broadcast	To inform that a Clan leader must be selected	Troop leader responsible for the process
	Broadcast	To send the information of each troop leader needed for the selection process	Troop leader information
	P2P	To inform the troop leader candidate to be selected to be the Clan leader	Troop leader information
	P2P	To inform a particular troop leader about its promotion	No

three kinds of patrols: MAS-Pack, MAS-Troop, and MAS-Clan patrols. Initially all IA-Scouts have an execution time equal to 0 ($\Gamma(a) = 0$), which makes them part of a MAS-Pack patrol.

Starting from the lowest position in the hierarchy, the ascending line of command is as follows: a MAS-Pack patrol member; a MAS-Pack patrol sub-leader; a MAS-Pack patrol leader; a MAS-Troop patrol member; a MAS-Troop patrol sub-leader; a MAS-Troop patrol leader; a MAS-Clan patrol member; a MAS-Clan patrol sub-leader; a MAS-Clan patrol leader; a Troop leader; a Clan leader.

As agents are incorporated into the system and, due to the fact that they are at this moment beginners $((\Gamma(a) = 0))$, they are incorporated into an incomplete MAS-Pack, i.e. a patrol that does not have the maximum of eight members a patrol should have. Initially, when there is not a Scout in the CCS-Scout organization, the first agent to be incorporated into the system becomes the number 1 (leader) of the Clan. The second agent to join the system will be the leader of the first Troop. The next agent will be the leader of the first MAS-Pack patrol and so on until 6 more members are added to the system therefore completing the patrol. It is worth mentioning that, although eight is the maximum number of members a patrol can have according to Scouting, in CCS-Scout this is a parameter and therefore this value can be changed depending on run conditions such as, for example, the number of agents in the MAS.

When another agent needs to be incorporated into the CCS-Scout and all current patrols are full, it must form a new MAS-Pack and this requires selecting a leader. The new MAS-Pack leader is selected by using the probability presented in (3) and applied to the current MAS-Pack patrols'

sub-leaders. The same occurs when selecting a sub-leader for a new patrol, which is selected from the remaining members of each current MAS-Pack patrol. When the sub-leader of a patrol X is selected to be the leader of a new patrol Y, the new sub-leader of X is selected from the remaining members of X. This movement of agents results in vacant spaces on patrols that are later occupied by new agents added into the MAS.

Figure 2 summarizes the way in which IA-Scout agents in a CCS-Scout system are organized based on Scouting organization. Note that there is no limit to the amount and type of patrols of each troop and there is also no limit to the amount of troops in the clan. The CCS-Scout is really organized within a Clan with a single leader.

Furthermore, each node in the CCS-Scout cloud (either the client or service provider) is endowed with a MAS-Patrol, which means that any node has one or more IA-Scouts responsible for both requesting for the termination of services required as well as for providing the solution for requested services. Moreover, service providers that deal with the same subject or business are grouped in MAS-Troops so that all the collaboration needed between them is guaranteed because this is a natural process in CCS-Scout. These groups should be seen like consortiums of companies who help each other meet each other's

Figure 2. CCS-Scout basic organization

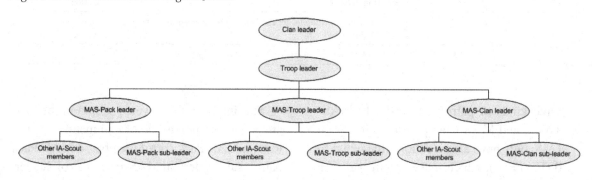

needs. Even different consortiums or MAS-Troops could collaborate if it was needed because they are organized in a MAS-Clan.

Initially, the entire CCS-Scout system could be disordered. In this case a process of self-organization is needed. In this regard, reference (Paletta, 2012a) contains a proposal of self-organization of a MAS-Scout based system that includes the way in which all leaders are selected. As CCS-Scout is derived from MAS-Scout, this proposal can be used without a problem.

Definition 9: *Court of Honor*: Is a tribunal constituted by Troop leaders that, as it happens in Scouting, it deals with the following matters as they happen in any patrol in CCS-Scout: rewards, promotions, and punishments.

Definition 10: *Promotion*: Is the process in which a specific IA-Scout is promoted from its current group to a higher level in the same or in another group. It is determined by calculating a probability of distribution inspired in the Boltzmann distribution (Metropolis et al., 1953). The energy functional $E_t(a)$ of an IA-Scout agent a at time t is defined as shown in (2).

$$E_t(a) = \alpha \times \Gamma(a) + \beta \times \mathrm{P}(a)$$
$$\alpha + \beta = 1 \tag{2}$$

$\mathrm{P}(a)$ represents the accumulation of merit / awards / medals received by agent a from the moment that part of the CCS-Scout started to form. The weights α and β are coefficients expressed in the range [0, 1] and used to establish a degree of importance between the "age" of the agent $\Gamma(a)$ and its "merits" $\mathrm{P}(a)$.

Either increasing the run-time of the IA-Scout agent or the awards the agent has received during its execution can be factors that contribute in augmenting the energy accumulated by the agent at any time t. Therefore, the difference or

change of energy increases between two instants of time t_1 and t_2 is required to determine the IA-Scout promotion. It can be logically inferred then that, the greater the difference in energy $\Delta E(a)$ the higher the probability that the agent will be promoted. An IA-Scout is selected to ascend a hierarchy level when *prob*(a to be promoted) > random(0, 1). Expression (3) is used to calculate this probability.

$$\Delta E_t(a) = E_{t2}(a) - E_{t1}(a)$$
$$prob(a \text{ to be promoted}) = 1 - e^{-\Delta E_t(a)} \tag{3}$$

$\mathrm{P}(a)$ is calculated based on the set of activities A_i an IA-Scout agent has accomplished since the last calculation of $\mathrm{P}(a)$ was completed. The aim is to reward those agents who have completed complex activities in a short period of time and to punish agents when simple tasks are performed during a long period of time. This is inversely proportional to the age of the agent. Expression (4) is used to calculate $\mathrm{P}(a)$.

$$\mathrm{P}(a) = \frac{1}{\Gamma(a)} \sum_{i=1} \frac{\rho(A_i)}{\tau(A_i)} \tag{4}$$

From time to time (based on the CCS-Scout parameter ϖ) by convening a court of honor, the patrol leaders have to consider the promotion of corresponding patrol members according to the ascending line of command mentioned before. Occasionally, a Troop might be without a leader so that, a leader must be chosen from all current MAS-Clan patrol leaders in the system. This process begins once one of these patrol leaders realizes that the troop has no leader and therefore initiates, through communication with the other patrol leaders, this selection process. The same situation occurs for electing the Clan leader, the highest authority in the CCS-Scout hierarchy.

Definition 11: *Selection*: Is the process in which IA-Scout leaders assign tasks or activities to IA-Scout members of the same group. This is made by using a strategy that combines the neighborhood expression used in the Kohonen neural network model (Kohonen, 1982; Kohonen, 1984) and the roulette-wheel selection algorithm (Holland, 1975). $\varphi(b)$ represents the quantity of times that any IA-Scout leader *a* receives a request as part of the communication between an IA-Scout and its leader from the corresponding IA-Scout member *b* being led by *a*. The $\varphi(b)$ numbers are counted for each leader. The idea is to calculate a probability in which *b* is selected depending on the difference between $\varphi(b)$ and $\varphi(b^*)$, *b** being the IA-Scout that has sent more requests and therefore has the bigger value of $\varphi(b)$. Therefore, this probability is directly proportional to their $\varphi(b)$. To do this, the Kohonen neighborhood expression $\Delta(b,b^*)$ is used (see expression (5)) aiming for those IA-Scouts that have sent more requests to have the higher probability of being selected, but also giving an opportunity to those IA-Scouts that have sent fewer requests and therefore have a lower probability of being selected. After that and by using these probabilities, the roulette-wheel selection algorithm performed by the leader is used to select the IA-Scout that will be assigned a specific task that has to be done. σ in (5) is a parameter of width that determines how great difference between $\varphi(b)$ and $\varphi(b^*)$ should be. It is recommended to start with a value of about 25% of the space to be measured and to gradually decrease the value over time.

$$\Delta(b,b^*) = \exp\left(\frac{-(\phi(b) - \phi(b^*))^2}{\sigma^2}\right)$$

$$prob(b \text{ to be selected}) = \frac{\Delta(b,b^*)}{\sum_j \Delta(b_j,b^*)} \quad (5)$$

Definition 12: *ID*: Is the CCS-Scout group (troop, patrol, and clan) form of identification that allows the differentiation of a group from the rest, like it happens in Scouting. This ID should be given during the creation of a new group. The corresponding leader of the new group is responsible to do so. Unlike in Scouting, where group names are mainly related to animal names (tiger, lion, squirrel, and so on), in CCS-Scout the name of each group is formed according to a numerical sequence based on the group's level in the organization. So that, the ID of the MAS-Clan is 1, the ID of an MAS-Troop is for example 1-1, 1-2, 1-3, and so on. In the case of MAS-Patrols, the character P, T, or C are added at the end of the ID to indicate if the patrol is related with a Pack (P), a Troop (T), or a Clan (C). Therefore, a valid ID for a MAS-Patrol is for example 1-2-1-T (a MAS-Troop patrol identified with number 1 depending on the Troop 2 of the Clan). Having an ID to differentiate one group from another is important for the communication process between IA-Scout agents.

Communication

Communication between agents in MAS is essential. What is more, service sharing in a CC is implemented by using IAs. In this regard, for communication to occur in CCS-Scout the following interactions between the agents that make up the system are needed: 1) between members of the same patrol; 2) between an IA-Scout and its leader; 3) between an IA-Scout leader and the members of the group in which he is the leader; 4) between patrol leaders, including the leader of the troop selected by the convening of a court of honor; 5) between troop leaders. Details of these five different CCS-Scouts' inter-agents' communication scenarios are presented below. First, it is important to mention that communication between IA-Scout agents in CCS-Scout systems is done through the exchange of messages between agents. Any message can be sent either to a particular IA-Scout by using its ID (peer-to-peer / P2P) or to all the current agents in the CCS-Scout system (broadcast). Note that broadcast messages allow simulating, a process that in Scouting is the blackboard that allows communication among Scouts. In order to know which agent is sending a message the message packet must have both, the sender's ID and rank, and the name of the group to which the sender belongs.

Communication between IA-Scout members of the same patrol is necessary for establishing the possible cooperation needed to solve a particular task assigned by the patrol leader. This exchange of messages is performed as follows: 1) IA-Scout a sends a message to all other members of the group to which a belongs to looking for cooperation; 2) IA-Scout b sends to a the confirmation that it will cooperate with a; a sends to b the task it wants b to carry out (this can be given to more than one agent, depending on the complexity of the task and on the decision taken by a; see Section 4.4 for details); 3) a can receive confirmation from other agents and, if it does not require more collaboration, it sends a response that cooperation is no longer required; 4) b sends to a an answer related with the task given to it by a.

Communication between an IA-Scout and its leader usually starts from a patrol member and ends with the clan leader. It is mainly carried out in order to periodically request activities to perform. This request is made only when the IA-Scout is without an activity/task at any given time or, in case it is a leader, when there is a member in its group without an activity/task. The request is also used to check that a leading group exists. In this regard, it is possible to have the following scenarios: 1) a patrol without a leader, for which the number 2 on the patrol takes the lead and it is necessary to wait for the next court of honor to elect a new number 2; 2) a troop without a leader, for which a court of honor must convene urgently (see communication between patrol

leaders below); 3) there is no leader for the clan and therefore a clan leader must be elected from current troop leaders (see communication between troop leaders below). Communication between an IA-Scout and its leader also occurs when the IA-Scout sends replies to its leader regarding the task assigned for it to solve.

Communication between an IA-Scout leader and the members of the group in which he is the leader is required for the assignation of tasks or activities starting from the Clan leader to the patrol members.

Communication between patrol leaders including the leader of the troop occurs in order to convene or convoke a court of honor. In this regard, any patrol leader is responsible to guarantee whether or not any of the patrol members has to be rewarded, promoted, or punished. To do this, and because leaders in general have all the information about satisfied activities, i.e. the level of complexity $\rho(A_i)$ of the activities and the duration of time $\tau(A_i)$ in which each activity A_i was completed, leaders must keep track of these statistics in the manner shown below.

By using expression (3) each leader calculates the probability of promoting each of its members. Once the number of members selected (i.e. *prob*(a to be promoted) > random(0, 1)) exceeds a parameter ϖ then corresponding patrol leader sends a message to the other patrol leaders to convoke a court of honor. Once the court of honor has been convoked each leader sends the best candidate that exists in their corresponding patrol to the rest. The best candidate is the one that has the highest probability of being promoted (expression (3)). In the case of the leader who convened the court of honor, it must select the best candidate from the list of ϖ members selected. After that, each leader has as many candidates as there are patrols in the specific troop, each candidate with its probability of being promoted. Therefore, in order to select the IA-Scout that should be elected according to each patrol leader a roulette-wheel selection algorithm is performed by each patrol leader. Information about the IA-Scout selected is then sent to the troop leader. Finally, once the troop leader receives all the candidates from the patrol leaders it makes the final decision based on the greatest number of votes or selections made in favor of a candidate. In the event of a tie, all IA-Scout involved are promoted. By using the IA-Scout's ID, the troop leader informs the corresponding patrol leaders about these promotions. It should be remembered that promotions might lead to the formation of other patrols.

Communication between troop leaders is necessary only when the Clan does not have a leader. In this regard, once a troop leader realizes that the Clan does not have a leader, the troop leader is responsible for the process of selecting a new Clan leader. For that, the troop leader sends a message to the rest of the troop leaders. The selection process is similar to what is explained above. Starting with the troop leader exchanging the candidates' corresponding probabilities of being promoted and ending with the counting of votes conducted by those responsible for the process, the Clan leader is elected. In this case, and due to the fact that there should be only one Clan leader, possible ties must be resolved randomly. The agent responsible for running the process is also involved in the election process and, unless it was selected, the process ends when it sends a message to the troop leader chosen informing it about its promotion.

On the other hand, in order to inform the account summary or balance statement of the services rendered among nodes in CCS-Scout by means of MAS-Patrols, and because all service's needs are handled by the MAS-Troop leader, these troop leaders maintain a table with account balances indicating how much to pay or reimburse each patrol leader. Troop leaders then hold a bag of money and make periodical collections or distributions of goods accordingly. To do that, the following two messages between IA-Scout troop leaders and IA-Scout patrol leaders have to be carried out:

- A P2P message from a patrol leader to its troop leaders aiming to ask the patrol leader balance account. This message does not have any data.
- A P2P message from a troop leader to the leader of one of its patrols responding the previous message. The corresponding data of this message has the details of the quantity that the patrol leader has to pay to the troop leader or get as reimbursement from it.

Furthermore, the manner in which debts between patrol leaders and troop leaders are settled is previously defined before the CCS-Scout system starts, for example, by using credits cards, paying for services rendered, and which items are free of charge.

Cooperation, Trust, Learning and Leadership

Cooperation is the process that occurs between IA-Scout agents aiming to accomplish a certain amount of activities. It is established through the communication between IA-Scout members of the same patrol. As part of this process, the calculation of the following two probabilities is necessary: 1) the probability to look for cooperation related to any activity; and 2) the probability of rejecting to cooperate in relation to a specific activity. The probability to look for cooperation related to any activity A_i is used by an agent a when it receives the assignment of a task $T = (A_1, ..., A_n)$ (see expression (6) as depicted in Box 2). This probability depends on the agent's age $\Gamma(a)$ (the younger a is the more help it will need), the complexity of the activity $\rho(A_i)$ (the more complex the activity is the more cooperation it will require), and the skills $\Pi(a)$ agent a has related to skills $\Pi(A_i)$ activity A_i requires (the less skills a has the more cooperation it will require). It is worth noting that $\Gamma(a) \neq 0$ (a has started executing before receiving any assignment).

Box 2.

$$\kappa(a, A_i) = \frac{\rho(A_i) * \left[\left|\Pi(A_i)\right| - \left|\Pi(A_i) \cap \Pi(a)\right|\right]}{\Gamma(a)}$$

$$prob(a \text{ has to look for cooperation related to } A_i) == \frac{\kappa(a, A_i)}{\sum_j \kappa(a, A_j)}$$

(6)

The probability of rejecting to cooperate in relation to a specific activity depends on the current workload $\omega(a)$ agent a has (the more workload a has, the more likely it is that a will refuse cooperation). Expression (7) in Box 3 shows the way this probability is calculated; $\hat{A}_i$ refers to activities that a is currently performing and A_i is the activity for which a has to decide whether to accept or reject in response to a request for cooperation.

The cooperation process between IA-Scouts follows the guidelines stated next (being a the agent which is assigned the task $T = (A_1, ..., A_n)$):
1) a must perform at least one activity A_i and this activity must have the highest level of complexity $\rho(A_i)$ from all activities of T; 2) a can look for collaboration with more than one other agent b at a time but only a single activity can be assigned to b; 3) any activity that a might be working on as a result of cooperation with any other agent b at time of receiving T has to be completed before starting to accomplish T; 4) probability shown in (6) is used to look for cooperation related to a particular activity; 5) an agent's decision about with which agent to cooperate is made randomly; 6) once a receives the assignment of T it rejects any cooperation requests coming from any other agent in order to give priority to the completion of T; and 7) in addition to the previous scenario, an agent can also refuse cooperation based on the amount of activities being undertaken and the amount of skills of the agent, for which the probability of rejecting cooperation shown in (7) is used.

As noted, depending on the current conditions of the patrol, an IA-Scout a may either get no help from another IA-Scout that can cooperate with it—for which a will have to perform all assigned activities—or a can get help from other agents in relation to all assigned activities, but at least one of them has to be necessarily performed by a.

It is important to emphasize that the cooperation mechanism is one of the most significant characteristics of the CCS-Scout proposal. The way in which Scouts cooperate with each other in order to achieve goals from activities that are conducted in groups is taken into account to define this mechanism. Unlike other proposals (in which the cooperation between agents is possible but without agents being able to learn) in CCS-Scout all agents clearly know: 1) with which other agents to look for cooperation; 2) how agents must cooperate with other agents; 3) how to distribute

Box 3.

$$\omega(a) = \sum_i \kappa(a, \hat{A}_i)$$

$$prob(\text{to reject cooperation related to } A_i) == 0.75 * \omega(a) + 0.25 * \kappa(a, A_i)$$

(7)

the activities of any task properly; 4) how agents have to communicate with each order in order to cooperate; and 5) how learning improves future cooperation between agents.

Trust is essential in Scouting and therefore it is also essential in CCS-Scout. Trust happens when, for example, an agent *a* assigns a task to a fellow patrol member *b* knowing that the duration in which *b* accomplishes that task as well as the quality of the response can help agent *a* in its promotion. Therefore, *a* trusts *b* to finish the assigned activities as soon and with the best quality as possible. Another example of trust is presented in the election process.

In CCS-Scout any IA-Scout must learn the necessary skills needed to perform the tasks. Therefore, the *learning* process is used to increase / add abilities to the set $\Pi(a)$ of any IA-Scout *a*. In this regard, for each skill s_i pre-defined in CCS-Scout and for each skill that can be part of $\Pi(a)$ there is a learning factor $\xi(s_i)$ that determines how much of the skill s_i (initially $\xi(s_i) = 0$ for all s_i) agent *a* has learned. Being $\xi(s_i)$ a factor measured between 0 and 1 where 0 indicates that the agent has not learned anything about s_i, the decision to add s_i to $\Pi(a)$ is given by the relation $\xi(s_i) > H$ where H is a learning factor level, another parameter of the CCS-Scout.

The learning process occurs as follows. Each time an IA-Scout agent *a* accomplishes an activity A_i, whether it belongs to a task assignment to *a* or whether A_i is related to the cooperation *a* has given to another agent, an adjustment factor $\Delta\xi(s_i)$ associated with the learning of all skills s_i related to A_i is calculated ($s_i \in \Pi(A_i)$). $\Delta\xi(s_i)$ is then applied to the accumulation factor $\xi(s_i)$ and relation $\xi(s_i) > H$ is evaluated. If the relational expression is true then s_i is added to $\Pi(a)$ indicating that *a* has learned the skill s_i. Expression (8) is used to calculate $\Delta\xi(s_i)$. It is assumed that 3 is the highest value for $\rho(A_i)$ and 0.1 the smallest number that $\tau(A_i)$ can have i.e. the learning constant λ ($0 \leq \lambda \leq 1$) is the maximum value $\Delta\xi(s_i)$ can have. Note that, as the agent's execution time $\Gamma(a)$ is

greater, learning is slower. Note also that this learning process was inspired by the Scouting slogan "learning by doing."

$$\Delta\xi(s_i) = \lambda \frac{1}{\Gamma(a)} \frac{\rho(A_i)}{30*\tau(A_i)} ; s_i \in \Pi(A_i). \quad (8)$$

Leadership is one of the basic principles of Scouting. Communication is a basic process needed to guarantee leadership. Leadership is guaranteed in CCS-Scout because all messages have the ID of the IA-Scout that is sending the message and because the ID has both, the number (rank) of the IA-Scout and knowledge of which group level the IA-Scout belongs to. All agents must obey orders that come from messages sent by other IA-Scouts with a higher rank. An example of this is the assignment of tasks.

Characteristics, Features, Principles, and Models

Does the CCS-Scout support all the characteristics, features, principles, and models associated to CC and indicated in the second section of this chapter? Let's do a brief review of each of these elements.

Because collaboration between patrols (or nodes) in the same troop (or consortium) and collaboration between troops in the entire CC system (or clan) is possible, all services or resources required can be satisfied giving to the clients the *illusion of infinite computing resources*. This collaboration process is carried naturally and automatically so that the *elimination of an upfront commitment by cloud users* is guaranteed. Clients request the completion of a service and they receive a response without knowing which node made it. Moreover, expression (1) defines the *ability to pay for use as needed*.

The following points offer a brief explanation related to the desired features of a cloud: 1) because the use of services in CCS-Scout by means of the collaboration process described previously can be carried out without human intervention, *Self-Service* is a feature present in CCS-Scout; 2) because the cost of the service is calculated based on the cost of just the activities included in the service and based on the skills needed to accomplish any activity (see (1)), clients will only pay for what is used and therefore the Per-*Usage metering and billing* feature is presented in CCS-Scout; 3) because CCS-Scout can grow without limit according to Definition 8 and because there are also no limitations in the collaboration process in the sense that all services required should be provided (no rejections), clients expect to be provided with any quantity of resources at any time and for that *Elasticity* is presented in CCS-Scout; 4) because CCS-Scout troops are associated with different kinds of businesses and because nodes of different troops can also collaborate with each other in the same way nodes of the same troop collaborate among them, services' requirements in CCS-Scout are highly customizable so that *Customization* is present as well.

Regarding the basic principles of CC, in CCS-Scout, providers form *Federations* in as much a quantity as they can organize in MAS-Troops. Moreover, all services in CCS-Scout enjoy of *Independence* because activities, skills and all other parameters related with them are encapsulated. On the other hand, the collaboration process between users and service providers that occurs in CCS-Scout guarantees the *Isolation* of the resources. CCS-Scout has also the abilities of *Elasticity* and *Business Orientation* because there are no limitations on the quantity and quality of services that can be demanded at any time. Finally, trust is presented in CCS-Scout because it is a Scouting principle, so that nodes in CCS-Scout *Trust* each other.

Furthermore, CCS-Scout not only provides ready-to-run services (clients do not have to wait for a requirement to be sent) but also provides the ability to deploy custom services (new services can be added at any time) as well as low-level virtualized resources (clients ask for services

unaware of who or how these services will be solved, clients just wait for the completion of the services). Therefore, there are no limitations in CCS-Scout for implementing the three service models that compose CC: *SaaS*, *PaaS*, and *IaaS*.

According to what is presented in this section, CCS-Scout is capable of implementing a CC system with all the characteristics, features, principles and models CC should have. Next section describes the scenario related with sharing medical information by using CCS-Scout.

Sharing Medical Information by Means of Using Ccs-Scout

The goal of this section is to present the details concerning the implementation of a CCS-Scout model aiming to share medical information. Let's call this model CCS-ScoutH. In this regard, describing the CC environment and the organization of its nodes is the first issue that must be dealt with.

In order to extend the benefit of sharing medical information worldwide, the CC environment to be implemented must have a global reach. Therefore, the representation of different countries must then be considered when organizing the nodes in the cloud. The best way to do this, in my opinion, is by taking advantage of existing structures. The World Health Organization[2] (WHO) is the best example and in the scenario presented in this chapter a node in the cloud representing the WHO will correspond to the MAS-Clan that CCS-ScoutH must have.

In this scenario then, nodes in the cloud, each of which depicts a country that is a member of the WHO and intends to be part of the CCS-ScoutH, represent the troop leaders in CC-ScoutH. Medical institutions or organizations, insurance companies, and other medical-related organisms are depicted in CCS-ScoutH by nodes that represent the patrols. Depending on the level of importance that these organisms have in their respective country (for example a ministry of health, an association of hospitals, etc.), these patrols could be MAS-Clan, MAS-Troop, or MAS-Pack.

Figure 3. A CCS-ScoutH organization example

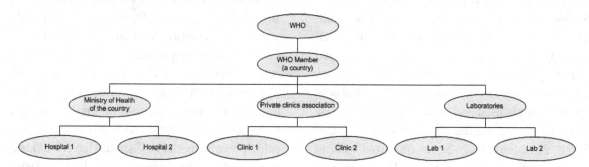

Finally, specific medical institutions like clinics, hospitals, doctors, labs, and so on may be the patrol members in CCS-ScoutH. Based on what was explained in the previous section it can be seen that the definition of the CCS-Scout hierarchical structure is very flexible. Therefore, the right structure of any troop in CCS-ScoutH (i.e. a country) is also flexible. Figure 3 shows an example in which any country member of the WHO is connected into the cloud. The Ministry of Health, a private clinics association, and laboratories of this country are also connected to the cloud as patrols. There are also two hospitals run by the Ministry of Health, two clinics that are part of the corresponding association, and two labs.

On the other hand, there are two tasks or services (see Definition 5) implicit in the CCS-ScoutH model to which all the nodes in the cloud must be able to respond:

1. EMR ← AskEMR(Patient ID). The goal of this service is to obtain and return the EMR that belongs to a person identified by the ID given as a parameter.
2. UpdateEMR(Patient ID, Data). The goal of this service is to add Data to the EMR that belongs to a person identified by the ID given as a parameter.

As different countries are being discussed, it is necessary that the CCS-ScoutH model takes into account the proper communication between the different nodes that are part of the environment. Therefore, the structure or format used to represent EMR should be a standard in the model. Note that except for some minor differences, medical information is common around the world so that the definition of a standard EMR format does not vary significantly (is not difficult to access, to understand). Something that has been done in relation to the above is to use XML[3], Olhede and Peterson (2000) may be consulted for more details.

However, an interesting question to ask is "Where is the Data associated with EMRs stored?" There is no constraining in CCS-Scout in general and in CCS-ScoutH in particular. Therefore, the model is flexible about the place where the data servers with the EMRs are located. Data can be in any of the nodes connected to the cloud including the MAS-Clan leader node. This is important for not having restrictions to be a part of the CCS-ScoutH model. For example, avoiding possible initial conditions (pre-conditions) that require transferring the existing data somewhere.

Each time a node in the CCS-ScoutH environment is asked to respond to the service AskEMR(Patient ID) the corresponding IA-Scout of the node looks first into the available data servers. If there is any data server associated to the node and information of the Patient ID is stored in that servers then the corresponding data is returned. Otherwise, the IA-Scout seeks for an answer from the other members for the same patrol, troop, or even clan if necessary. This is done through the cooperation process described in the previous section. Something similar happens with the service UpdateEMR(Patient ID, Data).

The patient's ID should be unique for every person worldwide; passport numbers or social security numbers can be considered as possible options. Another option would be to create the ID number automatically by using the CCS-ScoutH portal.

Another aspect of interest to take into account is related with the interfaces needed to interact with end users regarding the services provided by the CCS-ScoutH model. In this regard, there are Web client applications that form part of a CCS-ScoutH portal with minimal functions necessary to access at least the two services listed above. These applications can be existing applications related to the entity associated with the node or they are related to the CCS-ScoutH portal directly.

Following the steps of a possible scenario structured by using the model described above:

1. A patient P somewhere, is going to visit a medic.
2. P is attended by doctor D and because D is a member of one the CCS-ScoutH patrols, he or she can use his or her computer and Internet connection to get P's EMR by using the corresponding ID of P. This is done internally by the service request "EMR $\leftarrow$ AskEMR(Patient ID)" which causes the definition in CCS-ScoutH of the task T_1.
3. Through the internal processes of cooperation and compliance objectives of CCS-ScoutH, T_1 is solved and the response is received by D i.e. the EMR of P. The EMR could be empty.
4. Doctor D asks patient P to get a series of tests done.
5. P does the tests in the laboratory L. Because L is a member of one of the CCS-ScoutH patrols P's results can be added to P's EMR by using the service "UpdateEMR(Patient ID, Data)."

6. On a second visit of P to the doctor, D returns to seek P's EMR and he or she can not only review the tests results but also compare how values have changed in relation to other possible tests that P has done in the past.
7. At home, P wants to know about the tests results so that by using Internet, he or she uses his or her computer or mobile device (smartphone, tablet, etc.) to access the CCS-ScoutH portal and review the corresponding EMR.
8. Soon after, P moves to another country (or visits a country on a vacation) and he or she has to go to the hospital because of an accident. Once in the hospital and by using P's ID, the hospital personnel can obtain and review P's EMR looking for important medical information related to P like: blood type, allergies to any medications, and past surgeries among others.

Note the amount of benefits (different form the ones mentioned above) possible to gain by accessing the EMRs of a significant universe of people: it could be possible to make disease statistics by sex, age, geographic location, etc.; it could be possible to establish forums for and by different specialists to discuss difficult cases; doctors would have a way to find similar cases and analyze related information and therefore the information is a useful knowledge base for researching; this stand out among many other benefits that can be enumerated.

FUTURE RESEARCH DIRECTIONS

The following are some ongoing work related to what was presented in this chapter:

1. The definition of an XML-based universal standard structure to represent the EMRs. Having a standard structure to represent the EMRs is important in order to offer

a universal/uniform way to communicate and understand this data. It is interesting to consider XML because it is currently a well know standard.

2. The design of client-programs interfaces. Hospitals, clinics, labs, doctors, and even patients should have appropriate front-end programs to view and upgrade the EMRs. These programs could be both Web and desktop.

3. The definition of alternatives to organize the nodes in this cloud related to the medical sector. This chapter shows an option to consider for organizing nodes that focuses in the way scouts are organized. However, other options that take into account ideas coming from the medical sector could be useful.

4. Extending the benefits by defining new cloud services. The definition of new services supported by the architecture presented in this chapter could extend the benefits we can obtain from this software platform. For example, insurance companies can calculate customer's potential to have an accident.

5. The implementation of a real scenario. Having a real installation of CCS-ScoutH is necessary to adequately evaluate and evolve this HIS.

CONCLUSION

Sharing medical information is an issue that has been addressed continuously from a few years ago in response to the demands established by the healthcare sector. Sharing the Electronic Medical Records (EMR) associated to patients is one of the most representative examples of what type of medical information people want to share. By using the two technologies Cloud Computing (CC) and Multi-Agent System (MAS) this chapter described the model called CCS-ScoutH aiming to present another option, besides pre-existing works, for

sharing EMR worldwide. Moreover, theoretical aspects of Scouting are used to define the MAS-based framework in which CCS-Scout in general and CCS-ScoutH in particular was implemented.

Aiming to address the above, this chapter first presented the details of why CC is an adequate technology for addressing the problem and why MAS is an adequate technology for implementing CC. After that, the chapter focused on the particular experience called CCS-Scout that consists on combining MAS and CC by using Scouting principles. Finally the chapter described the CCS-ScoutH model as a solution for sharing the EMR medical information by combining CC, MAS and Scouting.

Although CCS-ScoutH has not yet been tested in real applications, it has been designed to be suitable for real medical sector environments where nodes in the cloud have to be organized and cooperation is needed. In fact, the experimentation and validation over simulated conditions were carried out to demonstrate that CCS-Scout in general can be successfully extended to real scenarios in current collaboration environments with no problems.

On the other hand, even though CCS-ScoutH was theoretically defined in this chapter to share EMR, there are no limitations on the kind of medical information necessary to share. Services can be easily adjusted to any kind of information.

REFERENCES

Ahuja, S. P., Mani, S., & Zambrano, J. (2012). A survey of the state of Cloud computing in healthcare. *Network and Communication Technologies*, *1*(2), 12–19.

Alley, D., Ahmed, T., Androvich, J., Archibald, S., Baker, A. S., Fultz, N., ... Wilson, K. (2012). The Cloud computing guide for healthcare. *Focus Research*, 1-22.

Armbrust, M., Fox, A., Griffith, R., Joseph, A. D., & Katz, R. (2009). *Above the Clouds: A Berkeley View of Cloud Computing*. Reliable Adaptive Distributed Systems Laboratory White Paper. Berkeley, CA: University of California.

Aylward, S. (2010). *Cloud computing in healthcare – Private, public, or somewhere in between*. The Official Microsoft Blog, New & Perspectives. Retrieved from http://blogs.technet.com/b/microsoft_blog/archive/2010/06/28/cloud-computing-in-healthcare-private-public-or-somewhere-in-between.aspx

Baden-Powell, R. (1908). Scouting for Boys. London: Windsor House, Bream's Buildings, E.C. (First published ed.), C.A. Pearson.

Blaisdell, R. (2013). *Cloud computing advantages for the healthcare industry*. Retrieved from http://webcache.googleusercontent.com/search?q=cache:http://www.rickscloud.com/5-cloud-computing-advantages-for-the-healthcare-industry/

Bollineni, P. K., & Neupane, K. (2011). *Implications for adopting cloud computing in e-Health*. (Unpublished Master's Thesis). School of Computing, Blekinge Institute of Technology.

Botts, N., Thoms, B., Noamani, A., & Horan, T. A. (2010). Cloud Computing Architectures for the Underserved: Public Health Cyberinfrastructures through a Network of HealthATMs. In R. H. Sprague, Jr. (Ed.), *43rd Hawaii International Conference on System Sciences* (HICSS) (pp. 1-10). Honolulu, HI: IEEE.

Brust, C., & Sarnikar, S. (2011). Decision Modeling for Healthcare Enterprise IT Architecture Utilizing Cloud Computing. In *Proceedings of 17th Americas Conference on Information Systems* (AMCIS). Association for Information Systems.

Buyya, R., Yeo, C. S., Venugopal, S., Broberg, J., & Brandic, I. (2009). Cloud computing and emerging IT platforms: Vision, hype, and reality for delivering computing as the 5th utility. *Future Generation Computer Systems*, *25*(6), 599–616. doi:10.1016/j.future.2008.12.001

Deng, M., Petkovic, M., Nalin, M., & Baroni, I. (2011). A Home Healthcare System in the Cloud-Addressing Security and Privacy Challenges. In *Proceedings of IEEE International Conference on Cloud Computing* (CLOUD) (pp. 549 - 556). IEEE Computer Society.

Dimitrova, M., Lozanova, S., Lahtchev, L., & Roumenin, C. (2012). A framework for design of cloud compatible medical. In *Proceedings of the 13th ACM International Conference on Computer Systems and Technologies* (CompSysTech) (pp. 195-200). Ruse, Bulgaria: ACM.

Ekonomou, E., Fan, L., Buchanan, W., & Thuemmler, C. (2011). An Integrated Cloud-based Healthcare Infrastructure. In *Proceedings of IEEE Third International Conference on Cloud Computing Technology and Science* (CloudCom) (pp. 532-536). Athens, Greece: IEEE.

Guo, Y., Kuo, M., & Sahama, T. (2012). Cloud computing for healthcare research information sharing. In *Proceedings of the 4th IEEE International Conference on Cloud Computing Technology and Science* (CloudCom) (pp. 889-894). Taipei, Taiwan: IEEE.

Harris, B. (2012). 5 ways cloud computing will transform healthcare. *Healthcare IT News*. Retrieved from http://www.healthcareitnews.com/news/5-ways-cloud-computing-will-transform-healthcare

He, C., Fan, X., & Li, Y. (2013). Toward Ubiquitous Healthcare Services with a Novel Efficient Cloud Platform. *IEEE Transactions on Bio-Medical Engineering*, *60*(1), 230–234. doi:10.1109/TBME.2012.2222404 PMID:23060318

Holland, J. (1975). *Adaptation in natural and artificial systems*. Ann Arbor, MI: The University of Michigan Press.

Hu, Y., Lu, F., Khan, I., & Bai, G. (2012). A cloud computing solution for sharing healthcare information. In *Proceedings of the 7th International Conference for Internet Technology and Secured Transactions* (ICITST) (pp. 465-470). London, UK: ICITST.

Jha, S., Katz, D. S., Luckow, A., Merzky, A., & Stamou, K. (2011). Understanding Scientific Applications for Cloud Environments. In R. Buyya, J. Nroberg, & A. Goscinski (Eds.), *Cloud Computing: Principles and Paradigms* (pp. 345–371). Wiley. doi:10.1002/9780470940105.ch13

Khansa, L., Forcade, J., Nambari, G., Parasuraman, S., & Cox, P. (2012). Proposing an intelligent cloud-based electronic health record system. *International Journal of Business Data Communications and Networking*, *8*(3), 57–71. doi:10.4018/jbdcn.2012070104

Kohonen, T. (1982). Self-Organized Formation of Topologically Correct Feature Maps. *Biological Cybernetics*, *43*, 59–69. doi:10.1007/BF00337288

Kohonen, T. (1984). *Self-Organization and Associative Memory*. Berlin: SpringerVerlag.

Kuo, A. M. (2011). Opportunities and Challenges of Cloud Computing to Improve Health Care Services. *Journal of Medical Internet Research*, *13*(3), e67. doi:10.2196/jmir.1867 PMID:21937354

Kuo, M. H., Kushniruk, A., Borycki, E., Lai, F., & Dorjgochoo, S. Altangerel, & Jigjidsuren, C. (2012). A cloud computing based platform for sharing healthcare research information. In *Proceedings of the 13th International Conference on Collaboration Technologies and Systems* (CTS) (pp. 504-508). Denver, CO: CTS.

Li, W., Yan, J., Yan, Y., & Zhang, J. (2010). Xbase: Cloud-enabled information appliance for healthcare. In I. Manolescu, S. Spaccapietra, J. Teubner, M. Kitsuregawa, A. Leger, F. Naumann, A. Ailamaki, & F. Ozcan (Eds.), *13th International Conference on Extending Database Technology (EDBT 2010)*, (vol. 426, pp. 675-680). ACM.

Lupşe, O. S., Vida, M. M., & Stoicu-Tivadar, L. (2012). Cloud Computing and Interoperability in Healthcare Information Systems. In P. Lorenz & P. Dini (Eds.), *The First International Conference on Intelligent Systems and Applications (INTELLI 2012)* (pp. 81-85). IARIA.

Mell, P., & Grance, T. (2009). The NIST Definition of Cloud Computing. *National Institute of Standards and Technology*, *53*(6), 50.

Metropolis, N., Rosenbluth, A. W., Rosenbluth, M. N., Teller, A. H., & Teller, E. (1953). Equations of state calculations by fast computing machines. *The Journal of Chemical Physics*, *21*(6), 1087–1091. doi:10.1063/1.1699114

Ming, L., Shucheng, Y., Yao, Z., Kui, R., & Wenjing, L. (2013). Scalable and Secure Sharing of Personal Health Records in Cloud Computing Using Attribute-Based Encryption. *IEEE Transactions on Parallel and Distributed Systems*, *24*(1), 131–143. doi:10.1109/TPDS.2012.97

Mohan, T. S. (2011). Migrating into a Cloud. In R. Buyya, J. Nroberg, & A. Goscinski (Eds.), *Cloud Computing: Principles and Paradigms* (pp. 43–56). Wiley. doi:10.1002/9780470940105.ch2

Olhede, T., & Peterson, H. E. (2000). Archiving of care related information in XML-format. *Studies in Health Technology and Informatics, 77,* 642–646. PMID:11187632

Paletta, M. (2012a). Self-Organizing Multi-Agent Systems by means of Scout Movement. *Recent Patents on Computer Science, 5*(3), 197–210. doi:10.2174/2213275911205030197

Paletta, M. (2012b). MAS-based Agent Societies by Means of Scout Movement. *International Journal of Agent Technologies and Systems, 4*(3), 29–49. doi:10.4018/jats.2012070103

Paletta, M. (2012c). Intelligent Clouds – By means of using multi-agent systems environments. In L. Chao (Ed.), *Cloud Computing for Teaching and Learning: Strategies for Design and Implementation* (pp. 254–279). Hershey, PA: IGI Global. doi:10.4018/978-1-4666-0957-0.ch017

Paletta, M., & Herrero, M. P. (2010). *An awareness-based learning model to deal with service collaboration in cloud computing. Transactions on Computational Collective Intelligence I (LNCS)* (Vol. 6220, pp. 85–100). Berlin: Springer.

Papakonstantinou, D., Poulymenopoulou, M., Malamateniou, F., & Vassilacopoulos, G. (2011). A cloud-based semantic wiki for user training in healthcare process management. In *Proceedings of the XXIII Conference of the European Federation for Medical Informatics* (MIE 2011) (vol. 169, pp. 93-97). Oslo, Norway: MIE.

Papazoglou, M. P., & Van den Heuvel, W. J. (2007). Service oriented architectures: Approaches, technologies and research issues. *The VLDB Journal, 16*(3), 389–415. doi:10.1007/s00778-007-0044-3

Pardamean, B., & Rumanda, R. R. (2011). Integrated Model of Cloud-Based E-Medical Record for Health Care Organizations. In *Proceedings of the 10th WSEAS International Conference on E-Activities* (pp. 157-162). WSEAS.

Rabi, P. P., Manas, R. P., & Suresh, C. S. (2012). Design and Implementation of a Cloud based Rural Healthcare Information System Model. *Universal Journal of Applied computer Science and Technology, 2*(1), 149-157.

Radwan, A. S., Abdel-Hamid, A. A., & Hanafy, Y. (2012). Cloud-based service for secure electronic medical record exchange. In *Proceedings of the 22nd International Conference on Computer Theory and Applications* (ICCTA) (pp. 94-103). Alexandria, Egypt: ICCTA.

Rao, G. S. V. R. K., Sundararaman, K., & Parthasarathi, J. (2010). Dhatri - A Pervasive Cloud initiative for primary healthcare services. In *Proceedings of the 14th International Conference on Intelligence in Next Generation Networks* (ICIN) (pp. 1-6). Berlin, Germany: ICIN.

Reese, G. (2009). *Cloud Application Architectures: Building Applications and Infrastructure in the Cloud.* Sebastopol, CA: O'Reilly Media.

Rochwerger, B., Vazquez, C., Breitgand, D., Hadas, D., Villari, M., Massonet, P., & Galán, F. (2011). An Architecture for Federated Cloud Computing. In R. Buyya, J. Nroberg, & A. Goscinski (Eds.), *Cloud Computing: Principles and Paradigms* (pp. 391–411). Wiley. doi:10.1002/9780470940105.ch15

Sarna, D. E. Y. (2011). *Implementing and Developing Cloud Computing Applications.* Boca Raton, FL: CRC Press.

Sobhy, D., El-Sonbaty, Y., & Abou Elnasr, M. (2012). MedCloud: Healthcare cloud computing system. In *Proceedings of the 7th International Conference for Internet Technology and Secured Transactions* (ICITST) (pp. 161-166). London: ICITST.

Vaquero, L. M., Rodero-Merino, L., Caceres, J., & Lindner, M. (2008). A break in the clouds: Towards a cloud definition. *ACM SIGCOMM Computer Communications Review, 39*(1), 50–55. doi:10.1145/1496091.1496100

Voorsluys, W., Broberg, J., & Buyya, R. (2011). Introduction to Cloud Computing. In R. Buyya, J. Nroberg, & A. Goscinski (Eds.), *Cloud Computing: Principles and Paradigms* (pp. 1–41). Wiley. doi:10.1002/9780470940105.ch1

Wang, X., & Tan, Y. (2010). Application of cloud computing in the health information system. In *Proceedings of International Conference on Computer Application and System Modeling* (ICCASM) (vol. 1, pp. 179-182). Shanxi, China: ICCASM.

Weerawarana, S., Curbera, F., Leymann, F., Storey, T., & Ferguson, D. (2005). *Web Services Platform Architecture*. Upper Saddle River, NJ: Prentice Hall.

Weiss, A. (2007). Computing in the Clouds. *Networker, 11*(4), 16–25. doi:10.1145/1327512.1327513

Wilson, D. (2012). *How to Improve Helthcare with Cloud Computing*. Hitachi Data Systems. Retrieved from http://docs.media.bitpipe.com/io_10x/io_108673/item_650544/cloud%20computing%20wp.pdf

Yu, W. D., Joshi, B., & Chandola, P. (2011). A service modeling approach to service requirements in SOA and cloud computing — Using a u-Healthcare system case. In *Proceedings of 13th IEEE International Conference on e-Health Networking Applications and Services* (Healthcom) (pp. 233 - 236). IEEE Xplore.

Zhang, R., & Liu, L. (2010). Security Models and Requirements for Healthcare Application Clouds. In *Proceedings of the IEEE 3rd International Conference on Cloud Computing* (CLOUD) (pp. 268-275). Miami, FL: IEEE.

KEY TERMS AND DEFINITIONS

CCS-Scout: The definition of a cloud computing system by using the MAS-Scout architecture.

Cloud Computing: A particular class of service oriented system focused on a wider distribution of the nodes that form part of the system.

Electronic Medical Record: A data structure used to represent the medical information related with a person or patient.

IA-Scout: A representation of an intelligent agent in the MAS-Scout system.

Intelligent Agent: A software entity capable of managing the knowledge it has in order to solve problems.

MAS-Scout: A Multi-Agent system focused on the principles of Scouting.

Multi-Agent System: The organization of more than one intelligent agent that has in some cases to work together to solve common problems or in other cases to compete to solve individual problems.

Service Oriented Architecture: A software architecture for distributed systems in which nodes communicate with each other by using services.

ENDNOTES

[1] http://www.w3.org/2002/ws/
[2] All countries that are Members of the United Nations may become members of the WHO by accepting its Constitution. Other countries may be admitted as members when their application has been approved by a simple majority vote of the World Health Assembly. Territories that are not responsible for the conduct of their international relations may be admitted as Associate Members upon application made on their behalf by the Member or other authority responsible for their international relations.
[3] http://www.w3.org/XML/

Chapter 9
Cloud Computing Location-Based Services for Quality Health Care Services Delivery

Jalel Akaichi
ISG-University of Tunis, Tunisia

ABSTRACT

This chapter proposes a cloud computing location-based services system able to query points of interest, according to mobile users' preferences and contexts, under dynamic changes of locations. The contribution consists of providing software as a service based on Delaunay Triangulation on road (DT_r) able to establish the Continuous k-Nearest Neighbors (CkNNs) on road, while taking into account the dynamic changes of locations from which queries, enhanced by users' preferences and contexts, are issued. The proposed software, implemented on a mobile cloud and exploited by mobile physicians for healthcare institutions localization and selection, considerably improves the quality of services provided for patients in critical situations by permitting real time localization of adequate resources that may contribute to save patients' lives.

INTRODUCTION

Emergencies due to heart problems, fires, road accidents, terrorist attacks, toxic releases, etc., lead frequently to human deaths and serious injuries. Physicians can rescue critical cases if they can reach rapidly their patients and convey them to the appropriate health care institutions. The main questions are then:

1. How to localize rapidly the suitable health care institutions?

2. Do identified health care institutions enclose the necessary and available medical resources able to fulfill the patients' and physicians' needs?

The answer to the first question falls under the context of the determination of CkNNs, which can be exploited as cloud services, useful for many critical applications such as in commerce, leisure, healthcare, etc. Indeed, there exist several techniques of effective treatment of this kind of queries in a space of static data. Recently, research

DOI: 10.4018/978-1-4666-6118-9.ch009

was focused on dynamic environments where the queries move on an unpredictable trajectory (e.g. mobile physician requests). The majority of the existing research assumes the metric of Euclidean distance; however, in the real world, the queries move in the road network where the measurement of interest is opposed to the Euclidean distance. Within this field, two principal conditions must be met for the determination of CkNNs. On one hand, the localization of the mobile query (e.g. a physician in his vehicle equipped with a mobile device and positioning system) and the localization of the static sites of interest (e.g. hospitals, emergency centers), are done with regard to the road network. On the other hand, the measurement of distance is defined as being the shortest way, and not the Euclidean distance, between the query point and the points of interest.

In this chapter, we propose a new method, to be implemented as a software as a service provided by a mobile cloud, aimed to deliver a valid result for the track of the kNNs. This approach ensures efficient updates for data and results of mobile queries. It permits, on one hand, the modeling of a road network through a triangulation and on the other hand, the restoration of a valid response for a continuous search of the kNNs (e.g. seek for me the three closest hospitals from my current position? Seek for me the two closest emergency departments from my current position?). The result of these kinds of queries is a set of points of interest (e.g. three hospitals, two emergency departments) localized in the road network map of a given town or village.

For a physician looking for necessary and available medical resources, this is not usually a sufficient response. In fact, more than determining the points of interest, the physician needs to distinguish whether these places have the necessary resources and whether these resources are available or can be made available. This constitutes an answer for the second question asked at the beginning of this introduction (Do identified health care institutions enclose the necessary and available medical resources able to fulfill the patients' and physicians' needs?).

Suppose that a physician usually travels from place to place, in a connected road network of a village or a town, to take care of his permanent and vocational patients who are geographically dispersed. The patients' states of health may vary and in time may become critical. The physician has to react quickly, as events are unfolding, to save his patients' lives. To achieve this objective, he must find the healthcare institution with the necessary medical resources in a reasonable time, while also taking care of his patient at home or work, or while travelling on one of the roads (e.g. in an emergency vehicle). This can be performed using mobile devices well equipped to query distant databases and to give efficient answers while moving. This can be ensured by cloud computing services able to provide efficient responses to location dependent queries triggered by mobile users such as physicians. Our proposed approach is able to help physicians to identify the nearest healthcare institutions or skilled staff. In fact, various queries can be sent to our system such as "find me the k-nearest health care institutions to my current position."

Answers to these requests are a set of points of interest which have to be displayed on the physician's mobile device screen. Moreover, while the physician is heading to the resulting points, he may browse the points' of interest contents, in order to have an idea about the medical resources available. He proceeds then to perform additional requests, leading to better decisions, such as making reservations for the needed medical resources (e.g. surgery room, medical hardware, etc.) at the point of concern (e.g. hospital), requesting some kind of skilled staff (e.g. specialized nurses, additional specialized physicians in surgery, etc.).

Nonetheless, selecting heath care institutions and browsing their associated medical resources and enquiring about their availability may take time and consequently threaten the patient life. The solution is to integrate physicians and patients contexts and preferences into the localization algorithm.

To perform the above scenario related to a mobile physician, we propose a cloud computing location based services constituted by the following main components:

- The first component would be a mobile device belonging to a given physician from which he queries the proposed pervasive system, in order to determine CkNNs adequate healthcare institutions.
- Secondly, cloud services able to answer the above requests based on a CkNNs engine taking as an entry a town's road network map enclosing points of interest, and physicians and patients' preferences. Answers to the physician's requests, in the form of filtered healthcare institutions are then displayed, as well as identified map pieces, on the physician mobile device screen.

If more than one point is determined after filtering based on users' contexts and preferences, the system has to display a comparative visualization of the chosen resources. This, obviously, gives the physician the ability to match his patient case with one of the ranked health care institution.

The goal of this chapter is to provide a solution based on a mobile cloud platform able to satisfy, anywhere and anytime, the mobile physician's localization requirements. We focus on one hand on identifying the needed points of interest; on the other hand we offer a solution for filtering identified points of interest, according to physician and patient contexts and preferences also stored and updated on the cloud.

The chapter is organized as follows. In section 2, we present the state of the art related to route guidance algorithms. In section 3, we depict in detail our route guidance software as a service

for CkNNs determination including users' preferences. In section 4, the route guidance approach is enhanced by users' contexts and preferences. In section 5, we describe the mobile cloud architecture where the route guidance approach constitutes its central component. In section 6, we present future research direction followed by final conclusions in section 7.

BACKGROUND

With the integration of the recent advances in mobile positioning systems and wireless telecommunications, Location Based Services (LBSs) contribute to the enhancement of the efficiency of pervasive systems which essentially provide spontaneous services created on the fly by mobile devices that interact by ad hoc connections (Bakhouya & Gaber, 2007). This is ensured by providing efficient responses for location dependent queries triggered by mobile users such as physicians in our case.

The majority of pervasive healthcare rescue systems are motivated by the purpose of the Management of the Emergency Vehicles (MEV) which is oriented to reduce the time from the reception of the notification of an incident to the arrival of the emergency vehicle on the incident scene. The two major components of MEV are emergency vehicle fleet management and route guidance destined to compute optimal routes in real-time.

Several systems for route guidance emergency calls are actually proposed. We describe in the following some of them.

In the first system (Murro, 2005), the author presents an overview of the GST optimized system. This is integrated into an Emergency Service Vehicle (ESV) and has like objective to handle route guidance in real time while taking into account the traffic information. The system aims to guide the ESV as fast and safe as possible to the incident point by facilitating the interaction between ESV and other road users. However, this system presents a high computational cost due to the use of Dijkstra algorithm (Dijkstra, 1959) as route calculator algorithm.

In the second system (Dimopoulou, 2006), the author describes a system composed of an ESV, a traffic management system, a Geographical Information System (GIS) and a lecturing program. The principal objectives of the system are reducing the time needed for arrival of the ESV to the place of the accident, reducing the overall time needed to transfer the patient of the trauma-centre, and offering care of high quality to en-route patients. This healthcare emergency system seems to be the best actual system referring to its efficient route guidance subsystem; however, its major shortcoming is the high cost of storage of information in the server related to the road traffic network (speed limits, direction of travel, detectors information, traffic parameters, etc.)

In the third system (Nygren, 2006), the author fixed as challenge, on one hand, the increase of safety and transport efficiency, and, on the other hand, the addressing of users (physicians, patients, etc.) needs. This proposed rescue system ensures an efficient monitoring and guidance of the ESV under a management of the traffic flow into what he calls sensitive zones. The multiple restrictions and requirements related to the access control and the 'parking' zones make this system very difficult to set up.

In order to achieve their distance computations, these systems are fundamentally based on route calculator algorithms. For that purpose, numerous of them have been proposed, in the literature, for the nearest neighbors' determination on road networks. Most of these algorithms are based on the computation of the distance from the query object to its nearest neighbor's points by using graph diagrams. We describe in the following the most important route calculator techniques found in the literature.

Branch and Bound Technique

This technique proposed in (Song & Roussopoulos, 2001) uses a branch and bound algorithm which builds a tree structure by pre-weighting chances to find an optimal solution in a particular branch of the tree. For that purpose, authors introduce situation evaluation heuristics which allow the determination of whether one solution is more advantageous than another. In particular, several points' requests are carried out at pre-defined example points on the way, by using the results of the previous example points in order to obtain borders for the search of the closest neighbors. This approach suffers due to its dependence with regard to the number of examples provided in the entry. In fact, if the number of examples is not high enough, the result may not be valid.

Voronoi-Based Network Nearest Neighbor Technique

Kolahdouzan and Shahabi (2005) proposed a solution to address CkNN's queries by using an approach called Voronoi-based Network Nearest Neighbor (VN3). This approach is based on the concept of the Voronoi Diagram (VD). The authors attempted to benefit from the properties of the VDs in order to design a Network VD (NVD). This diagram is defined for graphs where the objects are located on the links connecting the nodes of the graph. The distance between objects is defined as the shortest way rather than the Euclidean distance. Indeed, VN3 is summarized by the partitioning of the road network in areas (polygons) of Voronoi Network Voronoi Polygons (NVP) of the first order. Each polygon is centered by the point of interests (e.g. hospitals). The union of all the polygons forms NVP of the NVD. The basic idea adopted by the authors is that the NVP can be directly used to find the first nearest neighbor to a given point query q. It is sufficient to use an index structure to define the polygon which contains the query point and to restore the generator of the cell as being the first nearest neighbor in the road network. Thereafter, the suggested technique proceeds by an iterative process for the search of the next nearest neighbors. According to (Kolahdouzan & Shahabi, 2004), this is performed in two steps. The first one, which is a filter step, consists of generating a list of candidate points and inserting them into a lookup table. The second step is called the refinement step, which uses the list of the candidates previously generated in order to compute the distance between the point query q and a candidate point c. The total distance between q and c is computed by the formula dist $(q, c) = dist (q, ptq) \cup dist (ptq, ptc) \cup dist (ptc, c)$. The point having the minimum distance will be selected as the next nearest neighbor. In order to apply this method to the continuous search of the nearest neighbors, the authors propose two approaches. The first one, called examination intersection (IE), is based on the search of kNNs for all the splits points (points in the path where the nearest neighbor changes) in the way. The second aims to optimize the kNNs computing performance by carrying out calculation only for a pre-selected set of points in the way. The main disadvantage of this technique is that its performance degraded if k increased, the number of objects increased and the points of interest are concentrated in the same zone.

Most existing works, such in Yiu et al., (2011) are destined to solve query integrity problems in the Euclidean space where the distance between two objects is measured by a straight line. That is; the distance depends only on the locations of the two points. In Hu et al.,(2012) the authors propose a novel road network kNN query verification technique which utilizes the network VDs and neighbors to prove the integrity of the query result. The approach verifies both the distances and the shortest paths from the query point to its kNN result on the road network.

Incremental Network Expansion Technique

This Incremental network expansion (INE) based solution proposed in Papadias et al (2003) adopted a flexible architecture for Spatial Network Data-Base (SNDB) called incremental network expansion. It takes into account the Euclidean distance restrictions, the localization of the objects and the connectivity of the road network. This technique collects the space entities (e.g. emergencies sites) of the network and preserves Cartesian coordinates and connectivity between the nodes. INE includes an iterative process which takes in entry a road network and generates a graph associated to it. Formally, this technique carries out the expansion of the network on the basis of a query point q, and examines, in the graph's segments, the entities in the order they are met. The computation of distances is carried out by the application of the Dijkstra algorithm (Dijkstra, 1959). In fact, the algorithm starts by locating the segment which covers q, then, it seeks all the points of interest which are on the same segment. The search of the nearest neighbor is extended starting from the closest node to q. The second closest node to q is inserted in a queue Q. Once the expansion is done, if the search in another segment brings back no point, it will be then carried out starting from the node which is at the head of Q. The expansion is then realized incrementally for the entire graph. The major disadvantage of this technique is that it is applicable only for the search of dispersed points in space.

ROUTE GUIDANCE APPROACH SOFTWARE AS A SERVICE

The main purpose of this work is to propose a new guidance approach based on DT. This method, applied on road networks, is able to establish the CkNNs while taking into account the dynamic changes of locations from which queries are sent. The proposed solution, to be implemented as SaaS (Software as a Service), is a way of leveraging the Internet to consume localization services on demand. Physicians will share processing power, storage space, bandwidth, memory, and CkNN software.

Delaunay Triangulation Fundamental Properties

The DT is the dual of the VD. In a plan, two sites Si and Sj are connected by an edge, if and only if, the areas of Voronoi $V(S_i)$ and $V(S_j)$ which are associated to the latter sites, have a common edge.

Let's suppose that M is a point of space, and d is the Euclidean distance between two points. We define $V(S_i) = \{M / d(M, S_i) \leq d(M, S_j), \forall i \neq j\}$. The fundamental properties of the triangulation of Delaunay are as follows:

- The circle circumscribed with any triangle of Delaunay does not contain any site in its strict interior (property of the circumscribed circle) – reciprocally, if a triangulation verifies this criterion, it is Delaunay.
- An edge connects the closest sites.
- The DT maximizes the smallest angle.
- As any triangulation of n sites, the number of triangles is t=n–2, and the number of edges is e=2n–3. The Euler theorem stating that t–e+n =1 is thus respected.

In this context, the DT is used to model a road network made up of direct roads joining of the points of space.

Triangulation Construction

We decide to use a divide and conquer algorithm for the construction of the triangulation. It consists in dividing recursively the set of the sites that we have sorted in advance according to the collating sequence. This is completed according

to the increasing x-coordinates and, in the event of equality, according to the increasing ordinates. We then acquire elementary zones containing a low number of points (in general from 1 to 3) that we triangulate marginally and we merge, thereafter by pairs.

Nevertheless, this method is applicable only for Euclidean spaces. To resolve this difficulty, we leaned on the use of an extension of the method divide and conquer defined in Domiter (2004) who builds the DT geometrically while taking into account the real road distances separating the sites of interest. This algorithm, implementing the above extension, is optimal and has a complexity in the worst cases of $\theta(nlog(n))$. The use of the DT for this type of problem ensures an optimal algorithmic complexity at the level of construction with regard to the other geometrical techniques of space modeling. In fact, it offers an intuitive representation for the search for the closest neighbors. This is due to the fact that it permits connection between the closest points of interest; adding to that it maximizes the smallest angle. This facilitates the representation either of the points of interest concentrated in the same surface or dispersed in space. Indeed, it is considered as relevant for any distribution of points of interest on the network.

The Route Guidance Processing Method

Being given a set of points of interest P_i (for i ∈ 1...n) (e.g. emergencies sites), a user (e.g. mobile physician) moves on a way [S, E]; S being the starting point and E being the point of arrival. For example, this user executes a query in the point S such as: 'seek for me the three closest emergencies sites from my current position?' The response will be restored in the point q. A valid response for the query previously emitted will be a subset of points of interest such as three emergencies sites, for example.

The route guidance processing method based on DT_r takes as input a set of points of interest

P_i located in space, a set of edges E connecting every Pi's neighbors, a graph $G(P_i, E)$ representing DT with edges balanced by the distances of the shortest ways between the points of interest, a query point q, and the number k of closest P_i. It produces as output the list lst_{NN} of k-closest P_i.

Let's note that only the points that belong to the triangulation will be considered. In other words, the suggested technique doesn't take into account the case where the request point doesn't belong to any including triangle. The route guidance processing method is mainly performed in three steps enhanced and described below (Khayati & Akaichi, 2008):

- The point query localization ensured by the algorithm PQL.
- The first nearest neighbor determination performed by the algorithm R1NN.
- The expansion of the search of the second nearest neighbor to the (k-2)-nearest neighbors is achieved by algorithm ER2kNN.

Point Query Localization

There are several types of representation of queries by point and/or by window (Li et al., 2003). We are interested in this paper by the use of the point type which is considered as the more widespread type and the most largely used in the context of search of the kNNs. Let's start to announce property 1, which is useful for the point query localization.

Property 1

A point and its closest neighbor always define a Delaunay's edge. The demonstration of this property is given in one of our previous work (Khayati & Akaichi, 2008).

The previous property was defined by Delaunay for the construction of his Triangu-lation. Our method, described in detail through the algorithm PQL, is based on a first triangulation step leading to the localization of the point query

q in the graph representing the road network and balanced by real road distances. Consequently, this permits to minimize the space of indexing and thus to optimize the cost of execution of the PQL algorithm. Indeed, after carrying out a triangulation of the considered graph and being given the geometrical coordinates (x, y) of the point query q in it, we carry out the localization task in two steps.

Initially, we seek the triangle which contains the request q. Once the point query q is localized in a triangle resulting from the triangulation, this latter undergoes a transformation process which consists in dividing recursively the triangle into sub-triangles. A first transformation consists in building a triangle by joining the mediums of the enclosing triangle. A second transformation consists of subdividing the built triangle into three sub-triangles using a well-determined orthocenter.

We proceed then, to a localization of the point query q with regard to the sub-triangles of the enclosing triangle. This step has as objective to ensure a valid result for any search query of the nearest neighbor located in the graph's triangles. A central function of the algorithm PQL is related to the localization task which allows to situate a given point query q with regard to a triangle T.

The above central function takes as an entry any triangle of the graph G and copies it in the triangles list in order to be processed. Thereafter a procedure tests whether the triangle in question contains the point query q or not. If not, the search will be extended towards the adjacent triangle in the same direction of the point query q. The localization task will be carried out to find the right triangle with a successive application of the central function for every triangle in the determined triangulation. It returns true if a point "p" is on the same side of a point "c" with regard to a line (a, b). This is determined by checking if, by projecting the coordinates of the points ("c" and "d") on the line (a, b), the resulting line (c, d) is at the top or bottom of the right-hand side of (a, b). A specific function determines if a point "p" is in or not in the triangle T. By applying these previous procedures and functions, the triangle including the point query q is determined. Once the localization done, we proceed to the search for the nearest neighbors.

First Nearest Neighbor Determination

In order to determine, in efficient manner, first nearest neighbor or 1NN, we introduce property 2.

Property 2

Being given a point query q located in a triangle T_1 of the graph, the nearest point of interest N_1 is one of T1's summits. A demonstration of this property can be found in our previous work (Khayati & Akaichi, 2008).

The current step consists in searching for the first closest neighbor N_1 of the point query q as well as the Influence Region (IR). We note that this region corresponds to a Voronoi cell $V(S_i)$ that the DT_r can easily find using the summit's incidences without having to store all the information concerning all the sites (adjacent cells, border points, splits points, etc.). We proceed then by searching N_1 in the triangle enclosing the point query q. Once N_1 is found, thanks to property 2, it is inserted into the list of the closest neighbors.

We then carry on by a recursive approach that aims to delimit the local influence region (polygon) of the triangle T_1 and to expand this region towards the adjacent transformed triangles which share the same summit N_1.

IR illustrates the search by region which delimits the area where the point query q can move without the occurrence of a change of the 1NN. For the first value of the 1NN found, the algorithm delimits a second region named expansion region (ER_1). The search for 2NN will be only restricted in ER_1 delimited by the incidentals summits to 1NN. This is ensured thanks to property 3 introduced in the next section.

Expansion of the Search from 2NN to kNN

In order to expand the search, we have to prove that the second nearest neighbor belongs inevitably to an adjacent triangle. This is clearly ensured by property 3.

Property 3

The second closest neighbor of q belongs to the adjacent triangles which share the same summit N_1. The demonstration of property is detailed in Khayati & Akaichi (2008).

Algorithm 1.

```
PQL /*Point Query Localization*/;
Input: Point query q, Graph G;
Output: Sub-triangle t_st; /*the sub-triangle containing q */
Begin
    Given G, apply the DT to G to divide this latter into triangles T_s with ref-
erence to property 1;
    Given T_s and q, find the triangle ts, in G, which contains the point query
q;
    Given t_s, transform ts into sub-triangles;
End.
```

This step is applicable for all the other incidental points to the first nearest neighbor (1NN) of the query point and for points that are not incidental to the 1NN. This means that the distance, separating each incidental point and the 1NN, is always inferior to the distance separating each not incidental point and the 1NN. We conclude that the second nearest neighbor (2NN) to a query point q, belongs inevitably to one of the adjacent triangles having 1NN as summit.

We have chosen to use a Local Minimum Spanning Tree (LMST) for the implementation of the expansion. Indeed, an LMST is a tree covering the local minimal weights in a specified area. This tree was proposed in (Li et al., 2003) with the aim to compute the LMST (each node calculates the MST neighbor's). An edge connecting two nodes u and $v \in V$ (V being the set of the nodes) belongs to the LMST, if and only if, u is the direct neighbor of v in the LMST. We consider the LMST(G) as the sub-graph LMST of a given graph $G = (V, E)$; E being the set of the edges in the graph.

In the following step, the expansion of the research space (ER_1) to a second adjacent expansion region (ER_2) is conditioned by the existence of an edge minimizing the network distance between the local covering minimum trees (LMST) from (j−1) NN and the jNN (for $j \in [3, k]$). Once this condition is verified, we expand the expansion region (ER_1) to an expansion region (ER_2) in which we seek the next nearest neighbor. ER_2 is obtained by expanding the ER_1 on the triangles which are adjacent to it and will be thus delimited by the determined summits.

An LMST has as objective to minimize the local minimum trees and to better integrate the updates. For these reasons, it will be applied to the balanced edges of the triangulation. Indeed, the LMST has as root point the first nearest neighbor 1NN. The edge connecting 1NN and any other point of interest Nj of the graph will be balanced by the distance of the shortest way between q and Nj. The same expansion procedure will be carried out to seek the following closest points of interest.

ENHANCING THE SOLUTION WITH PREFERENCES AND CONTEXTS

Running Scenario

Consider the case of a physician requesting for the nearest three hospitals in order to take care of a patient. After getting the answer for the emitted request and reaching the first hospital, he notices that the institution has an awfully long wait which is unbearable for the current medical case. He headed to the second hospital where he finds that this latter does not match with the patient and the medical requirements in terms of hardware and/or skilled staffs. He decided then to go to the third hospital which was unfortunately closed and/or the route leading to it is suffering from congestion caused by a traffic accident. The previous problems render the provided solution obsolete and consequently may lead to complications harming the patient state which has to be supported efficiently as quickly as possible.

The Approach Limits

The above scenario shows paramount limits which may affect the patient support and the physician duty. The limits of our approach are, essentially, due to the following main clustered causes:

- Patients' cases and related physicians needs are not personalized. In fact, if two physicians, taking care of two different patients enduring different medical cases, ask the same query around the same location, they will get the same answer. This latter is not necessary well-adapted to the medical cases to be supported.
- The only context that the approach cares about is patient and physician location. We think that other kinds of contexts must be taken into account in order to optimize the treatment of the patient. Examples of such contexts are current road and health care

institutions conditions, etc. In fact, having information about health care institutions such as hospitals and emergency centers, may give a great help to match patients' cases and physicians needs with medical hardware and skilled staffs present in health care institutions.

Overcoming the Limits

To overcome the above limits, we decided to link a component to our guidance system which has to provide the localization data. When the component gets the localization data, it filters the results so that to keep only those matching with various preferences and contexts classified as follows:

- Physician and patient preferences/contexts: Physicians have the ability to specify their preferences along with their context. For example, a physician may specify that whenever he is looking for a health care institution, he would like that the route guidance system take into account characteristics permitting to treat patients according to identified diseases and current patients' states. Using such preferences, the route guidance system has to check the appropriate context to provide a context-aware answer that is tailored to both the physician preferences and patient context described by his current state.
- Health care institution context: Health care institutions registered within our system provide their contexts described by their features including their services, equipment, human resources capabilities, operating hours, current waiting time, etc. In order to find a suitable health care institution for a certain patient, the route guidance system have to be able to match patient and physician preferences and contexts with the health care institution static and dynamic features.

- Environmental context: The environmental context describes the characteristics of the path starting from the point where the patient is sup-ported to the point where the health care institution is reached. It is accessed by the route guidance system to enhance the answer quality of queries issued by the physician. Examples of environmental context include current road traffic (i.e., estimated travel time through road segments), time, weather, etc.

The following algorithms R1NN and ER2kNN permit respectively to ensure not only the first nearest neighbor (1NN) determination and the expansion of the search from 2NN to kNN presented, but also the evaluation of the localized nearest neighbors.

In fact, when the research of 1NN succeeds to localize the 1NN, it evaluates it according to defined preferences and contexts by computing a value which is function of satisfied and unsatisfied characteristics.

The same task of evaluation is also performed through the expansion of the research from 2NN to kNN for each localization of iNN ($i>=1$). The result is then the stored in lst_{NN}. After the end of determination of all the nearest neighbors, lst_{NN} is sorted according the evaluation values and then provided to the physician who select the nearest neighbor ranked as first.

PUTTING ALL TOGETHER ON THE CLOUD

Pervasive computing provides tools to mobile care givers when and where it is needed regardless of their movements and activities, therefore supporting location and time independence. However, with mobility come its inherent problems such as resource scarceness, finite energy and low connectivity (Fernando et al., 2013). CkNN based applications are one of the type of mobile and

Algorithm 2.

```
R1NN /*Research-of-1NN*/;
Input: t_s, t_st, T_a;
Output: N1, IR;
Begin
    Given t_s an q, determine the 1NN of q with reference to property 2;
    Evaluate N_1 according to preferences and contexts;
    lst_NN:= N_1;
    Define the region in ts where N_1 for q is still invariant.
    Transform T_a into sub-triangles T_sa;
    For all adjacent triangles of t_s do
        For (i:=2; i!=k; i++) do
            Determine the polygon P_i in t_sa ⊂ T_sa where N_1 is still invariant.
            Determine IR which is the union of all the k adjacencies' polygons.
        End for
    End for
    ER_1:= T_a / ER_1 contains the union of all t_s's adjacent triangles.
End.
```

Algorithm 3.

```
ER2kNN /*Expansion of the Research from 2NN to kNN*/;
Input:  q, N_1, IR, lst_NN:={N_1};
Output: lst_NN;
Begin
    Given ER_1, construct the Local Minimum Spanning Tree (MST) of all the point
of interest in IR;
    For (i:=2; i!=k; i++) do
        If the edge minimizes the minimum distance of MST then
            Expand the region ER to the adjacency.
            Construct the Local MST of all the point of interest in ER_i.
        End if;
        Search for the i^th NN of q with reference to property 3.
        Evaluate N_i according to preferences and contexts;
        lst_NN:=lst_NN ∪ N_i;
    End for;
    Rank lst_NN according to evaluation results and present it to the user.
End.
```

real time applications that demand high levels of responsiveness, that in turn, demand intensive and timely available computing resources. Cloud computing, defined as the aggregation of computing as a utility and software as a service (Vogels, 2008) where the applications are delivered as services over the Internet and the hardware and systems software in data centers provide those services [6], is a good response for these up-to-date requirements.

The key strengths of cloud computing can be described in terms of the services offered by cloud service providers: software as a service (SaaS), platform as a service (PaaS), and infrastructure as a service (IaaS) (Carolan et al., 2009). Offloading physicians, patients, road networks, and health care centers data and computation associated to them such as CkNNs programs in cloud computing, is used to address the intrinsic problems in mobile computing and users new requirements, by using resource providers other than the mobile device itself to host the execution of mobile applications which is complex and expensive. In fact, health care givers are not able to support either the development of needed software, or their deployment and maintenance. Using an infrastructure where data storage and processing could happen outside the health care givers mobile devices is the best solution that can be offered nowadays. This kind of infrastructure is called mobile cloud on which intensive applications such as CkNN software can be executed on low resource mobile devices used essentially for triggering location based services as described in the above sections.

Cloud computing represents important means permitting to deploy and maintain health care services such those introduced above. It avoids the need for health care institutions and medical actors, such as physicians, to invest in hardware and software in order to process, store and distribute data. Instead medical institutions and physicians outsource some of their services to cloud providers. The cloud provider is responsible for providing the infrastructure, maintaining and supporting all the centralized equipment and software as well as ensuring data security and integrity. Three main models are present on the cloud computing scene: Infrastructure as a service, platform as a service, and software as a service. For the latter, physicians' and health applications are delivered as services over the Internet and acceded through mobile devices and/or desktop computers. Advantages are that there is no need for mobile physicians and health care institutions to buy a full license and pay only for use. Upgrading and applying security patches is undertaken by the cloud provider such the Ministry of health.

Our proposed system is mainly composed of five components: CkNNs' manager responsible for locating desired health care institutions for mobile physicians, Health care institutions' manager responsible for handling information about hospitals, emergencies, etc, physicians' manager which supports physicians information, patients' manager which handles patients' folders, preferences and contexts manager which stores, manages, and learns about physicians and patients' preferences and contexts, privacy and security manager which handles privacy issues related to patients and security issues involved by the system.

Moreover, other resources have to be integrated into the whole mobile cloud solution such as resource and cost managers (Fernando et al., 2013). The resource manager has the accountability to maintain connections and monitor physicians entering or leaving the cloud. The cost manager has to determine the physicians priorities (e.g.: battery conservation, fast execution, monetary gain) and by taking into account activities at hand, available resources, and required resources, come to a decision whether to offload or not. The CkNNs' manager dynamically partitions the required location based services, offloads the related produced jobs, and preserves the job pool.

Note that, all the above managers have to exchange information in order to ensure an adequate functioning in a real time environment and cost efficiency.

FUTURE RESEARCH DIRECTIONS

Using a cache containing previous responses of CkNNs' queries may reduce the time consumed by the evaluation performed on each localized iNN. This will be one of the tasks on which we will focus on in our future research work. Moreover, we will emphasize on further spatiotemporal characteristics and constraints in order to provide modeling, analysis and mining tools able to extract knowledge related to physicians' trajectories and activities. The aim is to improve quality of services having an obvious impact on patients' wellbeing.

CONCLUSION

In this chapter, we presented a mobile cloud solution for a mobile physician on the road. It is based on a SaaS route guidance approach which efficiently finds the nearest neighbors for mobile queries on road networks. We started by situating our problem in the context of route calculator algorithms, by presenting various search techniques for CkNNs intended for road networks. Based on the challenge to propose new route calculator software as a service that outperforms the existing algorithms, we have considered a new technique named DT_r. This method is based on DT for the representation of the network. Mainly, the treatment, applied to evaluate efficiently kNN queries, is based on network partitioning in order to find, by applying PQL, the 1NN neighbor in a triangle containing the point query q. Once the latter is found, a second algorithm called R1NN permits to delimit the region of influence (ER_1) in order to seek by adjacency, in the neighborhood of the second nearest neighbor. The expansion algorithm ER2kNN extends the region of expansion (ER_1) towards a second expansion region (ER_2) to ensure a valid result for the k–2 following the nearest neighbors from q. By the proposed solution, we

attempt to improve the efficiency of the physician's reaction in motion, in order to enhance his task of saving patients' lives. The scenarios performing the whole approach suppose that when points of interest are restricted following the physician's demand, they are sent back to a mobile device and displayed according to preferences and contexts.

Our proposed mobile cloud system is mainly composed by CkNNs' based on the above route calculator, and health care institutions, physicians, patients, preferences and contexts and privacy and security managers. It empowers mobile health care givers and institutions by providing a seamless and virtualized location based software rich functionality, regardless of their resources limitations and increasing needs. By consequence, all of this contributes to quality enhancement of health care delivery.

REFERENCES

Bakhouya, M., & Gaber, J. (2008). *Ubiquitous and pervasive application design*. Paper presented in IEEE International Conference on Pervasive Services, Proceedings of the 2nd Workshop on Agent-Oriented Software Engineering Challenges for Ubiquitous and Pervasive Computing (AUPC). Rome, Italy.

Carolan, C. C. A. J., Gaede, S., Baty, J., Brunette, G., Licht, A., Remmell, J., … Weise, J. (2009). *Introduction to cloud computing architecture* (White Paper). Academic Press.

Dijkstra, E. W. (1959). A note on two problems in connection with graphs. *Numeriche Mathematic, 1*(1), 269–271. doi:10.1007/BF01386390

Dimopoulou, E. (2006). *Implementation of an advanced spatial technological system for emergency situations*. Paper presented at FIG Workshop on eGovernance Knowledge Management and eLearning. Budapest, Hungary.

Domiter, V. (2004). Constraint Delaunay triangulation using plane subdivision. In *Proceedings of the 8th Central European Seminar on Computer Graphics*. Retrieved August 13, 2014, from http://www.cescg.org/CESCG-2004/web/Domiter-Vid/

Feng, F., & Watanabe, T. (2004). Search of continuous nearest target objects along route on large hierarchical road network. In *Proceedings of the 14th Data Engineering Workshop* (DEWS). Kaga City, Japan: DEWS.

Fernando, N., Loke, S. W., & Rahayu, W. (2013). Mobile cloud computing: A survey. *Future Generation Computer Systems*, *29*, 84–106. doi:10.1016/j.future.2012.05.023

Gaber, J. (2006). New paradigms for ubiquitous and pervasive applications. In *Proceedings of First Workshop on Software Engineering Challenges for Ubiquitous Computing*. Lancaster, UK: Academic Press.

Khayati, M., & Akaichi, J. (2008). Incremental approach for continuous k-nearest neighbors queries on road. *International Journal of Intelligent Information and Database Systems*, *2*(2), 204–221. doi:10.1504/IJIIDS.2008.018255

Kolahdouzan, M., & Shahabi, C. (2004). *Vornoi-based K nearest neighbor search for spatial network databases*. Paper presented at the 30th VLDB Conference. Toronto, Canada.

Kolahdouzan, M., & Shahabi, C. (2005). Alternative solutions for continuous K-nearest neighbor queries in spatial network databases. *Springer Science*, *9*(4), 321–341.

Li, N., Hou, J., & Sha, L. (2003). Design and analysis of MST-based topology control algorithm. In *Proceedings of the 22th Annual Joint Conference on the IEEE INFOCOM*. San Francisco, CA: IEEE.

Loke, S. (2007). *Context-Aware Pervasive Systems: Architectures for a New Breed of Applications*. Boca Raton, FL: Auerbach Publications.

Murro, A. (2005). *Architecture and interface specifications*. Paper presented at Architecture Workshop. Brussels, Belgium.

Nygren, N. (2006). *Cooperative freight and fleet application*. Paper presented at CVIS W2 Open Workshop. Brussels, Belgium.

Papadias, D., Zhang, J., Mamoulis, N., & Tao, Y. (2003). *Query processing in spatial network databases*. Paper presented at the 29th VLDB Conference. Berlin, Germany.

Song, Z., & Roussopoulos, N. (2001). K-Nearest neighbor search for moving query point. In *Proceedings of ACM SIGMOD*. Santa Barbara, CA: ACM.

Tao, Y., & Papadias, D. (2003). Time-parameterized queries in spatio-temporal databases. In *Proceedings of ACM SIGMOD*. San Diego, CA: ACM.

Vogels, W. (2008). A head in the clouds the power of infrastructure as a service. In *Proceedings of the 1st Workshop on Cloud Computing and Applications*.

KEY TERMS AND DEFINITIONS

Branch and Bound Method: Destined for finding optimal solutions of various optimization problems. It consists of a systematic enumeration of all candidate solutions discarding large subsets of unproductive candidates.

Context: Information used to characterize the situation of objects that are considered pertinent to the interaction between a user and a system.

Context-Aware Computing: The system's aptitude to adapt to shift situations and answer back according to the context of use.

Continuous k Nearest Neighbors' Search Method: A continuous search of the k Nearest Neighbors using real distances while moving on the road networks.

Delaunay Triangulation: A recursive algorithm for dividing a space into triangles making sure that the circle circumscribing the vertices of a triangle contains the vertices of no other triangle within it.

Location Based Services: Services offered through mobile devices enhanced with positioning technologies. Offered services take into consideration users' location.

Mobile Cloud Computing: A model in which applications based on mobile devices and positioning technologies are designed, and deployed by means of cloud computing technology.

Pervasive Computing: An innovative computing concept where computing tasks seem to be anywhere and anytime. It's performed using any mobile device, in any location, in any format, and at any time.

Positioning Technology: Used by positioning systems to determine the position of a mobile object in the real world.

Voronoi Diagram: The dual to the Delaunay triangulation, is a way of dividing space into a number of regions called Voronoi cells. In the Voronoi diagram, a set of points is specified in advance and for each point there will be a matching region consisting of all points nearer to that point than to any other.

Chapter 10
Message–Oriented Middleware on the Cloud for Exchanging E-Health Data

Piero Giacomelli
Spac SPA, Italy

ABSTRACT

Cloud infrastructure has been one of the latest technologies in the e-health sector. Despite many research studies focusing on the privacy of the e-health data stored on the cloud, the ways of exchanging e-health information between client and cloud have not yet been fully addressed. Moving from this initial consideration, in this chapter, the authors evaluate the possibility of using Message-Oriented Middleware (MOMS) for exchanging data between the cloud storage and the remote device used in telemedicine and remote monitoring software. The evaluation is done using a cloud testing environment and a low bandwidth connection modem and a simulation of 50 patients taking a 10 minutes 3Lead EGC test. Some possible future directions on this architecture are suggested as well as some possible improvements.

INTRODUCTION

The objective of this chapter is to describe the possibilities offered by using Message Oriented Middleware in telemedicine and remote monitoring application. Telemedicine and remote monitoring seem the only successful ways for the clinician to monitor and check the health status of the patients whose number is increasing. Above all the number of chronic patients that require a constant monitoring is increasing.

The problem of monitoring is not only related to the western countries but also affects the development ones. Recent studies, which were done by the CDC (CDC, 2013) suggest that, for example, in the US, 5.1 million people suffer from Chronic Heart Failure. So, a long term monitoring could be practically impossible. Moving to the China population, for example, 20 million people need constant monitoring. The remote monitoring applications are promising not only when we deal with big numbers but also when we deal with big distances. In development countries like Africa or Asia, in most of the cases direct clinician consultation is very difficult due to the difficulties and the lack of transportation. Telemedicine applications

DOI: 10.4018/978-1-4666-6118-9.ch010

used the well-established client server technology using a remote connection with the server using the TCP-IP and HTTP/HTTPS protocol. So, in general, we have some remote sensor devices, both hardware and software, that exchange medical observation with a central server, which is used as a repository for the collected data.

In the latest years the cloud paradigm entered the field of server side software technology. So, new telemedicine and remote monitoring applications have been created or re-coded using this new approach. However, as regards the communication layer, there has been no significant evolution on the use of Message Oriented Middleware.

Despite the specification is quite established in other fields as the financial one, surprisingly the use of Message Oriented Middleware in a cloud environment applied to the telemedicine field has not been yet fully studied. The use of MOMs in remote monitoring applications where the server is a cloud based one and the exchange of Electronic Health Records (EHR) is done using MOM infrastructure has never been discussed before.

The purpose of our study is to fill this gap. After a basic introduction, we will propose a simulation on the use of Message Oriented Middleware in a real-life chronic patient remote monitoring. We will detail a possible scenario where we have a 3Lead ECG device that sends data to a central cloud infrastructure. The communication is established using the Java Messaging Service (JMS) protocol, and an open-source implemented framework (HornetQ). The format of the message was similar to HL7 Observation messages. The core part of the chapter is focused on describing this infrastructure and on providing a simulation where 50 software coded devices send a 3Lead ECG to the cloud infrastructure. This simulation will describe a fully coded infrastructure based on low bandwidth transmission line, so to avoid simulation based on higher technologies. After a simple test, we will perform some evaluations of the results, based on some simple statistical data analysis. The statistical data analysis suggests that this approach could outperform the old client server technology using Web-services endpoints.

This very first try suggests that Messaging Oriented Frameworks and cloud infrastructures could be successfully integrated for exchanging medical data in telemedicine or remote monitoring environment. Some possible improvements to the overall architecture are suggested as well as some configuration adjustments to boost performance.

BACKGROUND

Despite the Moore law (Schaller, 1997) first postulated back in 1965, postulating a limit on the individual computing capacity of any computer both from the perspective of CPU, storage capacity, we have seen a computational growth mainly driven by the cloud computing paradigm. Even if the cloud computing involves a wide range of the technological aspect, and even if there is still no wide agreement on a single definition (Armbrust et al., 2010), we could argue that cloud computing is infrastructure both hardware or software that is able to connect various computational devices such as desktop, pc, high performance server, through a communication network.

The key idea is simple if we have a computational task so important in terms of computational power involved that we divide the full task into simpler tasks that are elaborated separately from a different machine.

The computational power of such an infrastructure at least on the paper is of higher magnitude than using a single machine for this purpose.

The cloud paradigm is only one step forward. Some older projects were in the production stage back in the last five years of the '90. The SETI@ Home (Seti 2013) project was probably the first distributed computational task that involved users outside the academic circle. The project consists in finding trace of extra-terrestrial transmission by scanning observational data coming from the Arecibo radio Telescope (Figure 1).

Figure 1. Arecibo radio telescope

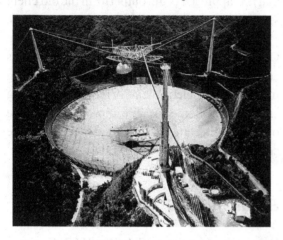

The data collected are too much and in continuous growth that a single machine would need decades to complete the analysis. So, instead of using one single powerful computer from a Web site volunteer, we could download some cheap consuming CPU software that performs the following actions:

- Download a portion of the data,
- Scan the download,
- Upload the outcome to the central server.

The project is still the largest project on distributed cloud computing. Even if (till now) no sign of extra-terrestrial intelligence has been found, a cousin project: the Great Mersenne Prime Search (Marlene 2013) has already reached some goals.

The project distributed the search of Mersenne prime numbers across many single pcs. In this case, the last Mersenne prime number found is the monstrosity M42643801 composed of 12837064 digits, which have been found in 2009 by an Intel Core 2 Duo (3 GHz) desktop pc.

But from these experiments, the main force that drove the cloud paradigm was, as usual, the commercial sector, in particular the rise of the social network paradigm and the raise of smartphone.

The creation of smartphones able to surf the Internet and access online data using apps, have practically doubled the number of possible devices that can access data across the World Wide Web using the HTTP protocol and the TPC communication layer. The first consequence was that every type of storage system, every repository, every RDBMS, connected with such high traffic Web sites, started growing exponentially.

So, the storage could not be thought as one single machine (no matter how powerful), but a Copernican change was needed about thinking such an infrastructure. Only to give the reader a hint we suggest looking at an infographic elaborated by Qmee in 2013 (Omee, 2013), resuming what is the amount of data exchange during one minute on the Internet by various high-traffic social network Web sites.

As one may see, we have, for example, YouTube Web site being uploaded with something like 72 hours of videos every minute. Twitter in its maximum peaks is able to manage 110,000 tweets per minute during the 2012 London Olympics Games.

It is interesting to notice that from this infographic are excluded Web sites containing adult content. There are no official studies because it is very hard to have access to adult content traffic from the major worldwide Web sites, even for research purposes. From one done only for evaluation purpose, it seems, for example, that the site x-videos stream is something like 50 gb of videos per second (ExtremeTech, 2013). But apart from these numbers it is a fact that as the bandwidth access becomes available to a larger part of the world, the traffic and storage capacity of a single Web site, needs to be sized to handle big numbers.

Only to solve the storage issue a whole new hardware/software approach has been taken by introducing the cloud paradigm. Basically, the idea is to share different tasks, like storage or by enforcing asynchronous calls, into a lot of different hardware. So, it does not matter how big the starting computational effort is. If we are able to divide it into a huge number of little tasks and then we assign every task a computation resource, it is only a matter of time before the job is completed.

Telemedicine applications started the latest years to couple with this new approach. But dealing with the cloud infrastructure for telemedicine or remote monitoring applications opened a whole bunch of particular questions that are now becoming object of research.

The first big issue that is to be raised when we deal with medical or physiological data is the security one. Electronic Health Records need to be treated in a very special way. The reason is clear as physiological data is transmitted from a remote device/sensor to a remote storage. That is, we need to assure that the whole transmission is

- **Safe:** So that it is not possible for a third-party entity to alter it in any way.
- **Recoverable:** Meaning that all transmissions even the ones that were not able to reach the final destination are recoverable.
- **Anonymized:** We need to guarantee that even in case of data are stolen it is not possible for a third-party malicious entity to reconstruct the association between the patient and his/her physiological data.

The first research on the e-health and the cloud focused mainly on the anonymization tasks (Löhr et al., 2010; Zhang et al., 2010; Guo et al., 2010). This was expected, because, on a cloud infrastructure, the medical records can be inaccessible even for an institution that uses them. So, for example, a UK hospital could use cloud storage that is on US territory for a telemedicine application and in most of the cases could even have limited administration rights on the storage itself.

Looking at the cloud side, we need to have a secure mechanism for storing Electronic Health Records (EHRs). Storing the sensitive data of patient health records, Cloud service providers and health care providers must ensure the privacy and confidentiality of the cloud-hosted data (Narayan et al., 2010). Apart from these major issues, there is also the protection of EHR medical data, which should be done according to regulation where the storage is. All these passages are needed because we need to assure as much as possible that a clinician takes medical decision based on displayed physiological data, and the data are the real ones that were recorded.

Just to give a practical example, let us image to use Amazon as a cloud infrastructure for storing purposes of an EHR coming from one country in EU. If the server infrastructure is based on the US territory, the storage of the EHR medical data is under the umbrella of the FED, so they should follow, for example, the Health IT Policy Committee recommendations, and in case of untrusted access to the cloud infrastructure Amazon should communicate it to the medical structure within 60 days.

But besides the storage another important issue is how one remote device transmits data to the cloud itself.

The traditional client /server approach to telemedicine coded the previous recommendations using technologies like FTP, HTTP and recently Web-services. Now we need to rethink the way of exchanging data with some key point in mind:

- Guaranteed safety and privacy of the transmitted data.
- Use the potential of the cloud infrastructure, like scalability, to avoid any data loss or corruption.

- Guarantee the fastest possible data transmission between device and cloud.

SIMULATING AN EGC CLOUD BASED MESSAGE ORIENTED MIDDLEWARE

As we claim in our introduction, we will propose the use of a Message Oriented Middleware for exchanging sensitive medical information data between remote monitoring devices and cloud infrastructure. By Message Oriented Middleware, we mean a software infrastructure that supports asynchronously the sending and receiving of messages. The storage of the messages is done using a queue infrastructure that is accessed asynchronously by a message producer and a message consumer.

Using such a structure, it has the main disadvantage of introducing a new layer of communication between the client and the server. But the introduction of such layer allows introducing the whole infrastructure:

- **Asynchronicity:** While one could implement asynchronous communication between client and server, the whole asynchronous management of the MOM is done by the intermediate layer.

Figure 2. The Message Oriented Middleware structure

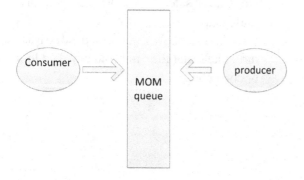

- **Routing:** In a particular condition, a message could be routed from the original queue to another one based on a condition.
- **Transformation:** Some message transformation could be done directly from the middleware layer.

In our case, we propose a Message Oriented Middleware implemented using JMS specification and HornetQ as a middleware layer to send HL7 messages from one device to a cloud infrastructure.

We will also do some statistical analysis to let the user better evaluate the performance.

However, before proceeding we have to describe the various actors for our proposed infrastructure. First of all MOMs do not have standards, even if the Advanced Message Queuing Protocol (AMQP) (Amqp, 2013) is an emerging standard that defines the format of the messages exchanged from the client to the server. The oldest implementation of the MOMs has been done with Java Messaging Service a set of Java API that implemented the MOMs in detail. The firstly implemented specification was JMS 1.0.2b that has been released back in June 2001. The current version is JMS 2.0 that has been released in March 2013. JMS is an interesting case because it does not specify the format of the message, so it is not fully interoperable like AMQP, but it has the advantage to code many kinds of information. In fact, JMS can be generic software without specification. So, instead, for example, of transmitting a single number as message we are able to transmit a whole object that can describe a measure. JMS has been successfully used and studied in a different environment.

Due to its extreme flexibility, the JMS implementation has been used for scheduling purpose (Vieira et al, 2003), P2P applications (Balsoy et al., 2002), large multi-agent and particle swarm optimization (Chiang et al., 2006 and even seismic networks (Olson, 2014).

The fastest, till now, framework implementing JMS is the HornetQ (2013). HornetQ is a MOM coded using the JMS specification 2.4 in the latest version (HornetQ 2.4.0 beta). We use this framework for the following reasons:

- It is licensed using the Apache software license v.2.0 (the source code fully available).
- The SPECJMS2007 test is the fastest JMS framework available on the production market, with an astonishing record of 8.2 million messages per second.
- The framework has a lot of features, and it is fully integrated with SSL. If it can use a secure socket layer channel to transfer messages. This permits secure transfer managed by a certificate that can be used to reduce the risk of a man in the middle (MIM) attack.
- The content of the message is a patient observed measure. This is a medical term but in any case it could be a piece of information containing data regarding patient health/mental status or real physiological data taken from a remote device/sensor. We include, in such a way, all measurements that are not directly related to golden standard rules for the treatment of patient health.

For example, for remote monitoring of patient with diabetes or Chronic Kidney Disease (CKD), the proteinuria and glucose tests are the most important values to monitor. However, the diet itself for these patients is equally important for prevention and monitoring purposes. In many telemedicine applications, we have remote glucometer that test the blood's glucose level while a pc or a tablet is in charge of sending data about the diet followed.

In our case, we are interested in monitoring the physiological data primarily because they are the most important as a primary source of evaluation. Secondly, because the human body provides a huge amount of information, it puts the system under stress. A simple 3-lead Electrocardiography (3L-ECG) could generate 3 single float number measurements every 300 milliseconds. Imagine multiplying this by 20 patients and an hour of measurement for each patient. So, we need a system able to transmit/receive billions of data with low latency. Even if we are not dealing with a life saving device, an ECG bad trace should alert, as soon as possible, an emergency unit to allow a fast hospitalization of the patient.

As we stated before a generic JMS message is a Java object that contains lot of information and can be tagged with many useful information. The interesting fact is that the body of the message; so the real content to be transmitted can be a generic Java object itself. So, we are not limited to transmit string or numbers but we can also transmit xml encoding and so on. This allows us to choose the right format for the content of the message.

Choosing the right protocol for messages containing physiological data can be a tricky task. For our test, we chose to use the HL7 protocol for creating messages of measurement of physiological data

The messages were exchanged using the HL7 protocol. Right now there is no ISO or industry standard for coding patient physiological data across different electronic devices. There are many consortium initiatives driven by the industry stakeholders that are dealing with building a standard. Unfortunately, there is not an agreement on which to use.

The HL7 (Health Level Seven International) (HL7, 2013) framework is a US ANSI standard for formatting Electronic Health Records and Electronic measurement between software and electronic devices. The standard defines much real world cases. In our analysis we are interested in HL7 coded messages regarding the ECG measurement. A patient physiological measurement is described using the HL7 standard as an observation result; the standard changed from version 2.x to version 3.x, as for version 2 the standard used a whole string to code the observation results, while in version 3.x the HL7 standard use xml codification. To give a short example, Figure 3 illustrates an HL7 2.4 observation message

The message is self-containing all the information encoded. In particular, we notice that we have the following information: ORUR01 is the type of Observation message. Every Woman Eve is the patient's last name and first name. Other data are: 1962-03-20 it the date of birth of the patient, but most importantly the measure was about the glucose level and it was evaluated in 182 mg/dl. Collateral information is the clinician that requests the observation, like Patricia Primary MD and the caregiver that took the measure was Howard Hippocrates MD.

As we argue that the major difference between HL7 Observation Request (ORU) version 2.x a 3.x is that while, in 2.x, the whole message was a long string, in 3.x the whole message is a formatted XML. We will not enter in the full detail of the message codification, but we point out some single tag of information that is represented in Figure 4.

The portion of code represents the observation of the same level of glucose we have seen previously. In this case, we also have some additional information like the interpretation range. Obviously, in terms of the size of a single message, the V3 version is much bigger than the previous version. But it is true that the XML is more interchangeable between different software systems and programming languages. The XML parsing library is present in almost all software; and it is not necessary to parse the whole message. To create random messages, we use the HAPI (HAPI,

2013) that is one of the most used Java libraries to create HL7 messages.

To make a test, near to the real-word problem, we publish an instance of the HornetQ standalone server into an AWS Free Usage Tier that is an Amazon virtual machine instance that Amazon offers as a testing environment for free. The hardware configuration is specified as below:

- 1 CPU,
- 512 Mb of ram,
- 1GB of data transfer per month.

We install on this machine a single HornetQ standalone server running a queue where all the messages are stored before being consumed. The client was a pc equipped with

- Ubuntu 12.10 (Quantal Quetzal) version (2Gb of RAM).
- Java Standard Development Kit 1.7.0.21.

To test, we use the TP/IP protocol using an old modem line without using an optic fiber channel. This could sound a little bit strange, considering the fastness of the growth of modern connectivity lines both for mobile devices and smartphones. However, while it is true that, in all modern countries, the growth of the speed of data transfer is growing rapidly, vast rural geographic areas find difficult to connect using modem GPRS network (Bouckaert et al., 2010). The PC was connected to the AWS storage using a 56K modem that was tested to have a mean line speed 112.6 Kb per sec-

Figure 3. An HL7 ORU glucose measurement v2.4

```
MSH|^~\&|||||20140113152039.012+0100||ORU^R01^ORU_R01|1|T|2.4
PID|||555-44-4444||ROSSI^ANNA^E^^^^L|GIACOMELLI|19730303|F|||via Roma 11^^VICENZA^IT^36100
|||||||AC555444444||67-A4335^0H^20030520
OBR|1|845439^GHH 0E|1045813^GHH LAB|15545^GLUCOSE|||200202150730|||||||||555-55-5555^PRIMARY^PATRICIA P^^^^MD
|||||||||F|||||444-44-4444^HIPPOCRATES^HOWARD H
OBX|1|SN|1554-5^GLUCOSE^POST 12H CFST:MCNC:PT:SER/PLAS:QN||^182|mg/dl|70_105|H|||F
```

Figure 4. An HL7 ORU glucose measurement v3.0

```
<observationEvent>
  <id root="2.16.840.1.113883.19.1122.4" extension="1045813"
      assigningAuthorityName="Laboratori Bianchi"/>
  <code code="1554-5" codeSystemName="LN"
        codeSystem="2.16.840.1.113883.6.1"
        displayName="GLUCOSE^POST 12H CFST:MCNC:PT:SER/PLAS:QN"/>
  <statusCode code="completed"/>
  <effectiveTime value="201312310837"/>
  <priorityCode code="R"/>
  <confidentialityCode code="N"
      codeSystem="2.16.840.1.113883.5.25"/>
  <value xsi:type="PQ" value="182" unit="mg/dL"/>
  <interpretationCode code="H"/>
  <referenceRange>
    <interpretationRange>
      <value xsi:type="IVL_PQ">
        <low value="75" unit="mg/dL"/>
        <high value="115" unit="mg/dL"/>
      </value>
      <interpretationCode code="N"/>
    </interpretationRange>
  </referenceRange>
</observationEvent>
```

ond. So, embedding the client software side into a device does require using a modem telephone line. This assumption makes the simulation close to most every telephone connection.

Considering the client software side, we coded one client that started instantiating on 50 different threads and so 50 different HL7 message senders. Every thread once started start sending three singles random values generated ECG HL7 ORU message version 3.0, every 300 milliseconds. The whole process was left up for 10 minutes to simulate 50 patients that did a home based 3 Lead EGC. The parallelism of the process is a key point as an ECG is taken according to medical protocols, and at the same time during the day. The request for all the patients to do the same measurement seems reasonable as most remote monitoring of the ECG is required at the same time, (for example in the morning).

So, the client configuration is only a small program that pushes hundreds of HL7 messages

to the HornetQ queue. To manage the performance test we also have to write a server side Java Messaging Server, HornetQ client consumer, which had been installed on the AWS server.

When the server side consumer starts, it connects itself to the queue EcgQueue and starts listening for new messages to arrive and stored into the queue. If a new message arrives the whole HL7 ORU message is extracted and stored into a single XML file of the repository. Because every message is tagged with a Unique Identifier, it is possible to find the time every step of the process was involved in.

HornetQ infrastructure allows fine-tuning the way the consumer and producers read and write messages to our queue containing the ECC measurements. Client and consumer were both fine-tuned as fast producer and fast consumer. This configuration means that both the client and the consumer write to and read from the queue, as fast as possible. This affects the dimension of the queue that starts to grow very fast, but we also expected that once reached a certain level of memory to be used, the consumer would prevent the extra increments on the queue itself. It is important to point out that we chose only one consumer and only one queue. Another possible interesting configuration would have been the one to one association between producer, queue and consumer. This means that instead of having 50 patients using the same queue for storing messages and one consumer, we could have created 50 queues one for each patient and 50 consumers, one for each patient. This could be more close to FDA specification for storing medical measurements. In this second configuration every patient stores messages on a queue only dedicated to him/her, if we have a runtime exception on one consumer, for example, the others are not affected. In our configuration a block of any kind of the unique queue could affect all the patients. For the sake of coding, we use the first configuration, even if we know that the second one is more promising in a real-world production system.

We were, as a result, interested in evaluating three different time frames for every message. To store the results in a manageable format on the AWS server we use an Oracle MySQL server installation, where we store the following information into a large single table:

- The message unique identifier.

- The time the message was sent by the client.
- The time the message was received by the server.
- The time the message was finally stored into the repository.

So, we have the first ten minutes sessions with 50 ECG simulators and one single queue with one single consumer. The resulting table (depicted in Figure 5) displayed the following information

So far, after the first, session we have that for every message sent we were able to collect the following information:

- Message ID.
- Time the message was sent.
- Time the message was received.
- Time the sent message was stored.

As one might notice, we also extracted the full corresponding date time format to correctly measure the difference in milliseconds between the measured times. So, for example,, we have that the columns sent, received and stored, which contains the integer number representing the corresponding time.

Using this information we were able to extract, using the Structured Query Language (SLQ), the following information:

Figure 5. MSQL table messages

ID	send	received	stored	send_s	received_s	stored_s
ID:19b2338d-422c-11e3-8e55-a796f5d7e6af	1383224292835	1383224293058	1383224293095	2013-10-31 13:58:12.0835	2013-10-31 13:58:13.0058	2013-10-31 13:58:13.0095
ID:19b6c76e-422c-11e3-8e55-a796f5d7e6af	1383224292865	1383224293105	1383224293144	2013-10-31 13:58:12.0865	2013-10-31 13:58:13.0105	2013-10-31 13:58:13.0144
ID:19b73c9f-422c-11e3-8e55-a796f5d7e6af	1383224292868	1383224293146	1383224293152	2013-10-31 13:58:12.0868	2013-10-31 13:58:13.0146	2013-10-31 13:58:13.0152
ID:19bf2be0-422c-11e3-8e55-a796f5d7e6af	1383224292920	1383224293170	1383224293184	2013-10-31 13:58:12.0920	2013-10-31 13:58:13.0170	2013-10-31 13:58:13.0184
ID:19c2ae51-422c-11e3-8e55-a796f5d7e6af	1383224292943	1383224293190	1383224293192	2013-10-31 13:58:12.0943	2013-10-31 13:58:13.0190	2013-10-31 13:58:13.0192
ID:19c3bfc2-422c-11e3-8e55-a796f5d7e6af	1383224292950	1383224293194	1383224293197	2013-10-31 13:58:12.0950	2013-10-31 13:58:13.0194	2013-10-31 13:58:13.0197
ID:19ce6e23-422c-11e3-8e55-a796f5d7e6af	1383224293020	1383224293208	1383224293211	2013-10-31 13:58:13.0020	2013-10-31 13:58:13.0208	2013-10-31 13:58:13.0211
ID:19d2daf4-422c-11e3-8e55-a796f5d7e6af	1383224293049	1383224293214	1383224293217	2013-10-31 13:58:13.0049	2013-10-31 13:58:13.0214	2013-10-31 13:58:13.0217
ID:19d76ed5-422c-11e3-8e55-a796f5d7e6af	1383224293079	1383224293226	1383224293230	2013-10-31 13:58:13.0079	2013-10-31 13:58:13.0226	2013-10-31 13:58:13.0230
ID:19ddb066-422c-11e3-8e55-a796f5d7e6af	1383224293120	1383224293231	1383224293234	2013-10-31 13:58:13.0120	2013-10-31 13:58:13.0231	2013-10-31 13:58:13.0234
ID:19e132d7-422c-11e3-8e55-a796f5d7e6af	1383224293143	1383224293236	1383224293240	2013-10-31 13:58:13.0143	2013-10-31 13:58:13.0236	2013-10-31 13:58:13.0240

- (The message was received - time message was sent) in mms.
- (Time sent message was received - time the sent message was stored) in mms.
- (Time the message was stored – time the sent message was received) in mms.

The result of this first server side elaboration was a data frame like the one in Figure 6.

Using the R framework (Ripley 2001) for statistical computing, we performed an analysis to evaluate the two delta times in milliseconds that we had after our first evaluation..

A first summary of the dataset considering the two delta times gave us the following outcome in milliseconds (Table 1).

The total number of correctly received and stored messages was of 3981684. The JVM estimated JMS size was of 50.2Kb.

The frequency can be seen in Figure 7.

On the other hand, considering the received storage delta we have the following summary (Table 2).

The corresponding frequency histogram is shown in Figure 8.

We also conducted a single test hypothesis of the mean of the send/receive value of delta. We found the following results:

- $t = 0.5276$, $df = 16199999$, p-value = 0.5977,
- Alternative hypothesis: true mean is not equal to 822,
- 95 percent confidence interval:
- 821.8510, 822.2588,
- Sample estimates:
- Mean of x,
- 822.0549.

With a two-side alternative, we found that the mean of the sent-/receive delta will be different from the mean value 822.

Figure 6. MSQL output with deltas

ID	delta send/receive	delta store/receive
ID:19b2338d-422c-11e3-8e55-a796f5d7e6af	223	37
ID:19b6c76e-422c-11e3-8e55-a796f5d7e6af	240	39
ID:19b73c9f-422c-11e3-8e55-a796f5d7e6af	278	6
ID:19bf2be0-422c-11e3-8e55-a796f5d7e6af	250	14
ID:19c2ae51-422c-11e3-8e55-a796f5d7e6af	247	2
ID:19c3bfc2-422c-11e3-8e55-a796f5d7e6af	244	3
ID:19ce6e23-422c-11e3-8e55-a796f5d7e6af	188	3
ID:19d2daf4-422c-11e3-8e55-a796f5d7e6af	165	3
ID:19d76ed5-422c-11e3-8e55-a796f5d7e6af	147	4
ID:19ddb066-422c-11e3-8e55-a796f5d7e6af	111	3

Table 1.

Min	1st Qu.	Median	Mean	SD	3rd Qu.	MAX
213	3410	6596	6598	3681.172	9785	12980

Figure 7. .Frequency distribution on milliseconds of send/receive deltas

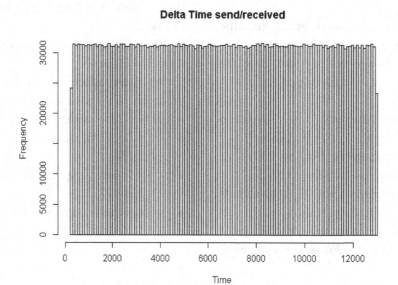

Table 2.

Min	1st Qu.	Median	Mean	SD	3rd Qu.	MAX
1	14	28	69	69.69	50	78

Figure 8. .Frequency distribution on milliseconds of received stored deltas

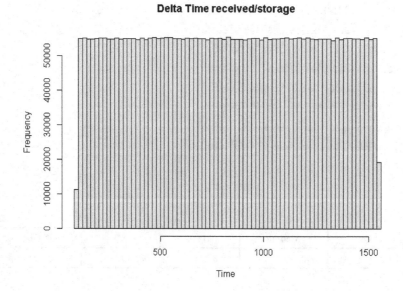

From our test, we noticed that even using low level hardware and low bandwidth device, the mean time a message is transferred from the client to the cloud storage using a Message Oriented Middleware is of 6 seconds. The 75% of the results stayed below a data transfer time between sending and receiving of 9 seconds. The results could seems not so promising, but we need to point out that we collect 50 ten minutes 3 Lead ECG using a low level hardware and a very poor broadband line between the client and the server. We also report the storage mean time and, in this case, the results are in line with the recent study on RDMS performance on the cloud (Sharma, 2012). Obviously, a great increase in performances would be to use a 3G or 4G network that are used by most of the western countries citizens by their smartphones. The size of a single JMS version 3.x, of the HL7 ORU specification, for a single ECG measurement, is of about 60Kb, but the amount of data to be transferred is not so high. In a realistic environment where we have 50 patients, every one of them was equipped with a single 3G line to send messages, the total amount of data to be transferred is very low and can be estimated in 15Mb over 10 minutes per patient. So, in this scenario, the speed of the line should not be bottlenecked. We also used the latest version of the HL7Message ORU specification, but as we stated before, a lot of the data contained in the message are of XML tag that are not information relevant to the measurement itself. Using a previous version the single message size decreases significantly.

Another improvement could be the use of multiple queues associated with the measurements. In our test, we created only one queue that stored all the messages coming from 50 different patients, with one consumer on the backend that parses and stores all the messages. But instead of this configuration, we could have 50 different queues, one for every patient and 50 consumers that acts in parallel by consuming the messages of only one single patient. This will distribute on the server side the load from one thread to multiple threads.

So, for a server this could be an advantage, in terms of performance on a single queue parsing.

Another interesting possibility offered by the HornetQ framework is to have a cluster configuration. So, instead of having one single instance of the server managing everything, we could have multiple servers that act like a whole sharing of one single queue, in a transparent way for the client. This kind of configuration is very powerful. In this case, the load of 50 consumers could be shared between different computing resources, allowing single, not so powerful machines to manage only a subset of the whole queue message consumption.

The advantage of using a Message Oriented Middleware, instead of classical client- server configuration or Web Services, is not only related to the frequency of message parsing. Message Oriented Middleware's also provide the opportunity to create a login mechanism and to use a secure socket layer (SSL) connection, allowing, with only some minimal configuration, only on the server side, to create an encrypted connection between the client devices and the server, reducing the risk of a man in the middle (MIM) attack. This kind of unauthorized data stealing is based on one machine that puts itself in a transparent way between the client device and the server. Once done, the machine starts to collect, at a low level, the data that are passed between the device and the server. Using a SSL connection, the data passed are encrypted (Mitchell et al., 1998). So, even if malicious software could dump, at a low level, the messages, it would be difficult to have access to the full content of the message.

FUTURE RESEARCH DIRECTIONS

In this chapter we presented a Message Oriented Middleware solution for transmitting clinical observations from remote patients to a cloud oriented infrastructure used for storing data. We used a simple scenario with 50 simulated patients, a low bandwidth transmission device and a cloud infrastructure hosted on the Amazon server farm. From our simple tests, we found that on this configuration we have a mean transmission speed of 9 seconds. Lots of research can be done on this direction to further explore the way Message Oriented Frameworks can be used in a cloud environment for high-frequency messaging exchange between different software platforms. Obviously, the first direction is the one involved in deciding, which is the best software architecture that can be used in such a context. As we have seen, the HornetQ framework allows very different architecture to attain different objectives, but still remains unclear which one would be the best for secure archiving, and fast responsive transmission between client and cloud based storage. Another interesting direction is the one involving messaging encoded with different specifications. Through this chapter, we used the Java Messaging Service specification, but in fact responsive environments AMQP are rising as a new standard to be used. One last word should be said about the adaptation of standards in using such frameworks. Right now there is no large 'agreed specification' to be used for transferring medical data between software systems. The US Food and Drug Administration (FDA) periodically publish a report with suggestions on how to implement this. Nevertheless, till now, no serious study on how the adaptation of MOMs to this suggestion has been done.

CONCLUSION

In this chapter, we illustrated a testing environment for using a Message Oriented Middleware in a cloud infrastructure, using HL7 messages coded as 3 lead ECG observations. We performed one single test on low-level hardware. The statistical analysis gives us a hint. The use of Message Oriented Middleware in cloud infrastructures, particularly in health related application, could impact on the speed and security the data, which are exchanged. We also performed a simulation

on 10 minute parallel 3Lead ECG of 50 patients using a cloud server with 512Mb of RAM, and a low level bandwidth device.

Despite this poor hardware, we had a mean time on sending and receiving HL7 messages of 6.5 second, which is in line with the modern Web-service technology. MOMs could efficiently compete with the actual way we exchange electronic health records between remote devices and storage units. We also point out some configuration improvements that could be easily tested in a lab environment, which could and should be the topic of further research.

REFERENCES

Amazon Free Usage Tier Website. (2013). *Amazon Free Usage Tier website*. Retrieved September 2, 2013, from http://aws.amazon.com/free

Amqp. (2013). *Official Amqp website*. Retrieved August 23, 2013, from http://www.amqp.org

Armbrust, M., Fox, A., Griffith, R., Joseph, A. D., Katz, R., & Konwinski, A. et al. (2010). A view of cloud computing. *Communications of the ACM*, *53*(4), 50–58. doi:10.1145/1721654.1721672

Bouckaert, J., Van Dijk, T., & Verboven, F. (2010). Access regulation, competition, and broadband penetration: An international study. *Telecommunications Policy*, *34*(11), 661–671. doi:10.1016/j.telpol.2010.09.001

CDC CHF. (2013). *Center of disease control chronic heart failure factsheet*. Retrieved September 2, 2013, from http://www.cdc.gov/dhdsp/data_statistics/fact_sheets/fs_heart_failure.htm

Chiang, F., Braun, R., & Hughes, J. (2006). A biologically-inspired multi-agent framework for autonomic service management. *International Journal of Pervasive Computing and Communications*, *2*(3), 261–276. doi:10.1108/17427370780000155

ExtremeTech. (2013). *Just how big are porn sites?* Retrieved September 2, 2013, from http://www. extremetech.com/computing/123929-just-how-big-are-porn-sites

Fox, G., Balsoy, O., Pallickara, S., Uyar, A., Gannon, D., & Slominski, A. (2002). Community Grids. In Proceedings of Computational Science—ICCS 2002 (pp. 22-38). Springer.

Giacomelli, P. (2012). *HornetQ messaging developers' guide*. Packt Publishing.

Guo, Y., Kuo, M. H., & Sahama, T. (2012). Cloud computing for healthcare research information sharing. In Proceedings of Cloud Computing Technology and Science (CloudCom), (pp. 889-894). IEEE.

HL7. (2013). *Official HL7 website*. Retrieved August 23, 2013, from http://www.hl7.org

HAPI. (2013). *Official HAPI website*. Retrieved September 2, 2013, from http://hl7api.source-forge.net

Hornet, Q. (2013). *Official HornetQ website*. Retrieved August 13, 2013, from http://www.jboss.org/hornet

JMS. (2013). *Official JMS specification*. Retrieved August 13, 2013, from http://www.oracle.com/technetwork/java/docs-136352.html

Löhr, H., Sadeghi, A. R., & Winandy, M. (2010). Securing the e-health cloud. In *Proceedings of the 1st ACM International Health Informatics Symposium* (pp. 220-229). ACM.

Mersenne. (2013). *Great Internet Mersenne Prime Search 2012*. Retrieved September 15, 2013, from http://www.mersenne.org/

Mitchell, J. C., Shmatikov, V., & Stern, U. (1998). Finite-state analysis of SSL 3.0. In *Proceedings of Seventh USENIX Security Symposium* (pp. 201-216). USENIX.

Narayan, S., Gagné, M., & Safavi-Naini, R. (2010). Privacy preserving EHR system using attribute-based infrastructure. In *Proceedings of the 2010 ACM Workshop on Cloud Computing Security Workshop* (pp. 47-52). ACM.

Olson, M. J. (2014). *Cloud computing services for seismic networks*. (Doctoral Dissertation). California Institute of Technology. Qmee. (2013). *Qmee infographic*. Retrieved August 13, 2013, from http://blog.qmee.com/qmee-online-in-60-seconds/

Ripley, B. D. (2001). The R project in statistical computing. *MSOR Connections*, *1*(1), 23–25. doi:10.11120/msor.2001.01010023

Seti. (2013). *Seti@home official website*. Retrieved August 13, 2013, from http://setiathome.berkeley.edu/

Sharma, G. (2012). Performance analysis of database on different Cloud computing environments. *International Journal of Advanced Computer Science and Information Technology*, *2*(2), 5.

Vieira, M. A. M., Viera, L. F. M., Ruiz, L. B., Loureiro, A. A. F., Fernandes, A. O., & Nogueira, J. M. S. (2003). Scheduling nodes in wireless sensor networks: A Voronoi approach. In *Proceedings of Local Computer Networks* (pp. 423–429). IEEE. doi:10.1109/LCN.2003.1243168

Zhang, R., & Liu, L. (2010). Security models and requirements for healthcare application clouds. In Proceedings of Cloud Computing (CLOUD), (pp. 268-275). IEEE.

KEY TERMS AND DEFINITIONS

Cloud Storage: A distributed virtual server side infrastructure for handling databases and repositories.

HAPI: An open source java framework for handling HL7 messages.

HL7: Global authority on standards on interoperability of health information.

Java Messaging Service: The java implementation of a Message Oriented Middleware.

Message Oriented Middleware: Software for sending and receiving messages between software in a synchronous or asynchronous way.

ORU message: The HL7 standard for the result of clinical observation.

Telemedicine: Use of telecommunication and information technologies in order to provide clinical health care at a distance.

Chapter 11
CoSeMed:
Cooperative and Secure Medical Device Sharing

Andreas Kliem
Technische Universität Berlin, Germany

ABSTRACT

E-health systems need to dynamically integrate heterogeneous types of medical sensors and provide access to streams of sensed medical data in order to properly support patient treatment. Treatment processes usually include several steps and medical departments, which means that sensors could be moved between networks of Care Delivery Operators instead of being reattached every time. Therefore, the authors propose a novel approach that allows sharing medical devices among different operators in this chapter. This means that each operator books a medical device as long as it delivers required data and is present in the operator's network, which the authors call the medical device cloud. Besides cost effectiveness, this approach can extend traditional cloud-based e-health systems, usually designed to share Electronic Health Records, by sharing the devices that emit the data. This mitigates judicial constraints because only the data sources and not the data itself are shared, and allows for more real-time access to mission-critical data.

INTRODUCTION

The evolution of Information and Communication Technology (ICT) in the healthcare domain is heavily influenced by upcoming distributed architectures that integrate and facilitate medical sensors in a ubiquitous fashion (Varshney, 2007). Streams of medical data emitted by integrated medical devices can support physicians in their decision-making process. However, a huge variety of heterogeneous sensors has to be considered in order to get a meaningful survey of a patient's condition. Treatment decisions often have to be made under time constraints, which require an aggregated view of the available data streams. Each stream utilized may differ regarding its specific characteristics, which might include real time requirements, used data formats and nomenclatures or, the communication protocol used by the medical device that provides the stream.

The resulting device integration and data aggregation problems often lead to proprietary

DOI: 10.4018/978-1-4666-6118-9.ch011

solutions. Medical device vendors gain flexibility in handling specific hardware requirements, protecting innovations or optimizing their products towards their design preferences. Additionally, market exclusivity can be achieved, which often forces Care Delivery Operators (CDOs) to be dependent on a vendor (i.e. vendor lock-in). However, proprietary solutions hinder the development of open and fully integrated e-health systems, which are required to efficiently deliver cost-effective health services. Moreover, the vendor lock-in problem is intensified, if the movement of medical devices is considered. Since each operator might rely on different solutions, interoperability cannot be achieved. Due to the aforementioned variety, interoperability in the e-health domain can only be achieved, if medical devices can be integrated at any required location regardless of the protocol (proprietary or standard-based) they are based on.

This leads to two options to design medical device integration systems. Either, try to implement all required protocols into one system or rely on standardization. Both options underlie serious obstacles. Although appropriate standards like ISO/IEEE 11073 (ISO/IEEE, 2004) or the Bluetooth Health Device Profile (Bluetooth SIG [BSIG], 2013) exist, the variety of medical devices and regarding requirements makes it difficult to achieve a widespread standardization in a reasonable time span (Buxmann, Weitzel, von Westarp & König, 1999). Moreover, even a lot of standards allow for vendor defined extensions, which again introduces proprietary parts. And, most standards rely on the definition of device profiles to express functionality needed for a certain kind of device. Due to the decreasing time to market, these profiles are changed or added rapidly, which requires to adapt the device integration system too. Implementing all required protocols into one system does not scale, since compute nodes, like smartphones or other embedded systems that are usually used as medical device integration systems underlie resource constraints and often do not allow to implement several protocol stacks in parallel. This raises the question, how a middleware for medical device integration systems can be designed, to achieve interoperability among several protocols, to fit to the rapidly changing requirements and, to be deployable on mobile embedded systems.

Apart from integrating medical devices, data availability has to be considered. Nowadays, treatment processes usually include several steps and institutions (i.e. CDOs), ranging from monitoring at home, emergency transportation or different hospitals, whereat each location might be managed by a different operator. If we assume that a patient is already equipped with a set of wearable medical devices that are organized in a Body Area Network (BAN), real time access to the emitted data could provide better knowledge to physicians. At each location the BAN can grow or shrink (i.e. new medical devices are integrated), in order to fit the set of medical devices to the current treatment situation. However, to prevent reattachment or replacement of the already given medical devices, it is required that the data streams can be accessed by every CDO that is involved in the treatment process. This means that handover processes and some kind of device access management have to be introduced, in order to share the medical devices among different networks and operators.

Based on these problem definitions, the major challenges for middleware architectures in the e-health domain are:

- **Medical Device Integration:** The process of medical device integration shall be organized in an autonomous and dynamic way. In order to integrate unknown or new medical devices in a Plug and Play fashion, the middleware shall allow for reconfiguration at runtime and hide the heterogeneity and complexity of transport protocols from the application layer.
- **Data Aggregation:** Proper data aggregation heavily depends on the characteristics and the semantic interoperability of the incoming data streams. Therefore, the

middleware shall provide capabilities to achieve semantic interoperability among heterogeneous data formats and to dynamically deploy and (re)orchestrate data utilization modules along streams of medical data.

- **Data Availability and Mobility:** Seamless monitoring of vital signs relies on the availability of the medical data streams. Since medical devices might be mobile and interconnected using wireless transports, the middleware has to cope with handover processes between different networks and aggregators, while application layer transparency shall be preserved.
- **Security and Privacy:** Due to the requirements of the application domain, data security and privacy has to be preserved. Vulnerabilities that arise out of the dynamically organized system design and the medical device mobility have to be analyzed and covered properly.

As shown in Figure 1, the approach I will present, extends the traditional way cloud computing concepts are adopted to the e-Health domain. Instead of sharing the data by using cloud computing in the sense of a shared data store for Electronic Health Records (EHR), I try to establish a cloud of medical devices, where the data sources are shared. The data availability and mobility problem are targeted by enabling each CDO along the treatment path of a patient to access the medical devices. A device integration middleware, that allows for dynamic reconfiguration during runtime and provides concepts to handle unknown or new device types, targets the underlying integration and interoperability problem.

BACKGROUND

As a result of the problem definition, the device integration middleware acts as a core enabler for the Medical Device Cloud features, because it

Figure 1. The Medical Device Cloud approach

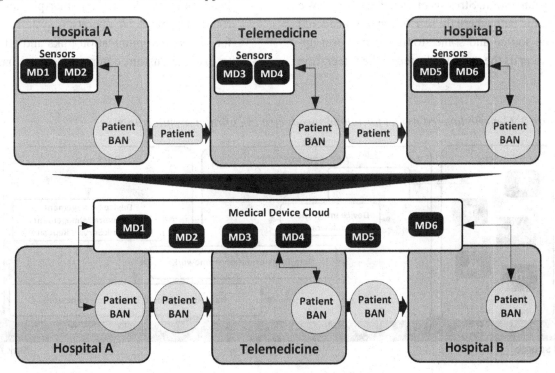

ensures interoperability among participating Care Delivery Operators. Therefore it is necessary to discuss general concepts of device integration architectures. As the approach allows to integrate devices based on different protocols and data formats, hiding the variety from the application layer is required. This refers to semantic interoperability and common data formats, which I will discuss briefly.

Following this description, I will introduce basic Cloud concepts related to the Medical Device Cloud approach. The analysis of the interaction of ubiquitous devices and Cloud Computing can be referred to as Cyber Physical or Vehicular Cloud approaches. Additionally, as the presented system is an extension to EHR Cloud Applications, sharing medical data via Cloud infrastructures will be discussed.

Device Integration

Integrating (mobile) embedded devices and sensors involves several steps, like data transmission, data aggregation and processing as well as storage or visualization. Streams of data thereby follow a dynamic path where the sensor can be considered as the source and some storage or end user application as the sink. Each step in the integration

path can be realized by different types of devices, where the position in the path basically depends on two important properties: the offered mobility and the offered resources. The mobility property usually decreases towards the sink, whereas the offered resources like processing power or storage capabilities increase. As shown in Figure 2, this leads to a generic three layered model of device integration architectures, where the three layers can be defined as:

- **Devices:** A set of (wearable) devices offering (standard-based) data transmission and location-independent operation to allow for seamless monitoring. The devices (i.e. sensors) are usually highly resource constrained and do not offer any capabilities to execute custom components. Their main purpose is to sense the environment and transmit the results to higher layers.

- **Aggregation:** One or more (wearable) devices that offer higher functionality in order to manage and integrate devices, aggregate data and transmit results to a backend. Devices in this layer (e.g. smartphones or routers) provide an operating system; offer several communication links and allow to execute custom components (e.g. parts

Figure 2. Generic layered model for ubiquitous device integration architectures

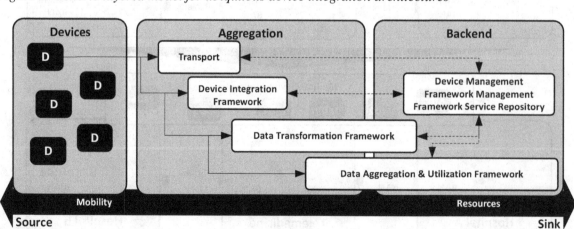

of the integration middleware). The main purpose of aggregation devices is to integrate sensing devices into a network and collect data from them. Dependent on the application domain, pre-processing or application layer components, like visualization, can also be placed at this layer.

- **Backend:** A backend primarily used by operating staff, offering persistent storage, monitoring and configuration capabilities, interfaces to higher level information systems (e.g. Hospital Information Systems for medical applications) as well as acting as an enabler (due to resource constraints in the device and aggregation layer) for security, mobility and interoperability enhancements. Components in the backend can be used to control and configure the behavior of aggregation layer devices (e.g. provide data collection plans or additional modules required to integrate a certain device).

In contrast to the OSI (ISO/IEC, 1994) layer model, the given layers are related to the devices and systems found at the respective position in the data path. This view allows for a more precise distinction between components related to the integration middleware and components related to data processing (i.e. application layer). However, this implies that the application layer can cross different layers of the given model. Based on the use case, application layer components might be present at both, the aggregation and the backend layer. I define application layer components as data utilization modules, where utilization refers to evaluation, presentation or storage for instance. Since the focus is on the device integration, utilization modules are treated as black boxes. A utilization module offers some kind of aggregation or processing service. These services are stored within the backend layer and the middleware shall provide a uniform execution framework that allows executing such a service where it is required (i.e.

at the aggregation or backend layer) and where the resource constraints are fulfilled.

Since device integration architectures deal with several diverse data sources, the architectural model is somehow related to the ETL (Extract, Transform, Load) or Data Integration process. This is reflected by several mandatory components. The aggregation layer integrates the sensing devices and therefore is required to host a transport and a device integration component, that allow to establish a connection to required devices and collect data from them, which refers to the extract process. The load process is related to store the data into the end target (e.g. a database) and therefore refers to the data utilization part at the backend, which as mentioned deals with storage and interfaces to information systems. Similar to the application layer components, the transformation component can cross both, the aggregation and backend layer. This is due to the fact, that transformation at the aggregation layer is only required, if a utilization module is deployed at this layer too. Otherwise, transformation at the aggregation layer would introduce unnecessary overhead. Finally, device management and a framework management component provides knowledge about the sensing devices and allows to configure the aggregation layer in order to fit to the current requirements.

In the following section I will have a deeper look at the transformation component and its theoretical basis, which can be referred to as semantic interoperability.

Semantic Interoperability - ISO/IEEE 11073

Semantic interoperability refers to a common understanding of the incoming data streams among all actors in the system (Heiler, 1995). A common nomenclature and a canonical data format give the opportunity for interoperable applications that are not affected by replacement of medical devices. Nowadays, replacement of a medical device often leads to adaption processes of an interface application (e.g. GUI) for instance, because in most cases the interface developer has to build directly upon the incoming data format. To bear on standardization and common nomenclatures at the application interface layer is no opposition to the already mentioned obstacles regarding standards at the device integration layer. While it is difficult to achieve interoperability at the device integration layer by constraining each vendor towards one standard, the benefits of semantic interoperability at the data processing or application layer can still be achieved by using data transformation approaches.

The canonical data format and the underlying nomenclature have to be chosen carefully. Important requirements are a sufficient coverage over the domain of context, the possibility to rapidly adopt user defined types (i.e. mechanisms for terminology management) and, a data exchange format suitable for mobile environments. Therefore we decided to rely on the ISO/IEEE 11073 family of standards, which is also promoted by the Continua Health Alliance (Continua Health Alliance [CHA], 2013). It not only provides a huge nomenclature, but also allows to model medical devices with an object oriented Domain Information Model (DIM) approach. This is an important capability, because it allows to store and share medical device configurations and functionalities among Care Delivery Operators (CDOs) participating in the Medical Device Cloud. This common way of describing a device, enables our middleware to automatically integrate and handle new device types. The extensibility of the nomenclature given by already established terminology management mechanisms, allows to model a huge variety of different medical devices, even if for instance a proprietary device is not completely covered by the nomenclature.

Development of the ISO/IEEE 11073 family of standards (x73) started in 1982 in order to provide interoperability and Plug and Play functional-ity for medical devices. The main application domains of the first versions were hospital and clinical environments. Due to the dissemination of mobile and wearable medical devices, effort was made on improving the original standard towards Telemedicine and Personal Health Device (PHD) environments (Yao & Warren, 2005), (ISO/IEC/IEEE, 2010). The following parts out of the x73 standard family are important for our approach:

- **11073-10101 Nomenclature:** A basic nomenclature to enhance semantic interoperability by providing a common meaning of numeric values throughout components in the system.
- **11073-10201 Domain Information Model (DIM):** Describes an object-oriented self-descriptive approach to model medical devices, their configuration and, capabilities.
- **11073-20601 Optimized Exchange Protocol:** Defines the transformation of a x73-DIM to an interoperable transmission format optimized for PHD environments.
- **11073-104xx:** Device specializations composed of a subset of available classes and services in the Domain Information Model. Each medical device in the Cloud has to be described by such a specialization. If a proprietary device is not covered with the existing specializations, a new one can be defined.

In terms of x73, medical devices are called agents and devices in the aggregation layer (e.g. a smartphone) are called managers. The basic concept of medical data exchange is to establish a connection between an agent and a manager and to create a local copy of the agent's DIM at manager side by using a service and communication model. The invocation of defined services allows the manager to keep its local copy up-to-date, if new measurements are provided by the agent. The manager provides the recorded data to higher application layers (e.g. GUI components). However, as we only rely on x73 towards the application layer, the main task is to transform the incoming data streams into the x73 format. This means that for each integrated medical device, a kind of virtual manager has to be created by the integration middleware.

The nomenclature defined in ISO/IEEE 11073-10101 (ISO/IEEE, 2004) (i.e. medical data information base (MDIB)) provides a common data dictionary applicable to a broad range of vital signs ranging from intensive care (e.g. ECG) over laboratory to common parameters, like weight or blood pressure. In x73 the nomenclature is primarily used to specify attributes that can appear in data streams (i.e. protocol data units) and are not statically defined. This allows communication partners to get a common semantic understanding of the exchanged data. An entry (i.e. term) in the nomenclature basically consists of a term code and a human readable reference identifier. For efficiency reasons, all nomenclature terms are organized in partitions (e.g. dimensions), where each partition has a set of private term codes that allow for vendor specific extensions. Using terminology management concepts like the Rosetta Terminology Management (RTM) (IHE International [IHE], 2013b), project started by the IHE (IHE International [IHE], 2013a), allows us to extend the nomenclature in case of proprietary devices that are not completely covered.

Besides the nomenclature, x73 defines a Domain Information Model (DIM), which consists of several classes and attributes that are used to model medical devices in an object-oriented fashion. Each class and attribute is referenced using nomenclature codes, thus interoperability is ensured through preserving the same semantic meaning among different implementations. A model of a medical device (i.e. agent) is composed of a set of objects that refer to the data sources accessible by manager devices. The set of objects and corresponding attributes is usually defined by device specializations that correlate to an actual medical device (e.g. blood pressure monitor). Each specialization picks out a defined set of objects and attributes available in the DIM to realize its intended functionality. Important for the approach to be presented is, that specializations define a static (e.g. system type) and dynamic (e.g. measurement value) set of attributes. If an aggregating device has predefined knowledge about the DIM of a specialization, only the dynamic attributes have to be exchanged and can be merged into the existing static part of the DIM later. Therefore each incoming proprietary data stream to be transformed has to be matched against a device specialization available in x73 or subsequently added to our system. Measurements encoded in the stream have to be translated by a transformation module to x73 attributes and merged into the DIM as dynamic attributes.

CLOUD COMPUTING IN E-HEALTH

The adoption of Cloud Computing concepts for the e-Health domain both raises opportunities and challenges. Evolving concepts like Electronic Health Record (EHR) Clouds, that allow to share patient data and help making the data available, or governmental initiatives and research funding for Cloud based e-Health services (EU, 2013), show that Cloud Computing already found its way into the healthcare domain and is not just a concept under discussion any more. Apart from the serious privacy and security issues related to sharing health records in clouds (Löhr, Sadeghi & Winandy, 2010), the availability of the data is of crucial importance. The data distributed by EHR Clouds usually was recorded in the past, which means that the history of a patient is reflected. However, as our approach just covers the real time data (i.e. the data currently emitted by the patients sensors), a hybrid architecture composed out of both, cloud based EHR sharing and medical device sharing, is required to allow for proper treatment decisions. Therefore I will shortly discuss the fundamentals of EHR cloud approaches.

As mentioned in the introduction, patient treatment nowadays is organized in a multi-tenant fashion, where multiple operators have to collaborate. Each participant in the treatment process must take knowledge about the patient's history and past treatments into consideration, while making own decisions. Knowledge about a patient is stored in patient records, where according to the HIMSS definitions (Garets & Davis, 2006) one has to distinguish between Personal Health Records (PHRs), Electronic Medical Records (EMRs) and Electronic Health Records (EHRs). A PHR should provide a complete summary of the health status and the medical history by gathering information from various sources, like EMRs or EHRs. These records are usually maintained by an individual (i.e. the patient) and allow to make the health status information available for those who are involved in the treatment process. EMRs are maintained by Care Delivery Organizations (CDOs) and are used to represent and document the health care services delivered to a patient by the maintaining CDO. In most cases each CDO hosts its own database to store EMRs. In order to share this knowledge between CDOs involved in a treatment process, EHRs can be used. An EHR is a subset of the knowledge maintained within the EMRs of the involved CDOs. This means an EHR is used to provide the knowledge required for present and future health care decisions and to exchange this knowledge between participating CDOs. Based on the EMR definition, the primary purpose of an EHR Cloud Application is to obtain relevant knowledge from the EMRs located at different CDOs and to distribute it among involved health care providers. Therefore the main challenges for EHR Cloud Applications are related to security and privacy (Lounis, Hadjidj, Bouabdalla & Challal, 2012).

As most EHR Cloud Applications are organized in a patient-centric fashion and are based on community cloud service models, like the Microsoft HealthVault (Microsoft Corporation [MS], 2013), the security and privacy challenges seen from the patient perspective are reviewed first. As the content of an EHR usually is collected from several EMRs, it has to be defined how access to EMRs from inside the EHR application can be managed. In concerns of privacy, it has to be considered that a patient might only want to make parts of the EHR available to physicians that for instance are only involved in a specific subset of the overall healthcare services delivered during the treatment process. Another crucial requirement is the authenticity of the data represented by EHRs. It has to be ensured that the author (i.e. a physician or a CDO) can be verified, which basically refers to the process of data authentication (Devanbu, Gertz, Martel & Stubblebine, 2002). Treatment decisions based on altered or unauthentic data can cause serious damage to the healthiness of a patient. Seen from a physician's point of view, the capability to collect data from multiple EMR/EHR repositories in a scalable and secure way is important, since a physician might have to handle patients that are present in different EMR systems. This is somehow related to the EMR access management challenge. Moreover, gathering access to patient data stored in multiple CDOs, requires an access control model that involves multiple entities, since both the patient's as well as the respective CDO's authorization is required. Finally, ensuring the data integrity is important, since undesired changes to the data or any loss of information have to be avoided. This is a critical issue when considering multiple CDOs that are updating an EHR, as knowledge might get lost or loose accuracy, if update processes are not properly managed.

EHR Cloud Applications have to cope with the given challenges, in order to provide proper and accepted patient record sharing solutions and to benefit from the cost-effectiveness and availability offered by Cloud based systems. As proposed by Zhang and Liu (2010), the security and privacy challenges can be mapped to three core problems. Secure EHR collection and integration refers to the process of gathering all required knowledge to properly handle the current treatment situation, which also involves that only data related to the current problem is disclosed. Secure storage and access management of EHRs is related to the data authenticity challenge, since the collection of relevant EMRs requires that the resulting EHR is authentic and access can be granted properly. Finally, secure EHR usage models refer to trust between the involved CDOs and physicians (i.e. the consumers of the data), because each involved entity has to ensure that the source of the data can be verified. The main challenge in the next years will be to verify and implement such security models, in order to boost the widespread adoption of EHR Cloud Applications as one building block for the overall information dissemination problem in the healthcare domain.

In order to extend the EHR Cloud capabilities with access to real time data emitted by moving medical sensors, our approach assumes, that medical devices can be shared among CDOs. Therefore we treat medical devices as resources of data. A data resource is considered to be required, if it becomes visible to a CDOs network and emits data. A required resource can be booked and integrated, which refers to the Pay-as-you-go usage model common to Cloud Computing environments. The Medical Device Cloud can either be operated by a third party, a health insurance for instance, or it can be operated in a federated fashion, which means that each participating CDO deploys its own medical devices to the Cloud and allows other CDOs to book them. Treating medical devices as resources of data can be referred to as Information-Acquisition-as-a-Service, which basically was introduced by upcoming concepts like Cyber-Physical Clouds (Craciunas, Haas, Kirsch, Payer, Röck, Rottmann, Sokolova & Trummer, 2010), Vehicular Clouds or Mobile Cloud Computing (Gerla, 2012) respectively.

Cyber-Physical Clouds are based on a sensor virtualization approach. This means that each mobile sensor does not directly execute any application code, but rather hosts a virtualization engine that allows deploying virtual sensors to it. Physical sensors basically act as servers that move in space and execute virtual sensors (Kirsch, Pereira, Sengupta, Chen, Hansen, Huan & Vizzini, 2012). Virtual sensors can migrate between physical ones, which is referred to as cyber-mobility (i.e. moving between sensors hosts). Additionally, virtual sensors can move with their sensor host, which is referred to as physical mobility. Similar to regular Cloud Computing, this allows for efficient resource utilization and enables robust and safe execution of virtual sensors, since each virtual sensor can be isolated from each other. However, as sensors (i.e. medical devices) in the health domain are still very resource constrained, sensor virtualization is not suitable at the moment. Therefore, our approach defines a one-to-one mapping between a physical and a virtual sensor. If a CDO successfully booked and integrated a sensor from a different CDO, a kind of a virtual sensor exists in our backend architecture, which simply refers to a binding inside the device control component. This notion of a virtual sensor allows the application layer to treat the sensor as a regular one, which means that the origin, the owner, the vendor and even the concrete data protocol (semantic interoperability) are hidden by our middleware and the system just interacts with a virtual sensor of a defined type that emits data currently required.

Device Integration Architecture

In order to provide an overall understanding of the required components, I introduce the basic concepts of our architecture for a single operator environment first. I explain how to extend the approach towards the Medical Device Cloud in the next section.

As already introduced, the approach is based on the assumption, that each participating patient is monitored by a Body Area Network (BAN) composed of medical devices with at least one device acting as an aggregator (i.e. smartphone) present. The aggregating device hosts the device integration middleware. The BAN is organized in a fully dynamic fashion, which means that devices can enter or exit at any time without the need for manual reconfiguration. As shown in Figure 3, the architecture aligns to the general model discussed in the background section. In the following I will discuss the backend and the aggregation layer. As the devices layer just consists of a set of medical devices and we do not make any assumptions regarding the device properties (protocol, data format, etc.), no further explanation is required for this layer. A measurement profile to be defined by a physician describes which device types shall be

used at which time. After the aggregating device is bound to a patient, the corresponding measurement profile is loaded from the backend and the device integration process is started.

Backend Layer: Apart from general capabilities like patient management, monitoring, persistent storage or interfaces to Hospital Information Systems (HIS), that refer to the Data Utilization Layer, the backend layer primarily offers a Device Control Layer that is related to the device management component introduced in the background section. All devices currently used or known by an operator are registered in the Device Directory (DD). This means the DD is the central control point for distributing medical devices among the aggregators the operator is responsible for. Therefore, the DD offers two main services. First, it provides knowledge about a medical device, which allows each aggregator device to query all

Figure 3. Overview of the general system architecture in a single operator environment

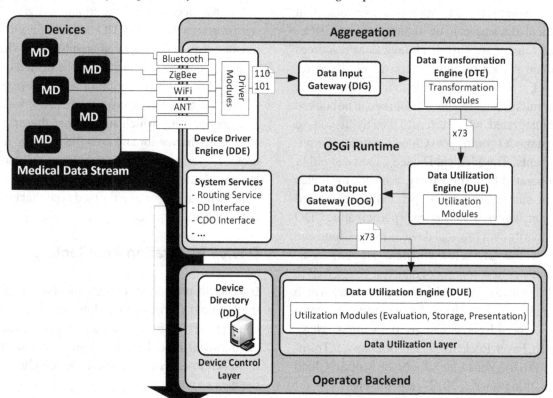

information required to integrate and handle a probably unknown device. Second, a device locking mechanism, that allows to dynamically bind a medical device to an aggregator, is implemented.

Each medical device entry in the DD contains some general information like the vendor, device type or state (e.g. location, time last connected). To support dynamic integration of unknown devices, the general information is extended by supporting modules and the device configuration. A supporting module can be either a device driver, a transformation module or a data utilization module. The integration middleware is able to load these modules during runtime, which means the middleware dynamically reconfigures itself to fit the current requirements. A device driver module refers to the transport component of the integration middleware and allows establishing a connection to a medical device. The resulting data stream might be in any (proprietary) format. Therefore, a transformation module can be loaded and deployed into the data transformation component. If required, the middleware can deploy data utilization modules too. However, as the main purpose is to integrate medical devices and provide the corresponding data streams, deployment and design of data processing or visualization modules is not in scope of this work. Besides the supporting modules, the device configuration is stored. The configuration basically refers to the static part of a x73 Domain Information Model (DIM) as introduced in the background section. Since the DIM is designed in a self-descriptive way, data utilization modules can properly process incoming data streams. If measurements are recorded from a medical device, the values are mapped to the dynamic attributes of the DIM and merged into the static part, that is loaded from the Device Directory. Besides general attributes like the system type, the static part of the DIM provides the semantics that allow to correctly understand and interpret the dynamic measurement attributes.

The second service offered by the Device Directory is a locking mechanism, that allows to bind a medical device to an aggregator (i.e. the patient the aggregator belongs to). This allows the system to dynamically distribute available medical devices among the patients. The effort required to deploy the system is reduced, since no manual interaction is needed if a device is added, replaced or, the measurement configuration is changed. If medical devices are considered as resources, the utilization is optimized, because sharing between patients is allowed. If an aggregator discovers a required medical device, it has to request an exclusive lock for this device from the directory prior to integrating it. A succeeded lock attempt results in a temporary binding between the medical and the aggregating device. The medical device only can be locked by another aggregator, if the current owner frees the lock or the lock timed out.

As the system manages concrete devices, a mechanism to uniquely identify them is required. Medical devices based on x73 already provide such a globally unique identifier, which is based on IEEE EUI-64. Medical devices not based on x73 have to provide an equivalent ID, which could be a concatenation of vendor and serial number. Which concrete values are used, depends on the device discovery process, since the aggregator must be able to extract the ID prior to actually integrating it.

Aggregation Layer: Aggregator devices like smartphones or routers are responsible to integrate medical devices and provide the data streams to the application layer (i.e. data utilization modules). Therefore, they host an OSGi (OSGi Alliance [OA], 2013) based middleware as shown in Figure 3. Because each component is designed as an OSGi bundle, the middleware can be reconfigured during runtime (i.e. device drivers or transformation modules can be reloaded). I will first discuss some general issues regarding aggregators and then introduce the main components of our middleware solution.

The given approach makes a clear distinction between medical and aggregator devices. This is because we do not allow to share aggregators among operators, which means that one aggregator always belongs to one operator, even if it is moved together with the devices it integrates (e.g. in case of a smartphone). Due to security reasons, most operators of medical IT-Networks cannot allow to dynamically integrate such aggregator devices, because they are not as resource constrained as medical devices, usually execute a complete operating system and are often targets of malicious attacks. Moreover, relying on shared aggregators to provide real time access to the medical data streams does not fit for every situation, since we cannot assume that a patient always carries his aggregator with one (e.g. emergency scenarios). Therefore an aggregator always transmits the data it records to the operator it belongs to.

Another important question is how to establish a relation between medical devices and patients. If a patient equipped with a medical device BAN enters a hospital for instance, it is unclear how the aggregator device in the hospital is able to identify, that all medical devices belong to the patient. Obviously, the aggregator is able to discover the medical devices, but cannot make any assumptions about the fact that they all belong to the same BAN or even more important that the medical devices belong to the patient. The hospital staff could equip each new patient with its own private aggregator that again loads the measurement profile and reintegrates all the medical devices based on that profile. However, this does not scale and intensifies possible conflicts, since the medical devices could be discovered by other aggregators and no relation between patient and medical device exists. This means that sharing medical devices is based on establishing new relations between medical devices, aggregators and patients. Therefore, we define two types of aggregator devices, bound and unbound ones:

- **Bound Aggregator:** These aggregators are manually bound to one patient, which means they are able to query the measure-

ment profile from the operator's backend and can establish initial pairings between medical devices and patients.

- **Unbound Aggregator:** Unbound aggregators can handle medical devices from different patients at the same time (e.g. to be used in environments with multiple patients present). To preserve a valid mapping between patient and medical device, unbound aggregators can only connect to sensors that are already bound to a patient (i.e. a lock exists in the Device Directory).

If an aggregator acts as a bound or unbound one has to be decided by the operator. In case a sensor moves between aggregators belonging to the same operator, the DD provides knowledge about active relations and allows integrating the sensor. But if the sensor moves between networks of different operators, a higher-level instance is required to allow for coordination between operators, which is discussed in the Medical Device Cloud section.

The integration of medical devices is handled by the Device Driver Engine (DDE) module. The basic idea of the DDE is to provide a framework for device driver execution that can be implemented on different platforms. Thus, every device vendor just provides one device driver module that complies to the specification of the DDE and therefore can be executed by each DDE implementation. Drivers are stored as supporting modules in the Device Directory and are loaded dynamically if a medical device is discovered. This allows the DDE to handle both proprietary and standard based devices while preserving resources, as only currently required drivers have to be loaded in the system. The DDE specification basically consists of three layers. A hardware abstraction layer hides the complexity of different transport protocols from the device drivers and allows for platform independence, because the driver modules only interact with well defined interfaces provided by the DDE and not with the actual transport protocol stack, that can differ from platform to platform. A discovery layer provides modules that allow discovering devices available through different transport protocols. This layer again consists of several modules that can be loaded during runtime. This is because some proprietary medical devices might rely on proprietary discovery mechanisms (e.g. broadcasts with special magic packets) and cannot be covered with general discovery modules (e.g. in case of Bluetooth). A session layer provides interfaces to the application layer, manages concrete device sessions (i.e. an established connection to a medical device) and reloading of required modules from the DD. If a medical device is discovered by the DDE, an event is generated and the application layer decides based on the measurement profile if the medical device is required. If this is the case, the DDE tries to acquire a lock from the DD. If the lock request succeeded, a session ID, which corresponds to the lock, is generated and the medical device is integrated by loading and instantiating the driver (if required).

The DDE wraps the recorded data and the session ID, into a data container that is forwarded to the Data Input Gateway (DIG). The session ID enables the DIG to identify the device type and configuration and to query the DD for required transformation or utilization modules to load. If a module has to be loaded depends on the configuration of the application layer (e.g. an app executed on the smartphone to display intermediate results) and on dependencies between the modules. A utilization module might depend on the respective transformation module, if the incoming data stream is not aligned according to x73. Based on the loaded modules the DIG performs the actual routing of the incoming data containers. Therefore it uses the routing system service that provides knowledge about the loaded modules as well as the required input streams and produced output streams. A common setup would be to first execute the transformation module and then forward the resulting x73 data containers to all registered data utilization modules.

Transformation modules are hosted inside the Data Transformation Engine (DTE). As mentioned in the Background section, the DTE allows us to achieve semantic interoperability at the application layer. Similar to the DDE, the DTE is able to dynamically load required transformation modules from the Device Directory. As shown in Figure 4, the approach behind the transformation modules can be referred to as template mapping (Sani, Polack & Paige, 2010). Compared to ontology mapping approaches, for instance, template mapping requires providing multiple pairs of templates and their mappings. However, as outlined in Ivanov, Kliem & Kao (2013), the approach is more lightweight and allows for better modularity and it fits to our device driver model. If a device driver module is provided by a vendor, a mapping module can be added easily. Ontology mapping would be the preferred approach, if an openly disclosed and documented abstract meta-model for each incoming data stream (proprietary or standard based) would exist, which is not the case for every vendor. Moreover, adoption of required technologies like the Web Ontology Language (W3C, 2012) or the Resource Description Framework is only partially supported or nonexistent for mobile and embedded systems usually, because of the required resources. The template mapping approach, therefore, fits to our general system model, because it allows to split the overall problem in a lot of lightweight modules and to deploy them if required.

After all registered utilization modules that perform manipulation on the incoming data stream were executed, the stream can be forwarded to the Data Output Gateway (DOG). The DOG then utilizes the CDO interface to transmit the stream to the backend. Communication between the aggregator and the backend is currently realized

Figure 4. Template Mapping example from a binary input stream to a x73 aligned output stream

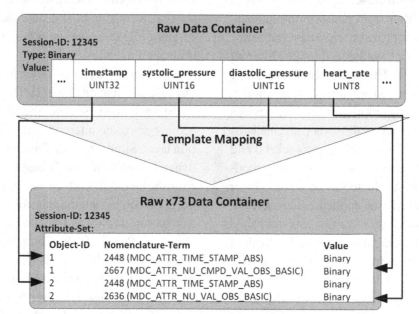

with Restful Web Services, because the required libraries are very lightweight and available for most mobile embedded systems.

Depending on the type of the medical device, the measurement profile and, the locking rules defined in the DD, the device might be unlocked if the measurement was completed. This allows to bind the device to a new aggregator (i.e. patient). Another instance of the aggregation middleware might be hosted at the backend, if further utilization modules have to be executed. This can happen, if two or more aggregators transmit data of one patient or complex algorithms are required to process the data.

In summary, the aggregator provides a lightweight middleware that is able to be reconfigured during runtime without any manual interaction. Therefore the middleware uses the knowledge about the available medical devices provided by the backend (i.e. the Device Directory). The next subsection will briefly discuss, how medical data streams are modeled.

Data Stream Representation

In order to model medical data streams, a data container format is introduced. Each component and module in the system expects a data container that provides a session ID. As already mentioned, the session ID generated by the Device Directory during the lock process allows to identify the corresponding medical device and to load additional modules from the backend, that are required to process the stream. Three types of data containers are defined:

- **Raw Data Container:** Contains the session ID, a type flag and a field with raw (proprietary) data emitted by the device driver. The type flag denotes the type of the raw data (e.g. binary, XML or text).
- **Raw x73 Data Container:** Contains the session ID, a timestamp denoting when the transformed values were recorded and a set of transformed data values aligned to fit

the x73 model. This means that, as shown in Figure 4, every entry is of the shape {object-ID - nomenclature-term - value}, where object-ID refers to the unique identifier of an object in the corresponding DIM and the value is aligned according to the x73 definitions.

- **DIM x73 Data Container:** Contains the session ID, an order ID and a set of data values aligned to fit the x73 model. In addition to the entry shape of the raw x73 data container, a timestamp and a Boolean flag, denoting whether the entry refers to a static or dynamic attribute in the DIM, is used. The order ID enables the data utilization

layer to preserve the correct order of incoming containers. For efficiency reasons, only the first container of one session contains the complete static attribute set.

A raw data container is emitted by the Device Driver Engine every time a new measurement is recorded from the medical device identified by the session ID. The included raw data field can be in any format as defined by the protocol spoken by the medical device. The Data Input Gateway acts as a dispatcher that redirects incoming data containers to the corresponding transformation or utilization module. Therefore it maintains a mapping table and has knowledge about all already

Figure 5. Medical Data Stream representation with a generic container format

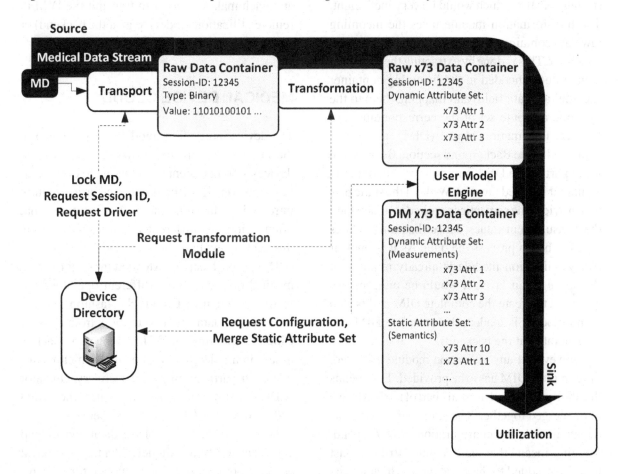

loaded transformation or utilization modules. If the required transformation module is loaded, the raw data container is forwarded.

As described in the last section, transformation could be realized through ontology mapping. However, we decided to use an approach based on specific modules (i.e. template mapping) for each medical sensor or group of sensors that refer to one standard (e.g. ANT+) (DII, 2013) instead of using a uniform transformation engine. This is because the medical data streams emitted by the transport layer can heavily differ. Some sensors produce pure binary values in a very efficient format (e.g. only a small set of ASN.1 encoded integers). Other sensors might produce only text formatted values. In case of a uniform transformation engine, these values first must be transformed to a format expected by the engine (usually XML), which would be very inefficient. The transformation module takes the incoming raw data container and transforms it to a raw x73 container. This is done by extracting the measurement values encoded in the incoming container (i.e. the raw data field) and mapping them to the dynamic attribute set of the corresponding x73 Domain Information Model (DIM), as already explained in the Background section. Because the static part of the DIM is missing at this step, the container is called raw x73. Without the static part that provides the semantics required to understand the measurement values, data utilization modules are not able to process the data. As it is unclear if any utilization module is already required at the aggregation layer, it would be unnecessary overhead to create the complete DIM at this step (if no module is loaded, the complete DIM can be generated at the backend).

However, if any utilization module is loaded, the complete DIM has to be provided. This means that the dynamic and the static part of the DIM have to be merged together. The static part is saved as the medical device configuration at the backend. Merging means that the dynamic attributes just have to be added to the static ones, which results

in a DIM x73 data container. One possible approach to supply the merged DIM is to exploit the object-oriented model provided by our x73 stack implementation. This layout directly refers to the standard's recommendations and is very easy to process. However, as the DIM x73 Data Container format is organized in an incremental fashion (only the first container includes the static DIM attributes) and the transmission of the whole object tree is rather expensive, we decided to use a table based representation similar to the Raw x73 Data container instead. Every row includes the x73 aligned attribute itself, the object-ID the attribute belongs to and a timestamp reporting when the attribute entry was changed. This way, each client (i.e. data utilization module) is able to restore the complete state of a DIM at any time of a valid session. Moreover, this table based approach makes it easier to transmit the DIM to remote utilization models (e.g. at the backend) or to store it to a database.

MEDICAL DEVICE CLOUD

The device integration middleware presented in the last section already allows sharing medical devices among patients that belong to one operator. However, most treatment scenarios require introducing different medical institutions that often belong to different operators. Therefore, this section explains how the Device Directory (DD) approach can be extended in order to share medical devices among different operators and to treat them in a Cloud like fashion as pure resources of data. Related to the introduction of Cloud Computing for E-Health, the approach is based on a federated architecture, which means that each participating Care Delivery Operator (CDO) deploys his own devices into the Cloud and allows other CDOs to book them.

The main prerequisite of a medical device cloud is the capability to uniquely identify a medical device among all participating operators. Therefore, we simply extend the Device Directory by implementing a Global Device Directory (GDD). As shown in Figure 6, the GDD acts as a negotiator between different operators and provides a global registry of all devices available in the Medical Device Cloud. If a medical device is discovered inside a CDOs network and the respective aggregator decides to integrate the device, a lock request is sent to the CDOs local DD. If the operator does not find the medical device in his local DD, the GDD has to be queried. The GDD then provides all necessary modules (e.g. device driver, transformation module) required to integrate the device. A medical device not registered in the local DD, implies that a different CDO owns the device. Each operator participating in the Medical Device Cloud acts as the device master for the medical devices he owns. In order to temporally transfer the access rights, the discovering operator has to enter a negotiation phase with the device master. The GDD maintains a master entry for every device known, which allows to identify the master for each medical device. The negotiation phase is similar to the device locking process described in

the previous section. Instead of granting the lock to an aggregator, the master grants the lock to another operator (i.e. a local DD). According to the sensor virtualization definition in the background section, a succeeded lock request results in a temporally binding of a physical medical device to virtual one present in the local device directory of the CDO. This notion of a virtual medical device hides the Cloud complexity from the using CDO, since it is not important who owns the physical device and which concrete device type is used, as long as the resulting data streams aligns to the definitions in the local Device Directory and the expected format. The virtual device entry in the directory provides all necessary knowledge (x73 configuration, device driver, transformation module) to properly handle the integration and the resulting stream.

Besides granting access rights, withdrawal has to be considered. If the medical device is moved to another aggregator, the protocol described leads to an access request at the master. One could assume that the medical device already left the network of the previous CDO and therefore can be integrated

Figure 6. Medical Device Cloud infrastructure

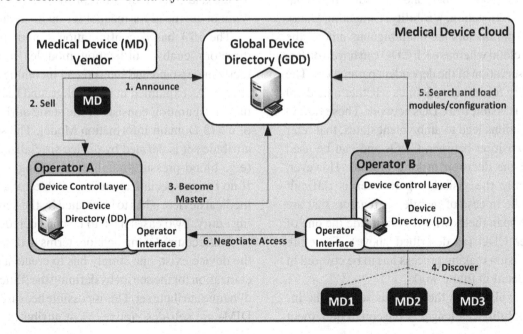

without any conflicts. But this assumption does not hold in case of nearby located or overlapping operator networks. A typical scenario for overlapping networks is a mobile aggregator (e.g. smartphone) that belongs to the Telemedicine operator and is carried into the range of a hospital operator network. The mobile aggregator still holds an active connection to the medical devices (i.e. the BAN or the patient), but the hospital physician needs access to the data streams. As a result, the master is always required to withdraw active locks prior to granting access to new operators.

The problem of overlapping networks results in a decision making process. The owning CDO needs to decide when to withdraw and grant locks. One approach is to simply rate participating CDOs according to their criticality. A hospital for instance, would get a higher rating than a Telemedicine-provider for instance and therefore be allowed to take the lock. This approach involves a lot of manual configuration and might not be fine grained enough (e.g. in case of a transition between the Telemedicine-provider and a practitioner). Another approach is to introduce a state model for medical devices. A medical device in the Cloud can be represented by global parameters (device owner and lock owner) and CDO dependent parameters (Location, Visibility, Collecting Data). Global parameters are unambiguous among the whole cloud whereas each CDO can have a different observation of the dependent parameters. The visibility for instance defines whether a medical device is visible to a CDOs network. These variant observations lead to ambivalent states, that refer to a transition between CDOs and can be used during the decision making process. However, especially the visibility parameter is difficult to handle in case of mobile aggregators that are able to span their own network inside the one of another CDO (as described above). Therefore the decision making process has to be covered in more detail in future work.

As explained in the previous section, the interoperability challenge, as the core requirement in order to allow CDOs to share medical devices independent from the model or vendor, is covered with distributing knowledge about a device through the Device Directory structure. Every CDO in the medical device Cloud is therefore enabled, to reconfigure its aggregation layer middleware according to the current needs. I will briefly explain how devices can be deployed to the Cloud in the next section.

Medical Device Deployment

Deployment of a medical device to the Cloud takes two steps. First the device has to be announced to the Global Device Directory. In case of a new device type or model, the supporting modules (device driver and transformation module) and the x73 aligned configuration have to be supplied. The second step is to define the device owner (i.e. the master). If the device was already announced by the owning CDO, this step is unnecessary. Otherwise, if the device was announced by the device vendor, for instance, taking the ownership can be protected by a predefined token, shared between the vendor and the CDO that bought the device. This model of vendor based device deployment, allows for a Plug and Play integration of medical devices, without any need for manual set-up procedures.

The x73 based configuration stored in the directory enables utilization modules to correctly understand and interpret an incoming data stream. As explained in the Background section, the configuration consists of the static attributes of a x73 Domain Information Model. The static attribute set is defined by device specializations (e.g. blood-pressure-monitor, weighing-scale). If no fitting specialization is available for a new medical device, it has to be created by the deploying entity. Two cases have to be considered:

If all required nomenclature terms to describe the device exist, one simply has to create a specialization for the sensor by defining the static and dynamic attribute set. This is possible because x73 DIMs are self-descriptive. Most attributes used

Figure 7. Deployment of medical devices and corresponding supporting modules

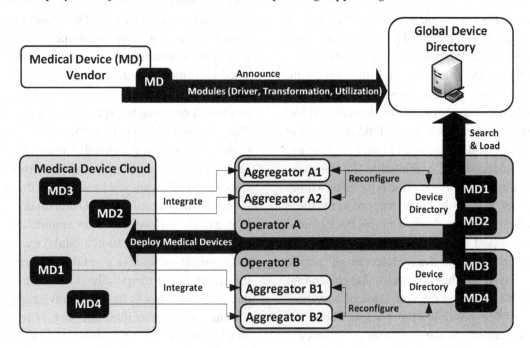

do not represent measured values. Rather they are used as a semantic description of the actual measurement attributes. This is underlined by the fact, that x73 compliant managers are able to operate with an agent (i.e. medical device) without having predefined knowledge about the DIM. Instead the DIM is exchanged during a configuration phase in this case. Therefore, data utilization modules can be designed in a generic fashion and deal with unknown specializations.

In the second case, if required terms are missing and cannot be composed of several existing ones (e.g. a missing Dimension), the required terms have to be added to private areas (i.e. vendor defined) in the available x73 partitions. This would allow for a uniform understanding within the medical institution that hosts one instance of the drafted architecture. Data exchange between medical institutions can be realized through transformation from x73 to HL7 (Health Level Seven [HL7], 2013) for instance. However, adding nomenclature terms involves adapting data utilization modules, which want to process data from the new sensor.

Terminology management as described in the background section could then be used to take the new terms to standardization.

SECURITY AND PRIVACY ISSUES

Privacy and security are core requirements in the healthcare domain. Therefore, common threats and possible attacks, especially the ones related to wireless sensor networks (e.g. Denial of Service, location tracking, eavesdropping or modification of medical data), have been discussed in several publications (Ko, Lu, Srivastava, Stankovic, Terzis, & Welsh, 2010;Ng, Sim & Tan, 2006). Besides threats related to the system performance and availability, a common classification can be found based on the principles confidentiality, integrity and authenticity (Marti, Delgado & Perramon, 2004).

Attacks related to confidentiality include eavesdropping, for instance, and basically are intended to get access to some kind of private information. This can be achieved by either intercepting the communication links or accessing stored data (i.e. attacking Hospital Information Systems). Eavesdropping of communication links is related to the entire data transmission chain. Regarding the device integration architecture, this includes the links between the devices and the aggregation layer as well as the links between the aggregation and the backend layer. Partala et al., (2013) analyzed threats related to the transmission chain. Their classification is based on a three tier model, that easily can be mapped to the three layered architecture defined in the Background section. Based on the possible threats and the distributed, multiple tier architecture of mobile e-health systems, they concluded that end-to-end security from the source to the sink of a medical data flow is not possible at the moment. Therefore, the vulnerability of tier 2 devices (i.e. aggregation layer) has to be further investigated in future work, since especially devices like smartphones are more frequently attacked in recent years. Because the device integration architecture allows for bound aggregators, that represent a concrete relation to a patient, data anonymization could be intercepted throughout the transmission chain. However, the security of our transmission chain is based on the protocols used. Since one of the main requirements was to provide interoperability among the Medical Device Cloud participants and allow to integrate sensors without restriction of used transport protocols, the system has to rely on the given security models provided by these transports (e.g. Bluetooth or Zigbee). The goal is, that the Device Driver Engine always enforces the usage of the highest level available for a certain transport. The transmission between aggregators and the backend layer is based on RESTful Web Services that can be encrypted using SSL. Since aggregators are bound to a CDO and not shared, the key distribution can be managed easily. A possible approach is to use PAKE (Password authenticated key exchange) protocols (Bellare, Pointcheval & Rogaway, 1992) during initialization of an ag-

gregator, where the password could be an internal patient ID assigned by the CDO. Apart from the bound aggregator issue mentioned, eavesdropping attacks are mitigated due to anonymization, since each medical stream is only identified by the session ID generated during the device lock process. A mapping between patient and medical data streams first happens at the CDOs backend. Confidentiality threats related to unauthorized access of stored data, are not in scope or this work, since the middleware just forwards the data to the information systems of a CDO and do not persist it at any step. However, if an application layer module (i.e. data utilization module) executed at the aggregation layer (e.g. a GUI application on the smartphone) temporally stores intermediate data, this issue has to be further investigated.

The second principle, integrity, is related to attacks that intercept the transmission or access stored data in order to modify the content. Even if the transmission chain is protected against eavesdropping, by encryption for instance, an attacker might still modify the data blindly. Therefore, mechanisms like redundancy codes, checksums or, message signatures are required. At the moment the middleware relies on the integrity mechanisms provided by the transports and the data stream representation does not include any application layer mechanisms that allow signing the contents. However, I plan to integrate this feature in the future. It is planned that the device directory component provides capabilities for key distribution and message signatures, since it already generates the session ID, which identifies a medical data stream.

The third principle, authenticity, can be covered with shared secrets, because an attacker usually tries to make the recipient believe, that the data comes from an authentic source. With regard to the devices layer, it has to be ensured, that no malicious device is injected (e.g. an attacker could emulate a device of a certain type) into the Cloud. The only requirement for an attacker is to guess a valid pair of medical device ID and medical device type, which can be achieved rather easily. However, since the architecture has to rely on the capabilities of the transport protocols used and cannot modify the application layer protocol (i.e. inject shared secrets) used by a medical device, it is difficult to achieve authenticity among the devices layer. The problem could be mitigated by heuristic approaches that for instance observe the movement and the emitted data of a medical device, which would increase the effort required to guess a valid sensor ID and type pair at the estimated location. Authenticity regarding the aggregation layer is related to the already mentioned key distribution and PAKE protocols used during the initialization of an aggregator.

An issue specifically related to the Medical Device Cloud approach is the federated structure and the resulting device sharing problem. As mentioned in the Medical Device Cloud section, reliable granting and withdrawal of device access rights is required. Reliable granting and withdrawal of access rights relies on trusted relationships between the participating CDOs as well as between a CDO and its corresponding aggregators. Trusted relationships between operators have to be established on the basis of contracts between the CDOs participating in the Medical Device Cloud. This can be either organized by a third party (e.g. governmental health ministry) or on a peer to peer basis. Since a medical device owner can always reject incoming device access requests, CDOs with unconfirmed identity can be handled properly. Trusted relationships between CDOs and aggregators are related to the authenticity principle discussed above.

If the chain of trusted participants is intercepted, by a malicious aggregator for instance, especially the withdrawal process of access rights could be damaged, because medical device release requests can be rejected unexpectedly or without any acknowledgement. With regard to the authenticity principle definition, we developed a security protocol based on a Public-Key-Infrastructure (PKI) and shared secrets (Kliem, Hovestadt & Kao,

2012). The protocol allows for reliable granting and withdrawal of device access rights even if a compromised CDO or aggregator does not release a revoked device. However, the protocol involves adaption of the communication protocols used by medical devices and the medical devices itself, which is difficult to achieve and contradicts our interoperability requirement. Therefore it has to be analyzed how such a global concept can be properly mapped to the actual communication protocol capabilities used in the system (e.g. Bluetooth provides PIN based models).

As mitigation to this problem, code signing concepts provided by the OSGi security layer can be used. Because each device driver module is an OSGi bundle, it can be signed and verified prior to be executed. Therefore, we integrate the medical device locking and unlocking process into the device driver bundles. We only allow bundles that are signed by the Global Device Directory operator to be executed. This means that only bundles that are signed and verified are involved in the medical device integration process.

FUTURE RESEARCH DIRECTIONS

Currently the proposed device integration architecture and the device deployment model is applied to a broader range of application domains. In the scope of the - Forschungscampus: Connected Technologies - project (Forschungscampus Connected Technologies [FCT], 2013) parts of the system are used to integrate devices in the Smart Home and Ambient Assisted Living (AAL) domain.

Related to the Medical Device Cloud application, future work primarily targets the decision models used to negotiate device access requests and the security issues mentioned. Especially scenarios where CDO networks are located nearby or overlap need to be investigated. Smooth handover processes are required to allow seamless monitoring if a medical device is moved between different aggregators, even in case the aggregators belong to the same CDO (e.g. in case of separated clinical wards). It has to be further investigated, how the authenticity principle can be properly reflected by the protocol agnostic system architecture.

Regarding the medical data stream processing, the dynamic placement of data utilization as well as transformation modules has to be analyzed. It is not necessarily required to host the transformation module at the aggregation layer, if no utilization is performed here. Moreover, based on the data input and output format description introduced by the generic container format and the knowledge provided by the device directory, utilization and transformation modules could be orchestrated dynamically along the data path. This also includes to consider multiple transformation modules that for instance allow to transform the stream to formats used inside clinical or EHR Cloud environments (e.g. HL7).

Finally, with respect to the increasing resources of embedded mobile devices, the system architecture can be extended towards hybrid devices, that both allow for data sensing and aggregation. This also involves network structures, where multiple aggregators or hierarchies of aggregators can be used to collect and pre-process the medical data streams.

CONCLUSION

I presented an approach for E-Health systems that allows for Plug and Play integration of medical devices in a protocol and vendor agnostic fashion. The fundamental basis is a middleware solution that can be reconfigured dynamically during runtime. This is achieved by maintaining a global registry of devices and providing knowledge (i.e. modules), that is deployed to the middleware if required.

The overall architecture allows sharing medical devices among different networks and Care Delivery Operators, which I defined as the Medical Device Cloud. Due to the movement of a patient and the resulting treatment process that can be composed out of different involved institutions (CDOs), the architecture might fit the requirements of current e-health systems in a more suitable way. Compared to common knowledge dissemination approaches in the E-Health domain (e.g. EHR Clouds), the presented approach is about sharing the devices (i.e. the data sources) instead of sharing the data themselves. Sharing data often underlies several judicial restrictions. Sharing devices can mitigate this problem and allow for further treatment process optimizations.

The presented approach aims to increase resource utilization and cost-effectiveness as well as data availability by applying the popular Cloud Computing Pay-as-you-go model to a set of medical devices that are able to move in space. Medical devices are considered as resources of data that can be booked by a CDO as long as they are visible and the CDO considers them to be required. Therefore, the system is an extension to the upcoming Electronic Health Record Cloud Applications. EHR Clouds provide the history of a patient by gathering patient records from several institutions that were involved in the treatment, whereas the Medical Device Cloud allows for real-time access to the data emitted by the patient's sensors.

REFERENCES

W3C. (2012). OWL 2 Web Ontology Language Document Overview (2nd Ed.). *W3C Recommendation*. Retrieved October 24, 2013, from http://www.w3.org/TR/owl2-overview/

Bellare, M., Pointcheval, D., & Rogaway, P. (2000). Authenticated key exchange secure against dictionary attacks. In *Proceedings of Advances in Cryptology—Eurocrypt 2000* (pp. 139–155). Bruges, Belgium: Springer. doi:10.1007/3-540-45539-6_11

Bluetooth, S. I. G. (BSIG). (2013). Health Device Profile. *Health Device Profile - Bluetooth Technology Special Interest Group.* Retrieved October 23, 2013, from https://www.bluetooth. org/en-us/specification/assigned-numbers/health-device-profile

Buxmann, P., Weitzel, T., von Westarp, F., & König, W. (1999). The standardization problem: An economic analysis of standards in information systems. In *Proceedings of the 1st IEEE Conference on Standardisation and Innovation in Information Technology SIIT '99* (pp. 57-162). IEEE.

Continua Health Alliance (CHA). (2013). About the Alliance. *About the Alliance - Continua Health Alliance.* Retrieved October 23, 2013, from http:// www.continuaalliance.org/about-the-alliance

Craciunas, S. S., Haas, A., Kirsch, C. M., Payer, H., Röck, H., Rottmann, A., et al. (2010). Information-acquisition-as-a-service for cyber-physical cloud computing. In *Proceedings of the 2nd USENIX conference on Hot topics in cloud computing* (pp. 14-14). USENIX Association.

Devanbu, P., Gertz, M., Martel, C., & Stubblebine, S. G. (2002). Authentic third-party data publication. In *Data and Application Security* (pp. 101–112). Schoorl, The Netherlands: Springer US. doi:10.1007/0-306-47008-X_9

Dynastream Innovations Inc. (DII). (2013). ANT+. *ANT+ Vision.* Retrieved October 24, 2013, from http://www.thisisant.com/company/

European Commission (EU). (2013). Living Healthy, Ageing Well. *Digital Agenda for Europe.* Retrieved October 24, 2013, from http:// ec.europa.eu/digital-agenda/en/life-and-work/ living-healthy-ageing-well

Forschungscampus Connected Technologies (FCT). (2013). Forschnungscampus Connected Technologies. In *Connected Living e.v.: Forschnungscampus.* Retrieved October 23, 2013, from http://www.connected-living.org/projekte/forsch-nungscampus

Garets, D., & Davis, M. (2006). *Electronic medical records vs. electronic health records: Yes, there is a difference* (policy white paper). Chicago: HIMSS Analytics.

Gerla, M. (2012). Vehicular Cloud Computing. In *Proceedings of Ad Hoc Networking Workshop (Med-Hoc-Net),* (pp. 152-155). IEEE.

Health Level Seven International (HL7). (2013). About HL7. *About Health Level Seven International.* Retrieved October 23, 2013, from http:// www.hl7.org/about/index.cfm?ref=nav

Heiler, S. (1995). Semantic interoperability. *ACM Computing Surveys, 27*(2), 271–273. doi:10.1145/210376.210392

International, I. H. E. (IHE). (2013a). Integrating the Healthcare Enterprise. *IHE - Integrating the Healthcare Enterprise* Retrieved October 23, 2013, from http://www.ihe.net/

International, I. H. E. (IHE). (2013b). PCD Profile Rosetta Terminology Mapping. *PCD Profile Rosetta Terminology Mapping - IHE wiki.* Retrieved October 23, 2013, from http://http://wiki.ihe.net/ index.php?title=PCD_Profile_Rosetta_Terminology_Mapping

ISO/IEC. (1994). Information technology - Open Systems Interconnection - Basic Reference Model: The Basic Model. In ISO/IEC 7498.1:1994(E) (pp. 1-68). ISO/IEC.

ISO/IEC/IEEE. (2010). ISO/IEC/IEEE Health Informatics–Personal Health Device Communication–Part 20601: Application Profile–Optimized Exchange Protocol. In ISO/IEEE 11073-20601:2010(E) (pp. 1-208). IEEE.

ISO/IEEE. (2004). ISO/IEEE Health Informatics–Point-Of-Care Medical Device Communication–Part 10101. In ISO/IEEE 11073-10101:2004(E) (pp. 0-492). IEEE.

Ivanov, D., Kliem, A., & Kao, O. (2013). Transformation Middleware for Heterogeneous Healthcare Data in Mobile E-health Environments. In *Proceedings of the 2013 IEEE Second International Conference on Mobile Services* (pp. 39-46). IEEE Computer Society.

Kirsch, C., Pereira, E., Sengupta, R., Chen, H., Hansen, R., Huang, J., et al. (2012). Cyber-physical cloud computing: The binding and migration problem. In *Proceedings of the Conference on Design, Automation and Test in Europe* (pp. 1425-1428). EDA Consortium.

Kliem, A., Hovestadt, M., & Kao, O. (2012). Security and Communication Architecture for Networked Medical Devices in Mobility-Aware eHealth Environments. In *Proceedings of the 2012 IEEE First International Conference on Mobile Services* (pp. 112-114). IEEE.

Ko, J., Lu, C., Srivastava, M. B., Stankovic, J. A., Terzis, A., & Welsh, M. (2010). Wireless sensor networks for healthcare. *Proceedings of the IEEE*, *98*(11), 1947–1960. doi:10.1109/JPROC.2010.2065210

Löhr, H., Sadeghi, A. R., & Winandy, M. (2010). Securing the e-health cloud. In *Proceedings of the 1st ACM International Health Informatics Symposium* (pp. 220-229). ACM.

Lounis, A., Hadjidj, A., Bouabdallah, A., & Challal, Y. (2012). Secure and Scalable Cloud-based Architecture for e-Health Wireless sensor networks. In Proceedings of Computer Communications and Networks (ICCCN), (pp. 1-7). IEEE.

Martí, R., Delgado, J., & Perramon, X. (2004). Security specification and implementation for mobile e-health services. In *Proceedings of e-Technology, e-Commerce and e-Service* (pp. 241–248). IEEE. doi:10.1109/EEE.2004.1287316

Microsoft Corporation (MS). (2013). Explore HealthVault. *HealthVault - Overview*. Retrieved October 23, 2013, from http://www.healthvault.com/us/en/overview

Ng, H. S., Sim, M. L., & Tan, C. M. (2006). Security issues of wireless sensor networks in healthcare applications. *BT Technology Journal*, *24*(2), 138–144. doi:10.1007/s10550-006-0051-8

OSGi Alliance (OA). (2013). About the OSGi Alliance. *OSGi Alliance*. Retrieved October 23, 2013, from http://www.osgi.org/About/HomePage

Partala, J., Keränen, N., Särestöniemi, M., Hämäläinen, M., Iinatti, J., Jämsä, T., et al. (2013). Security threats against the transmission chain of a medical health monitoring system. In *Proceedings of the 2013 IEEE 15th International Conference on e-Health Networking, Applications and Services* (pp. 218-223). IEEE.

Sani, A. A., Polack, F., & Paige, R. (2010). Generating Formal Model Transformation Specification Using a Template-based Approach. In *Proceedings of the 3rd York Doctoral Symposium on Computing* (pp. 11-18). York, UK: University of York.

Varshney, U. (2007). Pervasive healthcare and wireless health monitoring. *Mobile Networks and Applications*, *12*(2-3), 113–127. doi:10.1007/s11036-007-0017-1

Yao, J., & Warren, S. (2005). Applying the ISO/IEEE 11073 standards to wearable home health monitoring systems. *Journal of Clinical Monitoring and Computing*, *19*(6), 427–436. doi:10.1007/s10877-005-2033-7 PMID:16437294

Zhang, R., & Liu, L. (2010). Security models and requirements for healthcare application clouds. In Proceedings of Cloud Computing (CLOUD), (pp. 268-275). IEEE.

ADDITIONAL READING

Armbrust, M., Fox, A., Griffith, R., Joseph, A. D., Katz, H. R., & Konwinski, A. et al. (2010). A View of Cloud Computing. *Communications of the ACM*, *53*(4), 50–58. doi:10.1145/1721654.1721672

Asare, P., Cong, D., Vattam, S. G., Kim, B., King, A., Sokolsky, O., & Mullen-Fortino, M. (2012, January). The medical device dongle: an open-source standards-based platform for interoperable medical device connectivity. In *Proceedings of the 2nd ACM SIGHIT International Health Informatics Symposium* (pp. 667-672). ACM.

Bicer, V., Laleci, G. B., Dogac, A., & Kabak, Y. (2005). Artemis message exchange framework: semantic interoperability of exchanged messages in the healthcare domain. *SIGMOD Record*, *34*(3), 71–76. doi:10.1145/1084805.1084819

Boulos, M. N., Wheeler, S., Tavares, C., & Jones, R. (2011). How smartphones are changing the face of mobile and participatory healthcare: an overview, with example from eCAALYX. *Biomedical Engineering Online*, *10*(1), 24. doi:10.1186/1475-925X-10-24 PMID:21466669

Brito, M., Vale, L., Carvalho, P., & Henriques, J. (2010, August). A sensor middleware for integration of heterogeneous medical devices. In *Engineering in Medicine and Biology Society (EMBC), 2010 Annual International Conference of the IEEE* (pp. 5189-5192). IEEE.

Cayirci, E., & Rong, C. (2008). *Security in wireless ad hoc and sensor networks*. John Wiley & Sons.

Dagtas, S., Natchetoi, Y., & Wu, H. (2007, June). An integrated wireless sensing and mobile processing architecture for assisted living and healthcare applications. In *Proceedings of the 1st ACM SIGMOBILE international workshop on Systems and networking support for healthcare and assisted living environments* (pp. 70-72). ACM.

Fan, L., Buchanan, W., Thummler, C., Lo, O., Khedim, A., Uthmani, O., & Bell, D. (2011, July). Dacar platform for ehealth services cloud. In *Cloud Computing (CLOUD), 2011 IEEE International Conference on* (pp. 219-226). IEEE.

Hassan, M. M., Song, B., & Huh, E. N. (2009, February). A framework of sensor-cloud integration opportunities and challenges. In *Proceedings of the 3rd international conference on Ubiquitous information management and communication* (pp. 618-626). ACM.

Kindberg, T., & Fox, A. (2002). System software for ubiquitous computing. *Pervasive Computing, IEEE*, *1*(1), 70–81. doi:10.1109/MPRV.2002.993146

King, A., Procter, S., Andresen, D., Hatcliff, J., Warren, S., Spees, W., & Weininger, S. (2009, May). An open test bed for medical device integration and coordination. In *Software Engineering-Companion Volume, 2009. ICSE-Companion 2009. 31st International Conference on* (pp. 141-151). IEEE.

Kirn, S. (2003). Ubiquitous healthcare: The onkonet mobile agents architecture. In *Objects, Components, Architectures, Services, and Applications for a Networked World* (pp. 265–277). Springer Berlin Heidelberg. doi:10.1007/3-540-36557-5_20

Krumm, J. (Ed.). (2009). *Ubiquitous computing fundamentals*. CRC Press. doi:10.1201/9781420093612

Laukkarinen, T., Suhonen, J., & Hännikäinen, M. (2013). An Embedded Cloud Design for Internet-of-Things. *International Journal of Distributed Sensor Networks, 2013*. (pp. 13). Hindawi Publishing Corporation.

Yuriyama, M., & Kushida, T. (2010, September). Sensor-cloud infrastructure-physical sensor management with virtualized sensors on cloud computing. In *Network-Based Information Systems (NBiS), 2010 13th International Conference on* (pp. 1-8). IEEE.

KEY TERMS AND DEFINITIONS

Cloud Computing: Cloud allows to consume large amounts of resources, like computing, storage, or, software, over the Internet without the need for any long term contracts. Consumers do not have to be aware of the actual physical location or the physical system that provides the service. Cloud Computing is based on virtual infrastructures that allow to share physical infrastructures among several customers. This leads to a high degree of resource utilization and reduces costs. Customers rent and pay for virtual resources as long as they require them.

Electronic Health Record (EHR): A collection of health information or information about health services a patient received. It is associated with one individual (i.e. a patient). The purpose of an EHR is to share the health information among actors involved in the treatment process of a patient. Therefore, the necessary data is collected from Care delivery Operators that were involved in a patient's treatment process and maintain health information about this patient in their private information systems.

Interoperability: Allows actors in distributed systems to work together by providing a common understanding of the exchanged information. The general definition not only applies to information in the sense of data. It also includes components (e.g. devices) that can be integrated among different actors or replaced.

Mobile: Cloud Computing: An upcoming family of applications, where (embedded) mobile devices can be Cloud users and Cloud service providers at the same time. This on one hand refers to on-demand and real-time information dissemination and processing in peer-to-peer networks of mobile devices. On the other hand this can be considered as mobile resources that move in space and can be booked by consumers. The Cyber Physical Cloud approach extends this notion by adding virtualization to the mobile device domain. Physical mobile devices are servers that move in space and allow hosting virtual mobile devices.

Pay-as-You-Go: A popular billing model in the Cloud Computing domain. Related to Cloud Computing definition, it refers to the fact that customers just rent required resources as long as they consider them to be required, which means they just pay for the time they rented the infrastructure. Customers are not required to rely on long term contracts in order to access the resources they need.

Semantic Interoperability: A specialization of the general definition that is related to the understanding and interpretation of data that is exchanged for different actors of a system. Semantic interoperability provides a common understanding of the data, by using common nomenclatures and data formats. It targets the meaning of the data and not the packaging (i.e. syntax).

Template Mapping: An approach for data transformation between a source and a target model in order to achieve semantic interoperability. Template mapping assumes that for both the source and the target model instances exist (e.g. concrete medical device specializations). The predefined target instance then acts as a template, which is filled with dynamic values from the source instance (e.g. measurements).

Chapter 12
Cloud Computing for BioLabs

Abraham Pouliakis
University of Athens, Greece

Aris Spathis
University of Athens, Greece

Christine Kottaridi
University of Athens, Greece

Antonia Mourtzikou
University of Athens, Greece

Marilena Stamouli
Naval and Veterans Hospital, Greece

Stavros Archondakis
401 General Army Hospital, Greece

Efrossyni Karakitsou
National Technical University of Athens, Greece

Petros Karakitsos
University of Athens, Greece

ABSTRACT

Cloud computing has quickly emerged as an exciting new paradigm providing models of computing and services. Via cloud computing technology, bioinformatics tools can be made available as services to anyone, anywhere, and via any device. Large bio-datasets, highly complex algorithms, computing power demanding analysis methods, and the sudden need for hardware and computational resources provide an ideal environment for large-scale bio-data analysis for cloud computing. Cloud computing is already applied in the fields of biology and biochemistry, via numerous paradigms providing novel ideas stimulating future research. The concept of BioCloud has rapidly emerged with applications related to genomics, drug design, biology tools on the cloud, bio-databases, cloud bio-computing, and numerous applications related to biology and biochemistry. In this chapter, the authors present research results related to biology-related laboratories (BioLabs) as well as potential applications for the everyday clinical routine.

INTRODUCTION

"Leveraging cloud computing technology, bioinformatics tools, can be made available as services to anyone, anywhere, and through any device. The use of large bio-datasets, its highly demanding algorithms, and the hardware for sudden computational resources makes large-scale bio-data analysis an attractive test case for cloud computing" (Hsu, Lin, Ouyang, & Guo, 2013). Cloud computing is a rather new concept related to numerous computers that use Internet

DOI: 10.4018/978-1-4666-6118-9.ch012

infrastructure to communicate producing shared resources such as software, hardware and storage. Nowadays, cloud computing is not widely used for the various tasks related to medicine; however, there are numerous fields that are possible to be applied; thus cloud computing is an emerging field having the potential to change the everyday practice of medicine. The exception to this is the application of cloud for biology and biochemistry where cloud computing has been already applied, and there are numerous paradigms providing novel ideas and state of the art techniques, these paradigms stimulate as well future research in the based on the cloud environment

Within this chapter, we analyze the application of cloud computing technology for the use in the everyday routine of BioLabs, how to efficiently manage images, use applications, infrastructure, storage and processing power. Nowadays the Cloud is not used in the everyday routine of BioLabs, however, it has this potential, and we present the numerous benefits from applications in the modern BioLab. Additionally we provide a thorough bibliographical analysis of Cloud applications for research related to biology and biochemistry with emphasis on drug discovery, genomics and artificial intelligence. At the end of the chapter are presented future research directions according to the authors' views.

BACKGROUND

Selected basic knowledge background components are needed to approach the application of the Cloud on BigData produced by two medical and/or research laboratories related to medicine, namely the Medical Microbiology and the Clinical Biochemistry laboratories.

Medical Microbiology

Medical microbiology is a medicine branch related to the prevention, diagnosis and treatment of infectious diseases. Additionally, studies clinical applications of microbes for health improvement. Clinical microbiology is related to four kinds of microorganisms that may cause infectious diseases; bacteria, fungi, parasites and viruses.

Medical microbiology primarily focuses on the presence and growth of microbial infections in humans, their effects on the body and methods to treat these infections. Medical microbiologists primarily study:

1. Pathogen characteristics,
2. Transmission modes,
3. Growth mechanisms,
4. Infection mechanisms.

Via these studies a treatment can be proposed to physicians, therefore, medical microbiologists usually offer consulting services to physicians, by providing identification of pathogens and suggesting treatment options.

An additional branch of microbiology is related to the study of microbial pathology, mainly for non-pathogenic species in order to determine whether they can be used to develop antibiotics and other treatment methods. Finally, microbiology has other activities related to the population:

1. Identification of health risks related to the population.
2. Monitoring of the evolution of potentially virulent microbes.
3. Monitoring of the evolution of potentially resistant strains of microbes.
4. Education of the community.

5. Provisioning of assistance in the design of health practices.
6. Provisioning of assistance in the prevention and control of epidemics and outbreaks of diseases.

Clinical Biochemistry

Biochemistry is the science of chemistry applied in biology. Therefore, it is the study of chemical processes within and related to living organisms. During the last 50 years, biochemistry created a breakthrough in explaining living processes. Today almost all areas of the life sciences from botany to medicine are engaged in biochemical research. Nowadays the main focus of biochemistry is related:

1. To understand how biological molecules give rise to the processes that occur within living cells.
2. To study and understand how the processes occurring in single cells are related to whole organisms.
3. To understand how the information flow through biochemical signaling and the flow of chemical energy through metabolism, are related to the complexity of life and the related effects.
4. Biochemistry is also closely related to molecular biology and studies the molecular mechanisms by which genetic information encoded in DNA effects and creates life processes, thus molecular biology can be considered a branch of biochemistry, or biochemistry can be viewed as a tool for the study of molecular biology.

Biochemistry is also related with the structures, functions and interactions of biological macromolecules, these include proteins, nucleic acids, carbohydrates and lipids. These molecules are the structural components of cells and responsible for many of the functions associated with life. Cell chemistry is also dependent on the reactions of smaller molecules and ions, for example, water and metal ions (inorganic), or organic molecules such as the amino acids used for protein-synthesis. Biochemistry studies as well the mechanisms used by cells to harvest energy from their environment via chemical reactions (metabolism). These extremely important findings have direct applications in medicine and nutrition (a field closely related to medicine). Clinical biochemistry studies causes and cures of diseases and how to maintain health via nutrition, biochemistry studies as well the effects of nutritional deficiencies.

Obviously there is significant overlap of the activities related to the fields of Medical Microbiology and Clinical Biochemistry. However, if we consider a layered approach the first has the main focus on organisms while the second is related to the molecules of life.

THE CLOUD

Cloud computing is defined as a large number of computers connected through a network (nowadays the Internet), creating a system capable of executing an application on many computers and configuring virtual servers. Virtual servers do not have a physical presence and can be moved around and scaled up or down without to be noticed by end users, like a cloud, this is a possible origin of the term cloud computing. A second origin for the term perhaps is based on the diagrams used by telecommunication network designers; it is a common practice for network designers to use the cloud for networks that they do not wish to show in details; thus the network is sketched as a cloud that ensures delivery and flow of information from the origin to the destination and vice versa, it is quite a common practice that the network designers use a cloud to mention the Internet; therefore, the term Cloud may have an origin as computing facilities or services supplied through the Internet without caring for the details, i.e. where the machines are hosted and how many of these are used to deliver the service.

Cloud users are able to combine and use computing power on an as-needed basis, actually the computational resources that can be offered to the users seem limitless; thus cloud users can have as much processing power is required for their applications. Cloud computing, despite being a new trend related to Information and Communication Technology (ICT), has already showed numerous applications in medicine and health care improvement (Eugster, Schmid, Binder, & Schmidberger, 2013; Glaser, 2011; Kuo, 2011; Lupse, Vida, & Stoicu-Tivadar, 2012; Mirza & El-Masri, 2013; Patel, 2012; Rosenthal et al., 2010; Waxer, Ninan, Ma, & Dominguez, 2013; Webb, 2012). Actually it is forecasted that there will be an increase in the US cloud computing market for medical images approximately 27% by 2018 at a Compounded Annual Growth Rate (CAGR). This is mainly due to the growing volume of medical images and the increasing costs of the ownership for owning Picture Archiving and Communication Systems (PACS) (GlobalData, 2012).

This chapter presents the state of the art related to the application of the cloud for various fields related to Medical Microbiology and Clinical Biochemistry. Obviously the cloud is a very novel technology and has not been extensively incorporated in everyday practice of such laboratories, thus existing applications are rather limited. It also serves as a repository of ideas as we identify and propose potential applications, explore possible solutions for potential problems and finally promote the benefits of transforming traditional routine application of these laboratories into cloud based services.

Majors areas related to the application of the cloud include:

1. Data storage with an emphasis on image archiving and access.
2. Shifting of traditional Laboratory Information Systems to cloud based systems.
3. Support of Quality Control and Quality Assurance (QC and QA) using cloud hosted applications .
4. Shifting of training and proficiency testing services to the cloud and the benefits of this shift
5. Highlights for research using the cloud.
6. The application of virtual slides for microbiology both in everyday practice and research purposes.

Big Data and the Cloud

BigData is a term used to describe a collection of data sets being so large and complex that it becomes extremely difficult to process using the standard and on-hand database management tools or the traditional data processing software applications available. The challenges for BigData include data acquisition, clean-up, storage, search algorithms, data-sharing and transmission, data analysis and finally data visualization. The requirements to handle and process such large data sets is due to the additional information that can be derived from the analysis of a large set of related data, in contrast to the information that can be extracted from separate smaller sets with a similar amount of data. Simply for the same amount of information it is possible to extract more knowledge, this allows finding of correlations, to name a few, some of these are related to spot business trends, quality of research, disease prevention, legal issues related to citations and crime. Thus Big Data is tightly connected to the Cloud due to the fact that the required capacity to store them as well as the computing power required for processing in a reasonable time can be available from the Cloud.

Microbiology and Biochemistry are nowadays producing such a large volume of information, especially due to new types of molecular measurements, that traditional/standard software packages cannot handle and analyze (Dudley & Butte, 2010). Therefore, such information falls in the category of BigData.

However, not all data that occupy a large volume are considered big, for instance the elements of BigData are related to:

- The degree of complexity within the data set.
- The amount of value that can be derived from innovative vs. non-innovative analysis techniques.
- The use of longitudinal information supplements the analysis.

Thus, when defining, the size is not the primary characteristic of BigData, the most appropriate characteristic is the number of independent data sources (separate databases), each one having the potential to interact and be interconnected with one or more. Obviously Big Data cannot be processed by standard data management methods as usually there are inconsistent and unpredictable relations among the different data sources. Big Data have another attribute: they tend to be hard to delete, because they are not always private as they come from different and usually located in different places data sources.

APPLICATIONS OF CLOUD COMPUTING IN BIOLABS

Nowadays modern BioLabs are equipped with numerous modalities capable of performing medical tests and exchange data via networks as well as imaging systems capable of creating digital pictures. Furthermore, modern analyzers are supplied with blocks of biological samples and can perform multiple tests on each sample in parallel. The volume of data in a BioLab nowadays is enormous especially for places where research is conducted; i.e. the 1000 Genomes Project, which has about 200 terabytes of genomic data including DNA sequenced from more than 1,700 individuals, and available from the Amazon cloud (Amazon, 2013a), the data generation of "next generation" sequencing (NGS) which drives the efforts to turn to cloud computing as a solution to handling peak-time loads, without the need to maintain large clusters (Stein, 2010) or the DNA race (Schatz, Langmead, & Salzberg, 2010) that creates requirements for computational solutions to large-scale data management and analysis (Schadt, Linderman, Sorenson, Lee, & Nolan, 2010). The major cloud based applications for BioLabs, can be categorized as applications for the everyday of the medical laboratory and applications for the research laboratory, even though a clear border cannot be defined. The existing applications and the applications envisioned are presented in the sequel sections.

Information Systems for the Laboratories, Quality Issues, and Proficiency Testing

Laboratory information systems (LIS) are used to control the daily workflow of medical laboratories, to store data and communicate incoming and outgoing data and for the extraction of statistics for many varieties of inpatient and outpatient medical tests. LISs have been used in microbiology laboratories earlier than 1982 (Deshpande, 1982). Today it is rather impossible to operate a microbiology laboratory without an LIS (Georgiou, Callen, Westbrook, Prgomet, & Toouli, 2007; Georgiou, Prgomet, Toouli, Callen, & Westbrook, 2011; Toouli, Georgiou, & Westbrook, 2012).

The major features that laboratory information systems have included are management of sample check in, order entry, specimen processing, result entry, patient demographics and patient history. In short, a LIS tracks and stores all the information related to the patient's sample from arrival into the lab and stores the data for future retrieval. LISs produce reports for the tests they handle and statistics related to various aspects of the laboratory such as time for execution of examinations, sample volumes. Modern LISs are handling also storage and supplies (consumables) and can be directly linked to medical devices for direct transfer and storage of examination outcomes, usually via the HL7 protocol (Al-Enazi & El-Masri, 2013; Chronaki et al., 2012; Heymans, McKennirey, & Phillips, 2011; Oemig & Blobel, 2011; Yuksel & Dogac, 2011) to the LIS database.

Biomedical laboratories are heavily dependent on LISs and usually employ information technology (IT) personnel to manage the systems, i.e. the hardware and the software and additionally provide technical expertise and support, and are responsible in cases of infrastructure problems as well as optimize the systems to run mission critical applications, usually install and maintain multiple servers, RAID storage and disk arrays, dual communication lines, power backup systems etc. Cloud computing is changing this, since LISs can be partly or completely outsourced. Cloud computing has inherent all the resilience features required by modern microbiology and in general medical laboratories, additionally if LISs are operated via the Cloud, costs are reduced, by spreading costs associated with infrastructure ownership and support. Nowadays many laboratories are exploiting virtualization services, as they provide on-demand network access virtual servers, storage and applications. Definitely Cloud computing can minimize the cost for owning and managing in-house equipment and reduce required IT personnel. Finally cost reduction is not the only benefit; the set-up and configuration time for a new laboratory wishing to install a LIS hosted in the cloud is minimized due to the fact the cloud infrastructure is always available, in contrast installing physical servers in the laboratory requires time from the purchase order till the installation and configuration of the hardware and software.

Modern laboratories are obliged to adopt quality systems not only for their smooth operation and control but additionally for their "survival," since, in countries of the European Union; all laboratories should be accredited for all examinations performed by 2016. The favorite standard usually adopted by laboratories is ISO 9001, however, modern labs are obliged to follow other standards (such as ISO 15189 for accreditation) to ensure that they provide reliable examination results.

Quality control concepts for microbiology appear before 1970 (Harding, 1965a, 1965b), when quality control was mainly focused to microorganisms cultures. Later, between 1970 and 1980, the first publications appear in the literature stating the need to setup standards (Porres, 1974b), reference laboratories and reference data (Porres, 1974a). Nowadays, clinical microbiology laboratories are automated and are moving towards the molecular era. As a result, the requirements for standards and quality control and assurance have shifted (Kanungo, 2012; Underwood & Green, 2011; van Leeuwen & van Belkum, 2013; Wallace & MacKay, 2013). Today medical microbiology and clinical biochemistry laboratories are fully automated (especially the later), modern information management systems and LISs allow correlations to be performed just immediately after the release of the examination results, and the medical modalities (analysers) allow internal quality control. Data processing based on the stored information can be easily performed in real time or a later stage by the push of a button. Such information is important to acquire knowledge for lab quality and foresee forthcoming issues, allowing lab managers to initiate corrective actions for quality improvement. Cloud computing obviously can be of help for quality monitoring, as specialized software based applications may be developed and operated (Riquelme, Lorente, & Crespo, 2011; Vicentino, Rodriguez, Saldias, & Alvarez, 2009). The Cloud is able to provide centralized applications without restrictions of storage and application load, while additional benefits may be obtained as the quality data can be shared among numerous laboratories. Finally, enhancements of the applications can be immediately available to the laboratories, as there is no need for on-site deployment and time-consuming software installation procedures.

A concept closely related to quality is proficiency testing. BioLabs cannot be considered as qualified if the lab personnel is not proved to be proficient. For BioLabs, proficiency testing is not a new concept, as first publications appear from 1970 (Gavan & King, 1970). Pioneering in this field are the American continent countries such as U.S.A. and Canada (Richardson, Wood, Whitby, Lannigan, & Fleming, 1996; Whitby, Black, Richardson, & Wood, 1982; Wilson et al., 1977). The same applies to biochemical laboratories, especially for genetics (Hommes et al., 1990). Clearly a thorough bibliographic research was not able to prove that the Cloud has added to the field of proficiency testing for Bio-Labs, however, it is a promising technology for numerous applications. For example, proficiency testing nowadays for microbiology laboratories requires slide examination; virtual slides can be of help towards this trend and the advantages of the Cloud for storing and transmitting such large data are obvious.

Images Digital/Virtual Slides and Data Storage

Analysis of glass slides and Petri dishes to study bacteria cultures via the microscope or stereoscope is a part of the daily routine of the modern microbiology laboratory, thus nowadays microbiology laboratories are of need for digital images. Today, digitization of entire glass slides at near the optical resolution limits of light can occur in minutes. Furthermore, there are available systems capable for whole slide imaging. This boosted the application of digital slides (Rudnisky et al., 2007; Taylor, 2011). Digital imaging is unlocking the potential to integrate primary image features into high-dimensional genomic assays creating the opportunity for the application and use of these methods in clinical care and research settings. Virtual slides have variable sizes, ranging from a few hundreds of megabytes to over 1 gigabyte, depending on the magnification and the scanned area. The Cloud can offer advantages for the storage of these data. The cloud may provide affordable and adequate, maintenance-free, assured and easily expandable storage. However transfer of these data from/to the lab and the cloud may be an issue due to the asymmetric communication lines ADSL (Asymmetric Digital Subscriber Loop). ADSL lines have a high capacity of downloading (10ths of Mbits) and smaller capacity for uploading (hundreds of Kbits) this setting creates difficulties for the laboratory to upload massive data to the Cloud. However, the revolution in telecommunication networks may provide the required bandwidth via symmetric DLS lines, and automated slide scanning workstations may operate overnight and store unattended the virtual slide data.

Storage, archival and communication/transfer of images in the cloud allows the industry to manage data more efficiently and cost-effectively, while overcoming many of the technical challenges that data requirements pose (AT&T, 2012). The cloud enables hospitals to handle more efficiently data requiring large-bandwidth, use non proprietary formats and thus push the medical industry to globally accepted standards dropping competition barriers often placed by the medical industry. Additionally, the cost of ownership can be reduced, as system expansion is on a "pay when you need" model and the investments are protected since the product life can be extended through system-wide upgrades on a massive manner.

A BioLab wishing to store images and patient/examination records, today installs one and usually for high availability reasons more than one servers and disk arrays for high data throughput and failure protection. The Cloud has by design inherent the information protection property and availability characteristics. Thus, BioLabs may reduce dramatically all costs related to information and communication technology (ICT) infrastructure, as well as the associated costs for maintenance and licensing. Here the cloud acts as a LIS, and billing system simultaneously.

The issue of digital images, virtual slides and data storage is analyzed in greater detail in the chapter of the book, entitled "Cloud Computing for Cytopathologists," due to the fact that cytopathology laboratory routine work is heavily based on the examination of stained glass slides by humans, which is not the main way for working in the Medical Microbiology BioLab.

Cloud Computing for Research in BioLabs

In silico is an expression used to mean something performed on the computer or via computer simulation. The phrase has an origin back in 1989 and is an analogy to the phrases in vivo, in vitro, and in situ, these phrases refer to experiment done in living organisms, outside of living organisms, and where they are found in nature, respectively. Similarly in silico is used to define experiments performed in computers (silica is the basic substrate for the creation of microchips, the components used for the construction of computers). Modern Microbiology and Biochemistry research is heavily based on experiments performed in Silico (Dudley & Butte, 2010) and due to the production of Big Data, the Cloud has been extensively used and has the potential for a great number of new applications (experiments). Cloud computing according to cost analysis has the potential to be an alternative solution for computational biology (Angiuoli, White, Matalka, White, & Fricke, 2011; Dudley, Pouliot, Chen, Morgan, & Butte, 2010). The data generation rate related to sequencing requires such computing power that suggests Cloud computing as a solution. Nowadays Cloud based bioinformatics tools are available (see next paragraph), especially for high throughput

sequencing and genomics (Afgan et al., 2010) as well as for drug discovery, this has numerous practical and financial advantages (D'Agostino et al., 2013).

Cloud based tools for BioLab informatics. Today there are numerous bioinformatics tools such as Cloud-Coffee (Di Tommaso et al., 2010) and USM (Almeida, Gruneberg, Maass, & Vinga, 2012) based on MapReduce for Sequence alignment, CloudBurst for reference-based read mapping (Schatz, 2009), CloudAligner for short read mapping (Nguyen, Shi, & Ruden, 2011), SEAL for short read mapping and duplicate removal (Pireddu, Leo, & Zanetti, 2011), Crossbow to combine sequence aligner (Langmead, Schatz, Lin, Pop, & Salzberg, 2009), Contrail for de novo assembly (Schatz, Delcher, & Salzberg, 2010), Eoulsan for sequencing data analysis (Jourdren, Bernard, Dillies, & Le Crom, 2012), QUAKE for Quality-aware detection and correction of sequencing errors (Kelley, Schatz, & Salzberg, 2010), Myrna (Langmead, Hansen, & Leek, 2010) for the differential expression analysis for RNA-sequencing, FX RNA for sequence analysis (Hong et al., 2012), ArrayExpressHTS for RNA-sequence process and quality assessment (Goncalves, Tikhonov, Brazma, & Kapushesky, 2011), BioVLab being a virtual collaborative lab for biomedical applications (H. Lee et al., 2012), Hadoop-BAM for direct manipulation of NGS data (Apache Software Foundation, 2013; Niemenmaa et al., 2012), SeqWare: a scalable NoSQL database for NGS data (O'Connor, Merriman, & Nelson, 2010), PeakRanger a peak caller for ChIP-seq (Feng, Grossman, & Stein, 2011), YunBe a gene set analysis for biomarker identification (L. Zhang, Gu, Liu, Wang, & Azuaje, 2012), GATK being a Genome Analysis Toolkit (McKenna et al., 2010), Cloud BioLinux a pioneering virtual machine with more than 130 bioinformatics packages (Krampis et al., 2012), CloVR a virtual machine for automated sequence analysis (Angiuoli, Matalka, et al., 2011), PredictProtein (Kajan et al., 2013; Rost, Yachdav, & Liu, 2004) a suite of open source

Debian packages to predict protein structure, solvent accessibility, nuclear localization signals and intrinsically disordered regions. The Cloud has definitely had already provided numerous services to BioLabs, especially for research, this picture is expected to grow.

Molecular docking simulations for drug research and design. Computer technologies are of help toward drug design and discovery. One approach is the prediction based on theoretical computing molecular modeling to identify the three dimensional structure for new drug molecules, thus to find possible candidate compound solutions. Even though more than one trillion US dollars is invested in drug development, both prediction accuracy and drug identification time are not satisfactory (J. L. Chen, Tsai, Chiang, & Yang, 2013; Volkamer, Kuhn, Grombacher, Rippmann, & Rarey, 2012), since the prediction accuracy is less than 70%, and the drug discovery process takes tremendous computation time simply to find the possible drugs.

In silico molecular docking simulation is one of the main steps of Rational Drug Design (RDD) (Kuntz, 1992; S. Zhang, 2011). It is used to discover compounds by the computational examination of large databases of organic molecules for ligands that fit a binding site of the target molecule or receptor (usually a protein). The good ligand orientation and conformation inside the binding pocket (fitting) is computed in terms of specialized algorithms such as the free energy of bind (FEB) by software such as AutoDock (Abreu, Froufe, Queiroz, & Ferreira, 2010; Morris et al., 2009). However the computing resources to perform such simulation are huge; therefore, Cloud computing can be of help. Recently various research efforts have been conducted towards this direction. De Paris et.al. (De Paris, Frantz, de Souza, & Ruiz, 2013) proposed a cloud-based Web environment, called Web Flexible Receptor Docking Workflow (wFReDoW), which reduces the CPU time for the simulations. The simulations were based on a middleware built on Amazon EC2 cloud platform (Amazon, 2013b). The proposed methodology not only reduced the number of molecular docking simulations but additionally the middleware speeded up the docking experiments using the High Performance Computing (HPC) cloud. The experimental results showed a reduction in the total elapsed time of the simulations. Another research team (J. L. Chen et al., 2013) has employed methods based on Genetic Algorithms (GA) and tested their performance to solve the protein ligand docking problems. The test platform was an in-house developed parallel system (Cloud) composed of 16 virtual machines and the AutoDock software platform (Abreu et al., 2010; Morris et al., 2009). Their results illustrated that the proposed algorithm outperformed other docking algorithms in terms of both the computation time, and the quality of the result, i.e. better prediction accuracy. During the same time, another research team developed a new tool named Cloud-PLBS (Hung & Hua, 2013) a Web portal through which biologists can address a wide range of "questions" related to drug discovery and once again for Protein-Ligand binding site comparison. This tool was based on a combination of the already available platform/ algorithm SMAP (Ren, Xie, Li, & Bourne, 2010) and the open source project Hadoop (Apache Software Foundation, 2013) (a Cloud software platform). Concluding there are numerous efforts for the exploitation of the Cloud capabilities in drug design and discovery, actually, there are nowadays available several drugs discovered via similar methods, for example, Dorzolamide for the treatment of cystoid macular edema (Giuffre, 2006) and Amprenavir for HIV treatment (Goodgame et al., 2000), obviously new efforts to improving the protein –ligand problem solution quality and time via the Cloud will appear in the near future.

Enzyme research. Enzymes in biochemistry are molecules that catalyze the conversion of substrates into products within living organisms; thus enzymes are essential for the metabolism of life. The main characteristics of enzymes are:

- **Catalytic Power:** The ratio of the rate of an enzyme catalyzed reaction to the rate of the not catalyzed reaction, enzymes reduce the energy required for biochemical reactions thus they make reactions faster.
- **Specificity:** As enzymes perform specific actions and are selective to specific reactions.
- **Regulation:** Enzymes help avoid competing reactions from producing side products.

Enzymes are extremely important for the metabolism of components required for cell activities.

In terms of financial figures, the global market for industrial enzymes in 2012 was $3.3 billion and is estimated to reach by 2015 $4.4 billion (Huang, Lin, Chang, & Tang, 2013). In relation to enzyme research, the Cloud has been already applied successfully (Huang et al., 2013). In their research paper, Huang et.al. (2013), have proposed, designed and created a method based on a single execution file, this techniques allow the system to operate to any cloud platform supporting multiple queries. The aim of the tool was to identify one or more enzymes catalyzing one or more reactions, the method is based on the frequency of domain architecture. The authors examined the feasibility of the proposed method using a total of 1,664,839 protein data entries associated with more than one enzyme-catalyzed reaction; the ratio of the number of single enzyme catalyzed reactions to the number of the multiple enzyme catalyzed reactions was approximately 6:4. The authors tested their method via 20 runs of 5 fold cross validation. The accuracy of the method for single enzyme catalyzed prediction was about 90%, and estimation was less accurate for multiple enzyme catalyzed reactions. Via this method

requiring extreme computational power that can be provided by the Cloud, the authors, were able to identify if, for a specific reaction, there is available one or more enzymes catalyzing it, this is an extremely important issue both in biological sciences research as well as in the industry. Cloud services in this paradigm can supply a large scale memory space and computing power required to analyze the enzyme kinetic data.

Genetics. Technological advances for DNA sequencing have lowered the price for personal genome sequence (the 3 billion letters in our DNA) to under $20,000, while new sequencing methods are expected to lower it to less than 1,000$ (Davies, 2010). This has created a new challenge for scientists, related to the large databases required to host the increased data volume and obviously extreme CPU power for data analysis. Cloud computing seems to be the solution for both issues. A side effect of low costs in DNA sequencing comes from the offered opportunity that allows scientists to collect and analyze whole genomes for genome-wide association studies. As such, genetic data do have the potential to be more informative than standard medical records. In addition, the capability offered by cloud computing to access and analyzes such data sets, being supplied by scientific groups around the planet, necessitates either a paradigm shift in the way that science is done, and/or revised understandings of privacy and informed consent. A proposal by some researchers is to promote both shifts (Greenbaum & Gerstein, 2011).

Artificial Intelligence for BioLabs

In this section, we present and analyze applications of artificial intelligence for BioLabs; we focus on artificial neural networks as they are highly parallelizable; therefore they are ideal for implementation via the Cloud that supports the use of numerous interconnected multi-core computers.

A Short Description of Artificial Neural Networks (ANNs)

ANNs are complex computational models inspired by the human brain nervous systems that are capable of machine learning and pattern recognition (Duda, Hart, & Stork, 2001; Theodoridis & Koutroumbas, 2009). These models have the ability to learn from past experience in order to provide outcomes for new data. This capability of learning from a certain dataset makes the neural networks suitable for classification and prediction tasks in practical situations. Furthermore, neural networks are inherently nonlinear, which makes them more suitable for processing complex data patterns, in contrast to many traditional methods based on linear techniques. Historically, ANNs appeared in 1943 when McCullogh and Pitts proposed the idea of an artificial neuron. They proved that it was possible to construct an artificial network with some similarities to a biological neural network, using artificial neurons interconnected with each other, and by the use of mathematical algorithms governing their interactions. In 1949, Hebb proposed the idea of associative learning or Hebbian learning; according to Hebb, when an axon of a cell excites an interconnected cell repeatedly, then a learning mechanism should be applied in both cells; this mechanism should increase the efficiency of firing the second cell when triggered by the firing one. Later, in 1962, Frank Rosenblatt proposed an algorithm to train an ANN by changing the synaptic strengths in the links that interconnect neurons (see Figure 1 for a typical neuron schematic and functional diagram). Rosenblatt proposed an algorithm that altered the synaptic strengths each time the network gave a wrong answer, thus guided the system by "punishment." Unfortunately, later, Minsky and Papert showed that ANNs were not capable of solving extremely simple problems, such as the Exclusive OR (XOR) problem, as ANNs were capable of producing solutions to problems that were representing spaces capable of being separated by a single line. Unfortunately, this finding disappointed researchers and blocked research related to ANNs for the next 5 years, until Werbos introduced the idea of propagating the errors back to former layers of the network ("back propagation of the error algorithm") thus the XOR problem could be solved by more than one interconnected neurons each one implementing a separating line in the feature space. In addition, Hopfield et al., (Haykin, 1994) proved that asynchronous ANNs could find a minimum, using the "least energy"; thus via Hopfield's work ANNs gained the capability to solve, problems requiring minimization of the ANN output, and additionally developed a behavior mimicking capabilities of the human brain (Haykin, 1994). The typical structure of artificial neurons and a layered architecture of the ANN are depicted and explained in Figure.1.

Artificial Intelligence in Medicine and BioLabs: Do We Need the Cloud?

The application of artificial intelligence in medicine is not new (Karakitsos et al., 1996). During the last decades, various techniques have been used in medicine, involving either classical statistical models or more advanced techniques, such as neural networks (Cochand-Priollet et al., 2006; Karakitsos et al., 2011; Pantazopoulos et al., 1998; Varlatzidou et al., 2011).

Neural computing in microbiology has been considered one of the most rising research areas as the number of peer-reviewed scientific articles dealing with microbiology and NNs is constantly increasing the last two decades (Almeida & Noble, 2000). Especially in the area of predictive microbiology, ANNs have been studied for the modeling of microorganism growth (Hajmeer, Basheer, & Najjar, 1997), for classifying bacteria (Giacomini, Ruggiero, Calegari, & Bertone, 2000; Mouwen, Capita, Alonso-Calleja, Prieto-Gomez, & Prieto, 2006) either by supervised techniques as the back

Figure 1. Left: Schematic diagram of an artificial neuron, the inputs (i_1- i_N) are multiplied by the weights (ω_1- ω_N), the products are summarized in Σ block; finally the output is produced by the non-linear function, the output serves as either input to other neurons or as the ANN output. Right: Typical architecture of a feed forward ANN, data are supplied as inputs to the first layer of neurons (the input layer) where processing is performed, the results (outputs of the input layer) are then inputs of the second layer (hidden layer), in the same manner data are processed in each layer until they are processed by the output layer, the results of the last layer are the ANN outputs. It is usual to have one or more hidden layers of neurons.

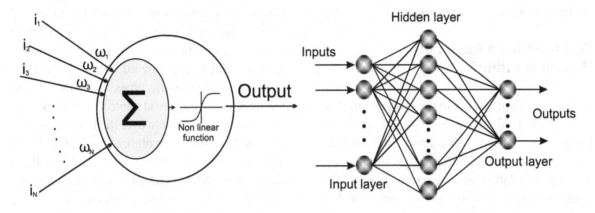

propagation neural network (Haykin, 1994) or unsupervised techniques such as the Kohonen Self Organizing Maps (Kohonen, 2001).

However, ANNs have disadvantages, rising mainly from their nature and construction process (see chapter Cloud computing for Cytopathologists). A typical cycle for the creation of a useful ANN system involves several, but typical steps

1. **Data Collection:** Obtaining the data that will be used to create the intelligent system.
2. **Data Preprocessing:** Depending on the type of the ANN system and algorithm that is selected data preprocessing may require.
3. **ANN Model Selection:** Choice of a suitable ANN type for the problem requiring a solution.
4. **Parameter Selection:** Configuration of the selected ANN parameters.
5. **ANN Training:** Identification of the ANN parameters that actually compose the solution to the problem.

6. **Evaluation:** Check the performance of the produced system on known and unknown data.

If the performance of the system is satisfactory then the produced ANN system can be used in a production environment: otherwise the procedure should start again from an earlier stage. This type of complexity and the requirement to run numerous systems and combinations of ANN types, architectures and parameters increases geometrically the required number of experiments and thus the required computing resources and computing time. Additionally the training procedure for several ANN types is computing "hungry," as it is not unusual that training of some ANNs can take weeks or even months of computer time.

Cloud computing has the capability to provide shared and on demand resources, thus can facilitate the production of ANN system via two ways, by increasing the number of experiments that can run and by decreasing the time of each experiment.

The second advantage of the Cloud in relation to ANNs is parallelism. ANNs are by their nature interconnected processing units (the neurons), therefore, neurons, or blocks of neurons, can be operational on separate cores and communicate their outputs to neurons hosted on other cores of the cloud; thus the cloud is an ideal environment to simulate, train and operate large scale ANNs.

Can the Cloud Assist the BioLab Routine?

Despite the Cloud is, not in the everyday routine of medical BioLabs, it is expected that such laboratories can benefit from the Cloud either by using cloud hosted centralized application for the hospital or by lab specific software systems. The main benefits of the cloud include increased data storage capacity, on the fly availability of new software capabilities as soon as they are available and immediately when required, professional system maintenance and security as well as access control and billing, reduced cost for infrastructures and maintenance, increased productivity.

Until now, BioLabs had to maintain the information and communication technology infrastructure either by own personnel of by hospital personnel managing centralized systems, thus the authority to decide which IT element could improve laboratory daily workflow in some cases was restricted. In the Cloud computing era, BioLabs are expected to use IT services without having to take control over the infrastructure. Cloud computing permits end users to use hardware and software stored remotely over the Cloud-based systems, without having to purchase them, but to apply a pay-per-use model. Thus small BioLabs are able to use infrastructures similar to very big laboratories, and to be competitive in a demanding business environment. Additionally Cloud services can be available over the Internet, thus data can be available to customers and BioLab services consumers without the need for expensive specialized communication channels.

Technical Issues, Problems and Benefits Related to Cloud Computing

The major issue related to cloud computing in the field of medicine is security, as data is stored remotely and transmitted usually via a public network such as the Internet. However, solutions to resolve these issues are available. Unauthorized access to patient data may be ensured by password based access and password control mechanisms, such as minimum password length, forcing the user to include specific types of characters and via mandatory biometric control. Data interception during transmission over the Internet may be secured by encryption algorithms, similarly for data storage into database systems. Additionally, at the service level there have been already proposed solutions for secure encapsulation (W. Zhang, Wang, Lu, & Kim, 2013). These shortcomings arising from the distributed nature of the cloud are surpassed by the advantages: database safety and long-term archival especially in the case of emergencies such as natural disasters can be ensured due to the distributed databases, single server failures are avoided by the use of two or more servers, the offered service efficiency, related to interconnection lines speed is obtained by use of multiple Internet service providers by the cloud owner, and finally increased load can be easily handled by adding more processing power to existing virtual servers, by splitting the application to run on multiple servers, either via load balancing or by the exploitation of multi-tier architectures and employing additional application and database servers.

FUTURE RESEARCH DIRECTIONS

The Cloud offers new computational paradigms related to BigData and analyses at scale, however, the application of the algorithms by a multiplication factor simply to handle the data volume and the increased computational load does not guarantee good results. Working in parallel and at scale has numerous limiting factors related to performance and the associated costs. One aspect requiring more research and efforts is the algorithmic factor and how to optimally exploit the available processing cores; the second aspect is related to logistics, including data locality, transfer speed and cost for networking, network quality (latency) as well as virtual machine start-up. The Cloud can give great benefits, but code refactoring and careful design of the utilisation of computational approaches is required. Cloud computing offers new capabilities but requires new ways of thinking and generates different performance-limiting problems (Kasson, 2013).

In the near future, it is expected that the cloud based research for drug discovery and other biochemistry related fields will continue to grow, simply because computer science has already proved the benefits of its application and because the requirements and needs of the industry are constantly increasing. For economy reasons, it is expected that BioLabs either autonomous or located in hospitals will migrate to Cloud-based LIS due to ease of availability, low cost of ownership and maintenance, as well as immediate adoption of improvements.

Research is the primary area that seems to be already "affected" by the Cloud; sequencing costs are continuously becoming lower, and nowadays it is possible and extremely easy for genomics researchers to acquire and have access to large amounts of data. But, the majority of laboratories has already become or will soon become, oversubscribed and underpowered, simply because it is not possible to store and process data in house in order to acquire knowledge from these. The lack of computational power to run exhaustive search algorithms, eventually, has already leaded numerous researchers towards cloud computing. This trend is expected to increase because of the cost factor, as well. Additionally, cloud computing provides the means for data sharing among research teams,

thus larger data sets can be exploited, and more robust results and conclusions can be obtained. This creates a need for future developments and applications related to standardize data formats and unified databases (J. Chen, Qian, Yan, & Shen, 2013).

Recently, biological applications started to be transformed into applications that exploit many cores of GPUs (Graphics Processing Units) in order to achieve better computation performance. There are already reported architectures specially designed for the BioCloud exploiting the "hidden" processing power offered by GPUs (Jo, Jeong, Lee, & Choi, 2013). The results are quite encouraging as they showed that such prototypes are highly effective for biological applications in the cloud environment. Other authors have adapted classical algorithms such as the Smith-Waterman (SW) algorithm for searches in sequential databases to identify the similarities between a query sequence and subject sequences (S. T. Lee, Lin, & Hung, 2013). The experimental results, indicated that the computational time can be improved by up to 41%. However, exploitation of GPUs for the cloud applications is very new field; future developments are expected.

CONCLUSION

Cloud computing has already extensively been used in the fields of biology and biochemistry with special emphasis on drug discovery where the concept of BigData combined with the storage and processing power provided by the Cloud has the potential to be fruitful. The Cloud has proved its added value and future applications are expected to be even more amazing.

For the everyday routine of medical laboratories, the Cloud capabilities have not up to now been fully exploited, however, it is expected that this picture will change, not only for isolated laboratories but for the IT services of complex hospitals. This is due to the fact that it has the potential to revolutionize the way bio-data can be stored, accessed, and processed.

Cloud based systems can improve data sharing among the various types of clinical laboratories by the exploitation of a model that saves resources and improves control and management. The storage and handling of the electronic file of a patient to a shared, however, secure place, not only saves paper and improves the concept of green medicine, but has the potential to promote medical data homogeneity in a global manner, thus facilitating BigData mining and new knowledge extraction.

Cloud along with BigData is a very new concept, which requires new ways of thinking and generates new scientific problems. However, this paradigm offers the possibility for unprecedented insight into biological functions.

REFERENCES

Abreu, R. M., Froufe, H. J., Queiroz, M. J., & Ferreira, I. C. (2010). MOLA: A bootable, self-configuring system for virtual screening using AutoDock4/Vina on computer clusters. *Journal of Cheminformatics*, *2*(1), 10. doi:10.1186/1758-2946-2-10 PMID:21029419

Afgan, E., Baker, D., Coraor, N., Chapman, B., Nekrutenko, A., & Taylor, J. (2010). Galaxy CloudMan: Delivering cloud compute clusters. *BMC Bioinformatics*, *11*(Suppl 12), S4. doi:10.1186/1471-2105-11-S12-S4 PMID:21210983

Al-Enazi, T., & El-Masri, S. (2013). HL7 Engine Module for Healthcare Information Systems. *Journal of Medical Systems*, *37*(6), 9986. doi:10.1007/s10916-013-9986-8 PMID:24154569

Almeida, J. S., Gruneberg, A., Maass, W., & Vinga, S. (2012). Fractal MapReduce decomposition of sequence alignment. *Algorithms for Molecular Biology; AMB*, *7*(1), 12. doi:10.1186/1748-7188-7-12 PMID:22551205

Almeida, J. S., & Noble, P. A. (2000). Neural computing in microbiology. *Journal of Microbiological Methods*, *43*(1), 1–2. doi:10.1016/S0167-7012(00)00200-1 PMID:11084224

Amazon. (2013a). *1000 Genomes Project and AWS*. Retrieved 22/12/2013, 2013, from http://aws.amazon.com/1000genomes/

Amazon. (2013b). *Amazon Elastic Compute Cloud (Amazon EC2)*. Retrieved 19/12/2013, from http://aws.amazon.com/ec2/

Angiuoli, S. V., Matalka, M., Gussman, A., Galens, K., Vangala, M., & Riley, D. R. et al. (2011). CloVR: A virtual machine for automated and portable sequence analysis from the desktop using cloud computing. *BMC Bioinformatics*, *12*, 356. doi:10.1186/1471-2105-12-356 PMID:21878105

Angiuoli, S. V., White, J. R., Matalka, M., White, O., & Fricke, W. F. (2011). Resources and costs for microbial sequence analysis evaluated using virtual machines and cloud computing. *PLoS ONE*, *6*(10), e26624. doi:10.1371/journal.pone.0026624 PMID:22028928

Apache Software Foundation. (2013). *Hadoop—Apache Software Foundation project home page*. Retrieved 23/12/2013, 2013, from http://hadoop.apache.org/

AT&T. (2012). *Medical Imaging in the Cloud*. Retrieved 26/08/2013, 2012, from https://www.corp.att.com/healthcare/docs/medical_imaging_cloud.pdf

Chen, J., Qian, F., Yan, W., & Shen, B. (2013). Translational biomedical informatics in the cloud: present and future. *BioMed Research International*, 658925.

Chen, J. L., Tsai, C. W., Chiang, M. C., & Yang, C. S. (2013). A high performance cloud-based protein-ligand docking prediction algorithm. *BioMed Research International*, 909717.

Chronaki, C., Pakarinen, V., Jalonen, M., Porrasmaa, J., Berler, A., & Tarhonen, T. (2012). HL7 CDA in the national ePrescription efforts of Finland & Greece: A comparison. *Studies in Health Technology and Informatics, 174*, 38–43. PMID:22491107

Cochand-Priollet, B., Koutroumbas, K., Megalopoulou, T. M., Pouliakis, A., Sivolapenko, G., & Karakitsos, P. (2006). Discriminating benign from malignant thyroid lesions using artificial intelligence and statistical selection of morphometric features. *Oncology Reports, 15*, 1023–1026. PMID:16525694

D'Agostino, D., Clematis, A., Quarati, A., Cesini, D., Chiappori, F., Milanesi, L., & Merelli, I. (2013). Cloud infrastructures for in silico drug discovery: Economic and practical aspects. *BioMed Research International*, 138012.

Davies, K. (2010). *The the revolution in DNA sequencing and the new era of personalized medicine*. New York, NY: Free Press.

De Paris, R., Frantz, F. A., de Souza, O. N., & Ruiz, D. D. (2013). wFReDoW: A cloud-based Web environment to handle molecular docking simulations of a fully flexible receptor model. *BioMed Research International*, 469363.

Deshpande, S. U. (1982). ILIS--An integrated laboratory information system: Biochemistry and hematology. *Clinical Chemistry, 28*(2), 271–276. PMID:7055947

Di Tommaso, P., Orobitg, M., Guirado, F., Cores, F., Espinosa, T., & Notredame, C. (2010). CloudCoffee: Implementation of a parallel consistency-based multiple alignment algorithm in the T-Coffee package and its benchmarking on the Amazon Elastic-Cloud. *Bioinformatics (Oxford, England), 26*(15), 1903–1904. doi:10.1093/bioinformatics/btq304 PMID:20605929

Duda, R. O., Hart, P. E., & Stork, D. G. (2001). *Pattern classification* (2nd ed.). New York: Wiley.

Dudley, J. T., & Butte, A. J. (2010). In silico research in the era of cloud computing. *Nature Biotechnology, 28*(11), 1181–1185. doi:10.1038/nbt1110-1181 PMID:21057489

Dudley, J. T., Pouliot, Y., Chen, R., Morgan, A. A., & Butte, A. J. (2010). Translational bioinformatics in the cloud: an affordable alternative. *Genome Medicine, 2*(8), 51. doi:10.1186/gm172 PMID:20691073

Eugster, M. J., Schmid, M., Binder, H., & Schmidberger, M. (2013). Grid and cloud computing methods in biomedical research. *Methods of Information in Medicine, 52*(1), 62–64. PMID:23318694

Feng, X., Grossman, R., & Stein, L. (2011). PeakRanger: A cloud-enabled peak caller for ChIP-seq data. *BMC Bioinformatics, 12*, 139. doi:10.1186/1471-2105-12-139 PMID:21554709

Gavan, T. L., & King, J. W. (1970). An evaluation of the microbiology portions of the 1969 basic, comprehensive, and special College of American Pathologists proficiency testing surveys. *American Journal of Clinical Pathology, 54*(3), 514–520. PMID:4918179

Georgiou, A., Callen, J., Westbrook, J., Prgomet, M., & Toouli, G. (2007). Information and communication processes in the microbiology laboratory--Implications for computerised provider order entry. *Studies in Health Technology and Informatics, 129*(2), 943–947. PMID:17911854

Georgiou, A., Prgomet, M., Toouli, G., Callen, J., & Westbrook, J. (2011). What do physicians tell laboratories when requesting tests? A multimethod examination of information supplied to the microbiology laboratory before and after the introduction of electronic ordering. *International Journal of Medical Informatics, 80*(9), 646–654. doi:10.1016/j.ijmedinf.2011.06.003 PMID:21757400

Giacomini, M., Ruggiero, C., Calegari, L., & Bertone, S. (2000). Artificial neural network based identification of environmental bacteria by gas-chromatographic and electrophoretic data. *Journal of Microbiological Methods, 43*(1), 45–54. doi:10.1016/S0167-7012(00)00203-7 PMID:11084227

Giuffre, G. (2006). Topical dorzolamide for the treatment of cystoid macular edema in patients with retinitis pigmentosa. *American Journal of Ophthalmology, 142*(4), 707–708. doi:10.1016/j.ajo.2006.06.042 PMID:17011883

Glaser, J. (2011). Cloud computing can simplify HIT infrastructure management. *Healthcare Financial Management, 65*(8), 52–55. PMID:21866720

GlobalData. (2012). *Snapshot: The US cloud computing market for medical imaging.* Retrieved 22/08/2013, from http://www.medicaldevice-network.com/features/featuresnapshot-the-us-cloud-computing-market-for-medical-imaging

Goncalves, A., Tikhonov, A., Brazma, A., & Kapushesky, M. (2011). A pipeline for RNA-seq data processing and quality assessment. *Bioinformatics (Oxford, England), 27*(6), 867–869. doi:10.1093/bioinformatics/btr012 PMID:21233166

Goodgame, J. C., Pottage, J. C. Jr, Jablonowski, H., Hardy, W. D., Stein, A., & Fischl, M. et al. (2000). Amprenavir in combination with lamivudine and zidovudine versus lamivudine and zidovudine alone in HIV-1-infected antiretroviral-naive adults: Amprenavir PROAB3001 International Study Team. *Antiviral Therapy, 5*(3), 215–225. PMID:11075942

Greenbaum, D., & Gerstein, M. (2011). The role of cloud computing in managing the deluge of potentially private genetic data. *The American Journal of Bioethics, 11*(11), 39–41. doi:10.1080/15265161.2011.608242 PMID:22047125

Hajmeer, M. N., Basheer, I. A., & Najjar, Y. M. (1997). Computational neural networks for predictive microbiology: Application to microbial growth. *International Journal of Food Microbiology, 34*(1), 51–66. doi:10.1016/S0168-1605(96)01169-5 PMID:9029255

Harding, H. B. (1965a). Quality control in microbiology. *Hospital Topics, 43*(10), 77–80. doi:10.1080/00185868.1965.9954565 PMID:5831293

Harding, H. B. (1965b). Quality control in microbiology: II. *Hospital Topics, 43*(11), 79–85. doi:10.1080/00185868.1965.9954597 PMID:5843067

Haykin, S. S. (1994). *Neural networks: A comprehensive foundation.* Toronto: Macmillan.

Heymans, S., McKennirey, M., & Phillips, J. (2011). Semantic validation of the use of SNOMED CT in HL7 clinical documents. *Journal of Biomedical Semantics, 2*(1), 2. doi:10.1186/2041-1480-2-2 PMID:21762489

Hommes, F. A., Brewster, M. A., Burton, B. K., Buist, N. R., Elsas, L. J., & Goldsmith, B. M. et al. (1990). Proficiency testing for biochemical genetics laboratories: The first 10 rounds of testing. *American Journal of Human Genetics, 46*(5), 1001–1004. PMID:2339686

Hong, D., Rhie, A., Park, S. S., Lee, J., Ju, Y. S., & Kim, S. et al. (2012). FX: An RNA-Seq analysis tool on the cloud. *Bioinformatics (Oxford, England), 28*(5), 721–723. doi:10.1093/bioinformatics/bts023 PMID:22257667

Hsu, C. H., Lin, C. Y., Ouyang, M., & Guo, Y. K. (2013). Biocloud: Cloud computing for biological, genomics, and drug design. *BioMed Research International*, 909470.

Huang, C. C., Lin, C. Y., Chang, C. W., & Tang, C. Y. (2013). Enzyme reaction annotation using cloud techniques. *BioMed Research International*, 140237.

Hung, C. L., & Hua, G. J. (2013). Cloud computing for protein-ligand binding site comparison. *BioMed Research International,* 170356.

Jo, H., Jeong, J., Lee, M., & Choi, D. H. (2013). Exploiting GPUs in virtual machine for BioCloud. *BioMed Research International,* 939460.

Jourdren, L., Bernard, M., Dillies, M. A., & Le Crom, S. (2012). Eoulsan: A cloud computing-based framework facilitating high throughput sequencing analyses. *Bioinformatics (Oxford, England), 28*(11), 1542–1543. doi:10.1093/bioinformatics/bts165 PMID:22492314

Kajan, L., Yachdav, G., Vicedo, E., Steinegger, M., Mirdita, M., Angermuller, C., … Rost, B. (2013). Cloud prediction of protein structure and function with PredictProtein for Debian. *BioMed Research International,* 398968.

Kanungo, R. (2012). Are clinical microbiology laboratories missing out quality control and quality assurance in laboratory management? *Indian Journal of Medical Microbiology, 30*(1), 1–2. doi:10.4103/0255-0857.93012 PMID:22361752

Karakitsos, P., Pouliakis, A., Meristoudis, C., Margari, N., Kassanos, D., & Kyrgiou, M. et al. (2011). A preliminary study of the potential of tree classifiers in triage of high-grade squamous intraepithelial lesions. *Analytical and Quantitative Cytology and Histology, 33*(3), 132–140. PMID:21980616

Karakitsos, P., Stergiou, E. B., Pouliakis, A., Tzivras, M., Archimandritis, A., Liossi, A. I., & Kyrkou, K. (1996). Potential of the back propagation neural network in the discrimination of benign from malignant gastric cells. *Analytical and Quantitative Cytology and Histology, 18*(3), 245–250. PMID:8790840

Kasson, P. M. (2013). Computational biology in the cloud: Methods and new insights from computing at scale. In *Proceedings of Pacific Symposium on Biocomputing,* (pp. 451-453). Academic Press.

Kelley, D. R., Schatz, M. C., & Salzberg, S. L. (2010). Quake: Quality-aware detection and correction of sequencing errors. *Genome Biology, 11*(11), R116. doi:10.1186/gb-2010-11-11-r116 PMID:21114842

Kohonen, T. (2001). *Self-organizing maps* (3rd ed.). Berlin: Springer. doi:10.1007/978-3-642-56927-2

Krampis, K., Booth, T., Chapman, B., Tiwari, B., Bicak, M., Field, D., & Nelson, K. E. (2012). Cloud BioLinux: Pre-configured and on-demand bioinformatics computing for the genomics community. *BMC Bioinformatics, 13,* 42. doi:10.1186/1471-2105-13-42 PMID:22429538

Kuntz, I. D. (1992). Structure-based strategies for drug design and discovery. *Science, 257*(5073), 1078–1082. doi:10.1126/science.257.5073.1078 PMID:1509259

Kuo, A. M. (2011). Opportunities and challenges of cloud computing to improve health care services. *Journal of Medical Internet Research, 13*(3), e67. doi:10.2196/jmir.1867 PMID:21937354

Langmead, B., Hansen, K. D., & Leek, J. T. (2010). Cloud-scale RNA-sequencing differential expression analysis with Myrna. *Genome Biology, 11*(8), R83. doi:10.1186/gb-2010-11-8-r83 PMID:20701754

Langmead, B., Schatz, M. C., Lin, J., Pop, M., & Salzberg, S. L. (2009). Searching for SNPs with cloud computing. *Genome Biology, 10*(11), R134. doi:10.1186/gb-2009-10-11-r134 PMID:19930550

Lee, H., Yang, Y., Chae, H., Nam, S., Choi, D., & Tangchaisin, P. et al. (2012). BioVLAB-MMIA: A cloud environment for microRNA and mRNA integrated analysis (MMIA) on Amazon EC2. *IEEE Transactions on Nanobioscience, 11*(3), 266–272. doi:10.1109/TNB.2012.2212030 PMID:22987133

Lee, S. T., Lin, C. Y., & Hung, C. L. (2013). GPU-based cloud service for Smith-Waterman algorithm using frequency distance filtration scheme. *BioMed Research International, 721738.*

Lupse, O. S., Vida, M., & Stoicu-Tivadar, L. (2012). Cloud computing technology applied in healthcare for developing large scale flexible solutions. *Studies in Health Technology and Informatics, 174*, 94–99. PMID:22491119

McKenna, A., Hanna, M., Banks, E., Sivachenko, A., Cibulskis, K., & Kernytsky, A. et al. (2010). The Genome Analysis Toolkit: A MapReduce framework for analyzing next-generation DNA sequencing data. *Genome Research, 20*(9), 1297–1303. doi:10.1101/gr.107524.110 PMID:20644199

Mirza, H., & El-Masri, S. (2013). National electronic medical records integration on Cloud computing system. *Studies in Health Technology and Informatics, 192*, 1219. PMID:23920993

Morris, G. M., Huey, R., Lindstrom, W., Sanner, M. F., Belew, R. K., Goodsell, D. S., & Olson, A. J. (2009). AutoDock4 and AutoDockTools4: Automated docking with selective receptor flexibility. *Journal of Computational Chemistry, 30*(16), 2785–2791. doi:10.1002/jcc.21256 PMID:19399780

Mouwen, D. J., Capita, R., Alonso-Calleja, C., Prieto-Gomez, J., & Prieto, M. (2006). Artificial neural network based identification of Campylobacter species by Fourier transform infrared spectroscopy. *Journal of Microbiological Methods, 67*(1), 131–140. doi:10.1016/j.mimet.2006.03.012 PMID:16632003

Nguyen, T., Shi, W., & Ruden, D. (2011). CloudAligner: A fast and full-featured MapReduce based tool for sequence mapping. *BMC Research Notes, 4*, 171. doi:10.1186/1756-0500-4-171 PMID:21645377

Niemenmaa, M., Kallio, A., Schumacher, A., Klemela, P., Korpelainen, E., & Heljanko, K. (2012). Hadoop-BAM: Directly manipulating next generation sequencing data in the cloud. *Bioinformatics (Oxford, England), 28*(6), 876–877. doi:10.1093/bioinformatics/bts054 PMID:22302568

O'Connor, B. D., Merriman, B., & Nelson, S. F. (2010). SeqWare Query Engine: storing and searching sequence data in the cloud. *BMC Bioinformatics, 11*(Suppl 12), S2. doi:10.1186/1471-2105-11-S12-S2 PMID:21210981

Oemig, F., & Blobel, B. (2011). A formal analysis of HL7 version 2.x. *Studies in Health Technology and Informatics, 169*, 704–708. PMID:21893838

Pantazopoulos, D., Karakitsos, P., Iokim-Liossi, A., Pouliakis, A., Botsoli-Stergiou, E., & Dimopoulos, C. (1998). Back propagation neural network in the discrimination of benign from malignant lower urinary tract lesions. *The Journal of Urology, 159*(5), 1619–1623. doi:10.1097/00005392-199805000-00057 PMID:9554366

Patel, R. P. (2012). Cloud computing and virtualization technology in radiology. *Clinical Radiology, 67*(11), 1095–1100. doi:10.1016/j.crad.2012.03.010 PMID:22607956

Pireddu, L., Leo, S., & Zanetti, G. (2011). SEAL: A distributed short read mapping and duplicate removal tool. *Bioinformatics (Oxford, England), 27*(15), 2159–2160. doi:10.1093/bioinformatics/btr325 PMID:21697132

Porres, J. M. (1974a). Quality control in microbiology: Utilization of reference laboratory data. *American Journal of Clinical Pathology, 62*(3), 407–411. PMID:4415417

Porres, J. M. (1974b). Quality control in microbiology: The need for standards. *American Journal of Clinical Pathology, 62*(3), 412–419. PMID:4472270

Ren, J., Xie, L., Li, W. W., & Bourne, P. E. (2010). SMAP-WS: A parallel Web service for structural proteome-wide ligand-binding site comparison. *Nucleic Acids Research, 38*, W441-444. doi:10.1093/nar/gkq400 PMID:20484373

Richardson, H., Wood, D., Whitby, J., Lannigan, R., & Fleming, C. (1996). Quality improvement of diagnostic microbiology through a peer-group proficiency assessment program: A 20-year experience in Ontario: The Microbiology Committee. *Archives of Pathology & Laboratory Medicine, 120*(5), 445–455. PMID:8639047

Riquelme, E., Lorente, S., & Crespo, M. D. (2011). Implementing a quality management system according to iso model in a Microbiology laboratory. *Enfermedades Infecciosas y Microbiologia Clinica, 29*(1), 72–73. doi:10.1016/j.eimc.2010.04.018 PMID:21193248

Rosenthal, A., Mork, P., Li, M. H., Stanford, J., Koester, D., & Reynolds, P. (2010). Cloud computing: A new business paradigm for biomedical information sharing. *Journal of Biomedical Informatics, 43*(2), 342–353. doi:10.1016/j.jbi.2009.08.014 PMID:19715773

Rost, B., Yachdav, G., & Liu, J. (2004). The PredictProtein server. *Nucleic Acids Research, 32*, W321-326. doi:10.1093/nar/gkh377

Rudnisky, C. J., Tennant, M. T., Weis, E., Ting, A., Hinz, B. J., & Greve, M. D. (2007). Web-based grading of compressed stereoscopic digital photography versus standard slide film photography for the diagnosis of diabetic retinopathy. *Ophthalmology, 114*(9), 1748–1754. doi:10.1016/j.ophtha.2006.12.010 PMID:17368543

Schadt, E. E., Linderman, M. D., Sorenson, J., Lee, L., & Nolan, G. P. (2010). Computational solutions to large-scale data management and analysis. *Nature Reviews. Genetics, 11*(9), 647–657. doi:10.1038/nrg2857 PMID:20717155

Schatz, M. C. (2009). CloudBurst: Highly sensitive read mapping with MapReduce. *Bioinformatics (Oxford, England), 25*(11), 1363–1369. doi:10.1093/bioinformatics/btp236 PMID:19357099

Schatz, M. C., Delcher, A. L., & Salzberg, S. L. (2010). Assembly of large genomes using second-generation sequencing. *Genome Research, 20*(9), 1165–1173. doi:10.1101/gr.101360.109 PMID:20508146

Schatz, M. C., Langmead, B., & Salzberg, S. L. (2010). Cloud computing and the DNA data race. *Nature Biotechnology, 28*(7), 691–693. doi:10.1038/nbt0710-691 PMID:20622843

Stein, L. D. (2010). The case for cloud computing in genome informatics. *Genome Biology, 11*(5), 207. doi:10.1186/gb-2010-11-5-207 PMID:20441614

Taylor, C. R. (2011). From microscopy to whole slide digital images: A century and a half of image analysis. *Applied Immunohistochemistry & Molecular Morphology, 19*(6), 491–493. doi:10.1097/PAI.0b013e318229ffd6 PMID:22089486

Theodoridis, S., & Koutroumbas, K. (2009). *Pattern recognition* (4th ed.). London: Academic Press.

Toouli, G., Georgiou, A., & Westbrook, J. (2012). Changes, disruption and innovation: An investigation of the introduction of new health information technology in a microbiology laboratory. *Journal of Pathology Informatics, 3*, 16. doi:10.4103/2153-3539.95128 PMID:22616028

Underwood, A., & Green, J. (2011). Call for a quality standard for sequence-based assays in clinical microbiology: Necessity for quality assessment of sequences used in microbial identification and typing. *Journal of Clinical Microbiology, 49*(1), 23–26. doi:10.1128/JCM.01918-10 PMID:21068275 van Leeuwen, W., & van Belkum, A. (2013). The European Journal of Clinical Microbiology and Infectious Diseases: Quality and quantity in 2013. *European Journal of Clinical Microbiology & Infectious Diseases, 32*(1), 1–2. doi:10.1007/s10096-012-1804-6 PMID:23263838

Varlatzidou, A., Pouliakis, A., Stamataki, M., Meristoudis, C., Margari, N., & Peros, G. et al. (2011). Cascaded learning vector quantizer neural networks for the discrimination of thyroid lesions. *Analytical and Quantitative Cytology and Histology, 33*(6), 323–334. PMID:22590810

Vicentino, W., Rodriguez, G., Saldias, M., & Alvarez, I. (2009). Guidelines to implement quality management systems in microbiology laboratories for tissue banking. *Transplantation Proceedings, 41*(8), 3481–3484. doi:10.1016/j.transproceed.2009.09.012 PMID:19857776

Volkamer, A., Kuhn, D., Grombacher, T., Rippmann, F., & Rarey, M. (2012). Combining global and local measures for structure-based druggability predictions. *Journal of Chemical Information and Modeling, 52*(2), 360–372. doi:10.1021/ci200454v PMID:22148551

Wallace, P. S., & MacKay, W. G. (2013). Quality in the molecular microbiology laboratory. *Methods in Molecular Biology (Clifton, N.J.), 943*, 49–79. doi:10.1007/978-1-60327-353-4_3 PMID:23104281

Waxer, N., Ninan, D., Ma, A., & Dominguez, N. (2013). How cloud computing and social media are changing the face of health care. *The Physician Executive Journal, 39*(2), 58-60, 62.

Webb, G. (2012). Making the cloud work for healthcare: Cloud computing offers incredible opportunities to improve healthcare, reduce costs and accelerate ability to adopt new IT services. *Health Management Technology, 33*(2), 8–9. PMID:22397112

Whitby, J. L., Black, W. A., Richardson, H., & Wood, D. E. (1982). System for laboratory proficiency testing in bacteriology: organisation and impact on microbiology laboratories in health care facilities funded by the Ontario Government. *Journal of Clinical Pathology, 35*(1), 94–100. doi:10.1136/jcp.35.1.94 PMID:7061723

Wilson, M. E., Faur, Y. C., Schaefler, S., Weitzman, I., Weisburd, M. H., & Schaeffer, M. (1977). Proficiency testing in clinical microbiology: The New York City program. *The Mount Sinai Journal of Medicine, New York, 44*(1), 142–163. PMID:300463

Yuksel, M., & Dogac, A. (2011). Interoperability of medical device information and the clinical applications: An HL7 RMIM based on the ISO/IEEE 11073 DIM. *IEEE Transactions on Information Technology in Biomedicine, 15*(4), 557–566. doi:10.1109/TITB.2011.2151868 PMID:21558061

Zhang, L., Gu, S., Liu, Y., Wang, B., & Azuaje, F. (2012). Gene set analysis in the cloud. *Bioinformatics (Oxford, England), 28*(2), 294–295. doi:10.1093/bioinformatics/btr630 PMID:22084254

Zhang, S. (2011). Computer-aided drug discovery and development. *Methods in Molecular Biology (Clifton, N.J.), 716*, 23–38. doi:10.1007/978-1-61779-012-6_2 PMID:21318898

Zhang, W., Wang, X., Lu, B., & Kim, T. H. (2013). Secure encapsulation and publication of biological services in the cloud computing environment. *BioMed Research International*, 170580.

KEY TERMS AND DEFINITIONS

Artificial Neural Networks (ANNs): Complex computational models inspired by the human brain nervous system, capable for learning and pattern recognition.

BigData: The collection of data sets so large and complex that it becomes difficult to process using on-hand database management tools or traditional data processing applications.

BioCloud: Bioinformatics via Cloud Computing.

Clinical Biochemistry: The science of chemistry applied in biology with medical consequences. Clinical biochemistry is synonymous with clinical chemistry and chemical pathology.

Clinical Microbiology: A medicine branch related to the prevention, diagnosis and treatment of infectious diseases, additionally studies clinical applications of microbes for health improvement. Clinical microbiology is related to four kinds of microorganisms that may cause infectious diseases; bacteria, fungi, parasites and viruses.

Cloud Computing: A large number of computers connected through a network, capable to run an application on many computers and to configure virtual servers, virtual servers do not have a physical presence and can be moved around and scaled up or down without to be noticed by end users, like a cloud.

In Silico: An expression used to mean "performed on the computer or via computer simulation," usually used for experiments conducted via computational systems.

Laboratory Information System (LIS): Or Laboratory Information Management System (LIMS) is a software-based system for the support of operations in a modern laboratory, such as workflow, sample tracking, data exchange interfaces. LIS systems are often capable of being connected with medical analyzers for automated extraction and storage of measurements.

Chapter 13
Cloud Computing for Cytopathologists

Abraham Pouliakis
University of Athens, Greece

Efrossyni Karakitsou
*National Technical University of Athens,
Greece*

Stavros Archondakis
401 Military Hospital, Greece

Petros Karakitsos
University of Athens, Greece

ABSTRACT

Cloud computing is changing the way enterprises, institutions, and people understand, perceive, and use current software systems. Cloud computing is an innovative concept of creating a computer grid using the Internet facilities aiming at the shared use of resources such as computer software and hardware. Cloud-based system architectures provide many advantages in terms of scalability, maintainability, and massive data processing. By means of cloud computing technology, cytopathologists can efficiently manage imaging units by using the latest software and hardware available without having to pay for it at non-affordable prices. Cloud computing systems used by cytopathology departments can function on public, private, hybrid, or community models. Using cloud applications, infrastructure, storage services, and processing power, cytopathology laboratories can avoid huge spending on maintenance of costly applications and on image storage and sharing. Cloud computing allows imaging flexibility and may be used for creating a virtual mobile office. Security and privacy issues have to be addressed in order to ensure Cloud computing wide implementation in the near future. Nowadays, cloud computing is not widely used for the various tasks related to cytopathology; however, there are numerous fields for which it can be applied. The envisioned advantages for the everyday practice in laboratories' workflow and eventually for the patients are significant. This is explored in this chapter.

INTRODUCTION

Cloud services (in modern tech jargon often referred as "the cloud") refers to a network of servers connected by the Internet or other network that enables users to combine and use computing power on an as-needed basis. Cloud computing is a novelty that rapidly showed tremendous opportunities for application in medicine and health care improvement (Eugster, Schmid, Binder, & Schmidberger, 2013; Glaser, 2011; Kuo, 2011; Lupse, Vida, & Stoicu-Tivadar, 2012; Mirza &

DOI: 10.4018/978-1-4666-6118-9.ch013

El-Masri, 2013; Patel, 2012; Rosenthal et al., 2010; Waxer, Ninan, Ma, & Dominguez, 2013; Webb, 2012). Actually it is forecasted that there will be an increase in the US cloud computing market for medical images approximately 27% by 2018 at a Compounded Annual Growth Rate (CAGR). This is mainly due to the growing volume of medical images and the increasing costs of the ownership for owning Picture Archiving and Communication Systems (PACS) (GlobalData, 2012).

Within this chapter, we analyze the state of the art related to the application of cloud computing services and infrastructure for cytopathology, identify and propose potential applications, explore possible solutions for potential problems and finally promote the benefits of transforming traditional applications of the cytopathology lab into cloud based services. The main areas related to the application of the Cloud for cytopathology include data storage with an emphasis on image archiving and access, the shift of traditional Laboratory Information Systems from laboratory or hospital hosting to cloud hosting, the benefits of cloud based services for the support of population screening and especially for cervical cancer screening that represents the major work load for cytopathology laboratories, the application of cloud applications for the support of Quality Control and Quality Assurance (QC and QA) of the modern cytopathology lab as well as the trends to shift the traditional proficiency testing for cytopathologists and the need for continuous medical education to e-services and why the cloud would be an appropriate choice. In this chapter, primary diagnosis and tele-cytology and tele-consultation issues are analyzed and finally we present research highlights for cloud based cytological image analysis and cytogenetics and genome analysis. Finally, issues and principles for virtual slides for cytopathology are presented, being a driving force for the application of cloud based services for cytopathology, both for the everyday practice and research purposes.

BACKGROUND

A cloud system is actually a network of computer servers offered under demand as a service. The system is designed to be flexible, scalable, secure and robust. Cloud systems usually provide software, data access, and data storage services provided by this interconnected grid of computers that permits sharing of resources through the Internet and works on a pay-per-use model.

Cloud systems are categorized into three different groups according to the offered service type:

- Infrastructure as a Service (IaaS), which means offering hardware, storage and physical devices over the Internet.
- Software as a Service (SaaS), which means offering software and hosted applications over the Internet.
- Platform as a Service (PaaS), which means offering the capability to deploy applications created using programming languages, libraries, services, and tools owned and supported by the provider.

For cloud computing, the user/consumer does not manage or control the underlying cloud infrastructure, but has control over the deployed applications. Clouds, according to their location of hosting, may be public, private, hybrid, and community, especially adapted to the medical field:

- **Public Clouds:** Are for general use. The cloud owners are responsible for information hosting; public clouds are rarely used in the field of medicine and in case of use, data are encrypted.
- **Private Clouds:** Are only for in-hospital use and are dealing with confidential patient data. The owners or the hospital premise are responsible for information hosting.

- **Hybrid Clouds:** Are hosting non confidential information on public Clouds and confidential information in a private domain.
- **Community Clouds:** Are hosting information among members of the same community. Laboratories and hospitals can create a community Cloud while sharing the same infrastructure and software.

Cloud computing, in the field of cytopathology, may provide precious Web-based services, which may be incorporated in the Laboratory Information System and become part of a Web-based Electronic Health Record. The modeling of this cloud system, maintained by one organization/institution may be of the SaaS, IaaS, or PaaS type, and can provide valuable services to the end users: cytopathologists, clinicians and even patients.

The main components of Cloud computing in the field of Cytopathology are the following:

1. **Applications:** The Cloud applications are hosted on servers that are remote from the user and can be run in real time from a thin client that hosts the application through a Web browser. The majority of Cloud applications are accessible via browsers. Thus there is no installation of the application, no maintenance required, and support issues are resolved because the software is hosted on a machine that is dedicated to that software, so there is minimal danger that the thin client could possibly influence the software. Cloud applications may be run as software as a service (SaaS), software plus service or data as a service. In Cloud applications, used by cytopathologists, the end users take advantage of some kind of "Software as a Service" for image reviewing, creating diagnostic reports, or patient billing.
2. **Client:** It is usually a Web browser such as Mozilla Firefox. In the mobile telephone environment, Apple's iPhone or Google's Android platforms some applications can be considered to run from the cloud. The client may also be a certain Web site such as Facebook, where there are many applications available for use. A Cloud client, in the field of Cytopathology, is the medium which cytopathologists use to access the Cloud via the Internet. Cloud client may be a computer or a Smartphone.

3. **Infrastructure:** Cloud infrastructure includes all computer hardware and the buildings containing it. The hardware consists of economic, mass produced server technology. The server environment may be running partial or complete virtualization, grid computing or paravirtualization technologies. Cloud infrastructure, in the field of Cytopathology, includes computer hardware and servers used for software running and data storage.
4. **Platform:** The cloud platform is referring to the way that applications can be deployed. In the field of Cytopathology, a well designed platform is an essential parameter for efficient application of laboratory's Cloud applications.
5. **Service:** Service refers to what users can reap from their cloud experience. To date there is a great amount of services for users wishing to take advantage of remote infrastructures such as cloud systems. Some of these services are unique, while others enhance services that are already available. A cloud service, in the field of Cytopathology, can be, without having to be limited to, either a Web-based image archiving system or a Web-based image gallery among others described in this chapter.
6. **Storage:** Storage devices are the first to fail on a computer. By using cloud technology, companies assure their data safety. In the case, there is an emergency situation, the chances of complete failure of all systems is very slim, due to the large number of computers working in the cloud environment. Cloud

computing, in the field of Cytopathology, enables, for example, the storage of large medical laboratory databases in the form of documents and image libraries, instead of physical storage at site (hospital or imaging center) which is much more expensive and difficult to maintain.

7. **Processing power:** The processing power that cloud computing is capable of has no boundaries. Cloud companies are willing to scale up their infrastructure if needed, so when there is a need for more processing power, it will be available on the fly. Due to Cloud computing immense processing power, companies do not have to worry about infrastructure purchasing or costs. Cloud computing, in the field of Cytopathology, can provide infinite processing power to all cytopathology laboratories at a very low cost.

POTENTIAL APPLICATIONS OF CLOUD COMPUTING IN CYTOPATHOLOGY

Modern cytopathology laboratories deal mainly with images as the routine cytological examinations are performed via the use of a glass slide and analysis with the microscope. However modern cytopathology laboratories perform additional examinations based on molecular techniques and immunocytochemistry methods. The modern cytopathology laboratory is equipped with numerous modalities capable of performing medical tests and exchange data via networks, imaging systems capable to create digital pictures of the slides or even virtual slides, which are complete slides in electronic format. The volume of data in a cytopathology lab nowadays is enormous.

The major cloud based applications that can be envisioned for the benefit of cytopathologists and the patients as well may be as follows:

Data Storage

Storing, archiving, sharing and accessing images in the cloud allows the industry to manage data more efficiently and cost-effectively while overcoming many of the legal, regulatory and technical challenges that data requirements pose (AT&T, 2012). The cloud enables hospitals to:

- Efficiently handle large bandwidth images.
- Use non-proprietary, standards-based, vendor-neutral architecture.
- Expand or contract storage capacity easily.
- Manage authentication, encryption and security protocols.
- Conduct efficient system-wide application upgrades.
- Extend the life of existing infrastructure/investments.

A cytopathology laboratory wishing to store many images and patient information files is nowadays obliged to install one or more servers and accompanying disk arrays, having poor or no earlier experience in its upkeep. A possible server crash may result to severe data loss. Furthermore, the server may require constant upgrades. These two reasons are good enough for a modern cytopathology laboratory to shift its data to the Cloud. By doing this, the laboratory reduces dramatically all costs related to server software and hardware, as well as the costs for maintenance and licenses. Here the cloud acts as a LIS, telecytology software, and billing unit. A patient may perform a cytological examination at a hospital or a private laboratory. Representative images of the case may be stored on a hybrid Cloud. If the patient performs another cytologic examination after some time, in another (and possibly distant ?) laboratory, he can provide the reporting cytopathologists direct access to the images stored in the Cloud. The cytopathologists can retrieve and merge the images on their workstation. The cytopathologists can make the final diagnosis after having reviewed the images of the first cytological examination.

Laboratory Information Systems

Laboratory information systems (LIS) are used to supervise many varieties of inpatient and outpatient medical tests. The major features that laboratory information systems are: management of sample check in, order entry, specimen processing, result entry and patient demographics as well as medical history. A LIS tracks and stores all the information related to the patient from arrival until he/she leaves and stores the data for future retrieval. LISs produce as well reports for the tests that handle and statistics related to various aspects of the laboratory such as time for execution of examinations, sample volumes etc. Therefore, a LIS can be defined as a series of computer programs that process, store and manage data from all stages of medical processes and tests. Modern LISs are networked and the various modern modalities (biomedical analyzers) having networking capabilities as well can automatically send examination results directly for storage, additionally barcode technology automates sample and patient identification.

Usually large laboratories have internal information technology (IT) personnel to handle hardware, software and provide technical expertise and support, and take care in cases of infrastructure lack as well as to optimize the systems to run mission critical applications. However, cloud computing is changing this picture. As there is pressure to meet timelines, to reduce costs, for example, by spreading costs associated with infrastructure ownership and support, many laboratories nowadays are exploiting virtualization capabilities that are basic characteristics of cloud computing, virtualization provides convenient and on-demand network access to a shared pool of configurable resources such as networks, servers, storage and applications, and definitely share the cost for owning and managing in-house equipment and personnel. In addition to cost reduction, the set-up and configuration time for a laboratory wishing to adopt a new LIS is minimal. Therefore, a cytopathology laboratory that does not have a LIS, but wants to start using a Cloud-based LIS may purchase a LIS system hosted in the cloud, configure it according to the needs, train the users and launch the application within a short time. Using a community Cloud, many hospitals can share standard software and save large amounts of money.

Screening Programs

Cervical cancer is one of the most common women mortality reasons in the world (Jemal et al., 2011). However it is a well studied disease with known natural history and can be prevented and treated if diagnosed in early stage. The key to prevention is the regular check of all women fulfilling specific criteria with test Papanikolaou; this process is called a population based cervical cancer screening program. As the involved population is very large, critical to the success of the program is the organization and quality control and assurance. Unavoidably a computerized information system supporting the program must be in place (Pouliakis, Iliopoulou, & Karakitsou, 2012; Pouliakis & Karakitsos, 2011). There are several important issues related to the software systems supporting screening programs where the application of cloud computing can be a solution:

- **Availability:** It is the ability to cope with, and if necessary recover from failures of the host server either due to hardware reasons or due to failure of the operating system and the application software, and to cope with hardware and maintenance activities that may cause downtime. The system availability is crucial for the program smooth operation, if the system is not operational the consequences range from missing appointments to canceled treatments. Hosting of such systems in a cloud ensures the high availability of servers, moreover as cloud services providers have multisite hosting and multiple Internet connection, the availability of connectivity is ensured as well.

- **Scalability:** Refers to the ability to spread both the system software and the load across multiple servers. Hosting the application in a cloud provider ensures that there will be plenty of CPU power available. By design, the virtual machines offered by cloud services providers are fault tolerant and utilize many servers that appear to the end user as a single machine, therefore the escalation of the application is easy to be performed via the use of additional servers either for hosting the application or for expanding the database.

- **Deployment and Problem Resolution:** Definitely deploying traditional application in end user computers is not anymore a choice for IT systems supporting screening programs, the chosen solution is central hosting the applications and preferably Web based applications hosted in the cloud. The benefits from this architecture are evident: the maintenance is easier and applied in a single place and bug fixes and improvements when applied are immediately available to the other users.

Quality Control and Assurance

There are many aspects related to the quality in cytology and how to control and assess, one of the fundamental methods is the correlation of the

cytologic and histologic answers (Izadi-Mood, Sarmadi, & Sanii, 2013). The concept is to evaluate the discrepancies, determine why occurred, and to ensure the appropriate patient care. The way cytologic and histologic correlation is performed, has changed over time. Years ago, it was just to collect all cases every few months and go through them. This is not any more an acceptable method because patients would not like to learn about a mistake a few months after it especially if this could have been corrected (Renshaw, 2011). The improvement of information systems and LIS in most cytologic and histologic laboratories, allows such correlations to be performed just immediately after the release of the examination results. Additionally, data mining either on-line or in a later stage may produce important knowledge for trends and problematic areas in the processes and therefore to initiate corrective actions for quality improvement. Additionally images based systems to evaluate the quality of classification systems such as the Bethesda System 2001 for reporting the results of cervical cytology (Solomon et al., 2002) have already been reported in the literature (Sherman, Dasgupta, Schiffman, Nayar, & Solomon, 2007). The cloud obviously can be of help for QC and QA as the related application may be developed and operated for such an environment, storage and application load will not be an issue and additional benefits may be obtained as the QC and QA application can be shared among numerous laboratories and rare cytological cases can be used by all participating labs.

Proficiency Testing

Proficiency Testing (PT) is not a new concept. European countries run tests for a variety of areas in pathology. In the United Kingdom, there are quality-assurance testing programs for a variety of areas called National External Quality Assessments Schemes; whereas, in the European Union, there is an aptitude test for cervical cytology that was created by the Committee for Quality Assurance, Trading, and Education (QUATE) (Demichelis, Della Mea, Forti, Dalla Palma, & Beltrami, 2002). The objective of the QUATE committee was to test each individual using the exact same slides to ensure equity of examination. Today there is published evidence that the results of proficiency testing by virtual slides is comparable to those of glass slides, thus computer-based testing can be equivalent (Demichelis et al., 2002; Gagnon et al., 2004; Stewart et al., 2007).

Additionally according to the International Academy of Cytology Task Force (Vooijs et al., 1998) the training programs for cytotechnologists and cytopathologists should provide instruction and experience in new technologies. Advantages of digital images for training include standardization of teaching sets and interactive capabilities, allowing educational feedback.

The position of the International Academy of Cytology Task Force in 1998: "Diagnostic Cytology Towards the 21st Century" is highlighted by the following:

- Computerized support/assistance devices aid in complete screening of the slide during training and provide feedback to cytologists on screening techniques.
- The subjective nature of cytologic analysis poses many challenges for implementation.
- There is concern for the value and validity of any large-scale formal testing programs.
- Locator and diagnostic skills are both critical in cytology, but assessment of each skill may occur in different ways using computerized technologies.
- Assessments should provide educational feedback to participants.
- The reliability or consistency of the testing event is critical.

- A valid and reliable correlation between work performance and performance on a proficiency test needs to be established.
- Any cytology proficiency test program should also be considered in the context of other laboratory quality assurance tools and the entire cervical cancer screening program.
- Regulatory agencies should evaluate entire laboratory performance, while each laboratory director should assume primary responsibility for evaluating and documenting the competency and daily performance of each practicing cytologist.
- Professional scientific organizations should take the lead in recommending methods and standards of performance assessment.
- A reliable method of correlating daily competency with results on PT is not yet established.
- Methods may evolve ever time using new technologies.
- The use of computerized techniques and images for assessment will require careful deliberation by experts as well as validation by practicing cytologists.
- Variables include diagnostic categories for testing, numbers of challenges per testing event, types of slide preparations and characteristics of the digital images.
- Availability of equipment and staff will affect the introduction of new technologies in different regions.

Definitely 15 years ago the International Academy of Cytology had foreseen, concluded and recommended the application of information technology in the field of proficiency testing, as a promising a solution to numerous issues. The trend for proficiency testing today is based on whole slide imaging. As a result, the advantages of cloud computing for storing and transmitting such large data are obvious.

Digital/Virtual Slides

Digital imaging in pathology has undergone a period of exponential growth and expansion catalyzed by changes in imaging hardware and gains in computational processing. Today, digitization of entire glass slides at near the optical resolution limits of light can occur in a few minutes additionally whole slides can be scanned in fluorescence or by multispectral imaging systems. Whole slide imaging has been successfully used in surgical pathology, but its usefulness and clinical application have been limited in cytology for several reasons, mainly the lack of availability of z-axis depth focusing as cytological samples in contrast to histological have a 3D structure. However nowadays, there are available systems capable for whole slide imaging with z-axis control. This boosted the application of digital slides for cytology (Al-Janabi, Huisman, Willems, & Van Diest, 2012; Fung et al., 2012; Ghaznavi, Evans, Madabhushi, & Feldman, 2013; Gutman et al., 2013; Hipp, Lucas, Emmert-Buck, Compton, &

Balis, 2011; Krishnamurthy et al., 2013; Rudnisky et al., 2007; Taylor, 2011; Wright et al., 2013).

Digital imaging is unlocking the potential to integrate primary image features into high-dimensional genomic assays by moving microscopic analysis into the digital age. This creates the opportunity for the application and use of these methods in clinical care and research settings. Digital whole slide imaging seems to be the future of cytopathology, probably sign-out of glass slides will be replaced by whole slide scanned images.

Virtual slide sizes are enormous, ranging from more than 500 Mega bytes and up to 1 Giga byte, depending on the magnification and the scanned slide area. The use of cloud has similar advantages as for the storage of standard cytological images, however with a few orders of magnitude more storage space requirements. The cloud can provide an affordable storage space, easily expandable and offering data storage assurance. Additionally no local maintenance by laboratory technicians is required. Transfer of such data volumes from/to the lab and the cloud is an issue. However the revolution in telecommunication networks, may provide the required bandwidth, and automated slide scanning workstations (see Figure 1) may operate overnight and store unattended the virtual slide data.

Figure 1. From left to right: Modern automated slide scanner capable of creating unattended up to 200 virtual slides, system for single slide scan with an automated stage, system for guided image capture for fluorescent microscopy

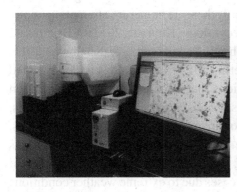 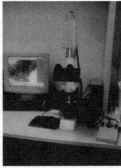 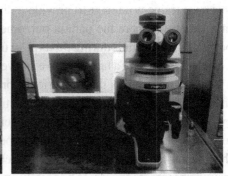

Continuous Medical Education, E-Learning

Over the past decades education has met the introduction of the Internet, radically changing the way humans learn and teach. As the evolution of information technologies, and telecommunications, made the World Wide Web (WWW) a low cost and easily accessible tool for the dissemination of information and knowledge, education could not be left outside. Various researchers have proved that the traditional learning theories can be applied in a Web-based learning system and moreover Web-based distance education, may improve education and support new educational systems, radically changing training in comparison to traditional learning (Garrison, Schardt, & Kochi, 2000). Medical science and medical education represents a major category of lifelong learning, as it is one of the most rapidly evolving sciences and new media offer an advantage for improvement, therefore the new developments and the constant growth of existing knowledge make continuous education vital for continuous medical education. In the field of cytopathology, teaching usually takes place in front of the microscope, supplemented by real-case presentations, didactic lectures and audiovisual materials. However it is not possible for all hospitals to provide microscopes dedicated for educational purposes and a smaller number of them possess multi-user microscopes, permitting simultaneous access to a high number of trainees.

A common technique for teaching cytopathology is via the exploration of ambiguous cases. In this case trainees attempt to provide a diagnosis in a situation where the patient outcome would be unaffected. Pitfalls during this type of training, i.e. false negative or a false positive answers, give a value to trainees, as they experience problems that should never happen in clinical practice. The cytopathology lab is the environment where training takes place in front of the microscope, being the means for knowledge delivery. Web-based training programs appears to be a really promising

solution; as the financial barriers, workplace and time restrictions, experienced by the traditional educational methods in cytopathology, can be eliminated. Additionally, Web-based learning systems can involve traditional learning methods and skills such as decision making, reasoning and problem solving, can be developed (Casebeer et al., 2003; Stergiou et al., 2009). Such skills are critical for the everyday medical practice of professionals.

Cloud computing seems that can become the means to give additional value, to the already available digital age education. Rich information becomes crucial for training; still images captures by the microscope do have limitations. The trainee experiences only a small part of the glass slide, and areas selected by experts. This constitutes a bias for the trainees of the digital era. The solution is obvious complete digitized slides. However, the storage and transmission of such large amount of data, despite being possible nowadays, faces a lot of difficulties. The rise and spread of cloud computing facilitate the elimination of both barriers, as storage is virtually unlimited, has low price and telecommunication infrastructure has a large capacity and is cheap as it is shared. Thus cloud computing and virtual slides seem to be the future of continuous medical education and eLearning for cytopathologists.

Tele-Cytology, Teleconsultation

Telecytology is the interpretation of cytological material at distance via the use of digital images. Historically there are numerous attempts to implement telecytology (Khurana, 2012; O'Brien et al., 1998; Thrall, Pantanowitz, & Khalbuss, 2011; Tsilalis et al., 2012). Telecytology is ideally suited to situations that often encounter transportation problems, such as countries with lots of mountains, islands or many dispersed cities and villages. In these situations due to weather conditions vehicles, ships or planes are unable to move and in many cases due to extreme weather conditions (snow, rain, winds) cities and villages are cut-off. However, telecytology has still limited applications and acceptance. This is mainly due to the challenges of making digital images of acceptable quality reproducing the biological material available on the glass slides, therefore, minimizing diagnostic errors due to the poor quality of the digital representation.

Two hypothetical examples of the use of cloud computing are:

Example1: A hospital has a cytopathology department that wishes to establish a system wherein images and virtual slides are available online and all cytopathologists can report remotely from outside the hospital. By using the hospital server, the users experienced many difficulties because of frequent LAN disruptions within the hospital network. By shifting the data to the Cloud, the cytopathologists will be able to access Web-based cytopathology software. Here, the Cloud enables a telecytology, teleconsultation application.

Example2: A hospital wants to cooperate in real time with a cytopathology laboratory in a remote location. They need to send images in real time from the center to cytopathologists at a nodal center and report the same. For this purpose, they push the images into the Cloud, enabling the cytopathologist to review images at a nodal center, without having to buy additional software and hardware. Here, the Cloud works as a gateway to the peripheral center wherein all its information is available on the Cloud.

Primary Diagnosis

Cytopathologists traditionally perform diagnostic tasks with minimal information; thus they are using other sources of information in order to improve the accuracy of their diagnoses (the triple test in breast fine-needle aspiration cytology, immunocytochemistry, or molecular tests such as flow cytometry for cervical cancer detection). The cloud represents a system of interconnected information systems, therefore, disconnected medical data sources, will be possible to be integrated. As more and more of patients' medical record could be available, the amount of information available to cytopathologists will increase. Cloud computing has the potential to make the entire medical record of a patient, accessible for review by a cytopathologist. However, the obligation of the cytopathologist to review such records is questionable and a subject for discussion (Renshaw, 2011), because at present there is no standard or a recommendation. Some questions are: should cytopathologist review admission notes for all cases? Should cytopathologists seek prior material from other laboratories that are mentioned in these notes if they were not sent for review by the clinicians? Should cytopathologists review imaging material? For example, reviewing mammograms to ensure that lesions under examination by cytopathologists, appear as well in the radiographic material, the ultimate goal is to ensure that cytological material is from the tissue appearing in the mammogram.

Despite the questions mentioned in the previous paragraph, it is a fact that there will be increasing access to more and more information, probably by means of cloud computing technology. Accessing all these data is obviously time consuming and in the most of the cases of no value, and this is a major reason for the previous questions related to the obligations of cytopathologists in the digital era. The answer is not clear; however, cloud systems have the capability to exploit advanced and intelligent search engines that may automatically identify important information and alert cytopathologists. These capabilities will remove the time barriers for the adoption of extensive health record examination. As a result, further evaluation and development of intelligent cloud based search engines exploiting artificial intelligence appears worthwhile. Computing power intensive algorithms seem to be easily a reality with cloud based services on demand.

Another aspect of primary diagnosis is related to homeworker cytopathologists. Virtual slide technology enables the digitization of complete slides; thus the diagnostic data can be now stored and transmitted, the barrier, in this case, being the large amount of data. Eventually cloud computing provides endless storage and fast communication channels, in this aspect, remote primary diagnosis could be a reality.

Research

The potential applications of cloud computing for research in cytopathology seem endless, due to the storage and mainly the availability of processing power. The major research fields envisioned are:

Cytogenetics: Large comparative genomics studies and tools require increasing computational power mainly because the number of available genome sequences constantly rises. Local computing infrastructures are likely to become not capable of coping with the demand for increased computational power and the associated cost. Therefore, alternative parallel computing architectures, toolboxes (Drozdov, Ouzounis, Shah, & Tsoka, 2011; Konganti, Wang, Yang, & Cai, 2013; Shannon et al., 2003) and in particular cloud computing systems, seem to be the solution to alleviate this increasing pressure. Nowadays many efforts and implementations are already available in the literature: existing comparative genomics algorithms (specifically the Reciprocal Smallest Distance-RSD algorithm) from local computing infrastructures have been redesigned for cloud environments in order to exploit their speed and flexibility (Wall et al., 2010). The results indicated that cloud computing environments may provide a substantial boost for the algorithm execution

time and problem solving with a manageable cost. However, the design and transformation of the RSD algorithm into a cloud application was not a trivial task. Technological advances for DNA sequencing have lowered the price for a personal genome sequence (the 3 billion letters in our DNA) towards under $1,000 (Davies, 2010). This creates a new challenge for scientists, the analysis of cohorts of cancer research and treatment. However, large databases are required due to the increased data volume and obviously extreme CPU power for their analysis. Cloud computing seems to be the solution for both issues. A side effect of low costs in DNA sequencing comes from the offered opportunity that allows scientists to collect and analyze whole genomes for genome-wide association studies. As such genetic data do have the potential to be more informative than standard medical records. In addition the capability offered by cloud computing to access and analyze such data sets, being supplied by scientific groups around the planet, necessitates either a paradigm shift in the way that science is done, and/or revised understandings of privacy and informed consent. A proposal by some researchers is to promote both shifts (Greenbaum & Gerstein, 2011).

Proteomics: Proteomics techniques can be used to identify markers for cancer diagnosis because the proteome reflects both the intrinsic genetic program of the cells, as well as the impact of the environment. Proteome analysis has been used in cytopathology for the identification of tumors in various organs: thyroid (Torres-Cabala et al., 2006), breast (Li, Zhao, & Cui, 2013; Sohn et al., 2013), gastric system (Fowsantear, Argo, Pattinson, & Cash, 2013; Lee et al., 2013; Uppal & Powell, 2013) and cervix (Yim & Park, 2006) as well as for response to treatment (Madden et al., 2009), One of the most promising developments from the study of human proteins is the identification of potential new drugs for the treatment of diseases.

Proteome research is mainly based on the assignment of unidentified spectra to peptides.

These methods, including tag-based and de novo searches, have a high computational cost and involve processing of large volumes of experimental spectra thus requiring computers with large storage capacity. These exhaustive identification attempts are rarely carried out in laboratories, due to the lack of computational power, and limited support by information technology specialists to run identification algorithms. Cloud computing is the ideal environment to perform such type of research. As a result, several attempts have been proposed and conducted by various researchers (Halligan, Geiger, Vallejos, Greene, & Twigger, 2009; Leprevost et al., 2013; Mohammed et al., 2012; Muth, Peters, Blackburn, Rapp, & Martens, 2013). Cloud computing allows laboratories to pay for compute time as per requirements, rather than investing on local server clusters.

Artificial Intelligence: The application of artificial intelligence in cytopathology is not new (Karakitsos, Stergiou, et al., 1996). During the last decades, various classification techniques have been used in medicine and especially in diagnostic cytology, involving either classical statistical models or more advanced techniques, such as neural networks (Astion & Wilding, 1992; Cochand-Priollet et al., 2006; Karakitsos, Cochand-Priollet, Guillausseau, & Pouliakis, 1996; Marchevsky, Tsou, & Laird-Offringa, 2004; C. Markopoulos et al., 1997; Pantazopoulos et al., 1998). More specifically, concerning cytology, these techniques have been applied to various organs, among others stomach(Chien et al., 2008; Karakitsos et al., 2004; Yamamura et

al., 2002), breast (Dey, Logasundaram, & Joshi, 2013; Ljung, Chew, Moore, & King, 2004; Ch Markopoulos et al., 1997; Wolberg, Tanner, Loh, & Vanichsetakul, 1987), urinary system (Karakitsos et al., 2005; Schaffer, Simon, Desper, Richter, & Sauter, 2001; Vriesema et al., 2000), cervix (Boon & Kok, 1993; Giovagnoli, Cenci, Olla, & Vecchione, 2002; Karakitsos et al., 2011; Kok, Habers, Schreiner-Kok, & Boon, 1998; Kok et al., 2001) thyroid (Haymart, Cayo, & Chen, 2009; Karakitsos, Cochand-Priollet, Pouliakis, Guillausseau, & Ioakim-Liossi, 1999; Rorive et al., 2010; Varlatzidou et al., 2011) and endometrium (Karakitsos et al., 2002; Pouliakis et al., 2013).

One of the major artificial intelligence technique/science is related to Artificial Neural Networks (ANNs). A typical cycle for the creation of a useful ANN system (see Figure 2) involves several steps

- **Data Collection:** Obtaining the data that will be used to create the intelligent system.
- **Data Preprocessing:** Depending on the type of the ANN system and algorithm that is selected data preprocessing may be required.
- **ANN Model Selection:** Choice of a suitable ANN type for the problem requiring a solution.
- **Parameter Selection:** Configuration of the selected ANN parameters.
- **ANN Training:** Identification of the ANN parameters that actually compose the solution to the problem.

Figure 2. Typical cycle for ANN system production

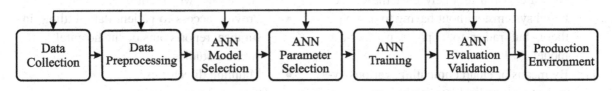

- **Evaluation:** Check the performance of the produced system on known and unknown data.

If the performance of the system is satisfactory then the produced ANN system can be used in a production environment otherwise the procedure should start again from an earlier stage. This type of complexity and the requirement to run numerous systems and combinations of ANN types, architectures and parameters increases geometrically the required number of experiments and thus the required computing resources and computing time. Additionally the training procedure for several ANN types is computing "hungry," as it is not unusual that training of some ANNs can take weeks of computer time. Cloud computing can provide a pool of shared resources available on demand thus can facilitate the production of ANN system both by increasing the number of experiments that can run and by decreasing the time of each experiment.

Impact of Cloud Computing on Cytopathology Daily Workflow

- **Knowledge of IT:** Until now, cytopathologists had total responsibility for the laboratory's IT infrastructure, by having the authority to decide which IT element could improve laboratory daily workflow. In the Cloud computing era, cytopathologists are expected to use IT services without having to take control over the infrastructure that supports it.
- **Costing:** Cloud computing permits cytopathology end users to use hardware and software stored remotely over the Cloud-based systems, without having to purchase them, but rather to apply a pay-per-use model.
- By means of cloud computing, various cytology and medical applications are deliv-

ered as a service over the Internet, which is named software as a service (SaaS software).
- **Integration:** Cloud computing can provide a software platform for laboratory information systems, remote image review software (telecytology) and billing software to cytopathologists, having remote access to all applications by using computers or tablets over the Internet.

How Does Cloud Computing Benefit the Cytopathology Department?

Cloud computing allows administrators of cytopathology departments to take advantage of virtual imaging possibilities without having to maintain any software or hardware. Cytopathologists only have to maintain a single central processing unit.

This system permits cytopathologists to focus on their diagnostic practice and not how or where the service is hosted or processed.

FEW CASES ILLUSTRATING THE ROLE OF CLOUD COMPUTING IN CYTOPATHOLOGY

Advantages of Cloud Computing in Cytopathology

Cytopathology laboratories can benefit from the Cloud by using it in order to:

- Store data,
- Increase productivity,
- Make new software and extra storage available as and when required,
- Provide access to patient data, billing, insurance, reports outside the hospital,
- Archive studies,
- Maintain directories,
- Conduct examinations,

- Maintain access control, manage billing, and keep audit trail for telecytology purposes,
- Decrease costs on infrastructure,
- Ensure system maintenance, performance, and security by professional agencies,

Shortcomings of Cloud Computing

In Cloud computing, protected patient data is stored remotely and is sent and received through the Internet. This makes the data vulnerable to security violations. However, solutions may be proposed. The main threats Cloud computing is facing are:

- New threats of data security and privacy, these threats, may be anticipated by data encryption during storage and transfer and connecting with the server usingencryption protocols.
- Unauthorized access may be anticipated by passwords and password control mechanisms and via mandatory biometric checks.
- Database safety and long-term archival process in case of emergencies and natural disasters have to be discussed with the Cloud computing service provider in detail.
- Server failures may be avoided by maintaining mirror servers.
- Efficiency of service, related to broadband speed may be ensured by the hospital co-operation with multiple Internet service providers to prevent disruption of service.
- Increased load can be easily handled by adding more processing power to existing virtual servers and/or by splitting the application to run on multiple servers, either via load balancing or by the exploitation of multi-tier architectures and splitting to one or more separate application servers and database servers.

FUTURE RESEARCH DIRECTIONS

It is expected that Cloud computing will be further exploited by cytopathology laboratories wishing to improve their quality standards. One of the major challenges of Cloud computing will be to resolve possible problems regarding data safety and security. A possible solution could be a multi-cloud approach with a key sharing mechanism (Mouli & Sesadri, 2013) and patient identification cross reference numbers (Kondoh, Teramoto, Kawai, Mochida, & Nishimura, 2013).

In the distant future, it is expected that the cytopathology departments will witness a large-scale migration to Cloud-based LIS due to ease of availability and low cost of ownership and maintenance.

In relation to the research activities, as sequencing costs are continuously becoming lower, nowadays it is not only possible but extremely easier for genomics researchers to have large amounts of data. The increasing availability of computational power according to Moore's law and the falling overhead for data storage, give to the scientists the opportunity not only to create and store large genetic data sets over the course of their research, but it is possible to process them. However, the majority of the laboratories have already become or will soon become, oversubscribed and underpowered in relation to the exploitation of data. Unavailable software and lack of computational power to run exhaustive search algorithms, eventually, will lead many researchers towards cloud computing to conduct their research. Alternatively much of the minable information may remain untouched, underutilized and not properly explored. As a bonus cloud computing provides the means for data sharing among research teams, thus larger data sets can be exploited, more robust results and conclusions related to rear diseases can be obtained.

CONCLUSION

Cloud computing promotes the concept of bedside cytopathology, point-of-care cytopathology, and instant cytopathology. It gives the cytopathologists, pathologists, physicians, and even patients the possibility to review images and medical data on any display device with a simple Internet connection.

Cloud computing is expected to provide flexibility to all cytopathology services, as it has the potential to revolutionize the way cytopathology data will be stored, accessed, and processed.

Cloud based systems can improve the telecytology field by providing a model to save resources and improve patients control and management. Also, having an electronic clinical history would save paper, physical space and would improve the clinicians and cytopathologists efficiency. The use of shared infrastructure would result in increasing medical data homogeneity, facilitating correlations and data mining.

REFERENCES

Al-Janabi, S., Huisman, A., Willems, S. M., & Van Diest, P. J. (2012). Digital slide images for primary diagnostics in breast pathology: A feasibility study. *Human Pathology*, *43*(12), 2318–2325. doi:10.1016/j.humpath.2012.03.027 PMID:22901465

Astion, M. L., & Wilding, P. (1992). Application of neural networks to the interpretation of laboratory data in cancer diagnosis. *Clinical Chemistry*, *38*(1), 34–38. PMID:1733603

AT&T. (2012). *Medical Imaging in the Cloud*. Retrieved 26/08/2013, 2012, from https://www.corp.att.com/healthcare/docs/medical_imaging_cloud.pdf

Boon, M. E., & Kok, L. P. (1993). Neural network processing can provide means to catch errors that slip through human screening of pap smears. *Diagnostic Cytopathology*, *9*(4), 411–416. doi:10.1002/dc.2840090408 PMID:8261846

Casebeer, L. L., Strasser, S. M., Spettell, C. M., Wall, T. C., Weissman, N., Ray, M. N., & Allison, J. J. (2003). Designing tailored Web-based instruction to improve practicing physicians' preventive practices. *Journal of Medical Internet Research*, *5*(3), e20. doi:10.2196/jmir.5.3.e20 PMID:14517111

Chien, C. W., Lee, Y. C., Ma, T., Lee, T. S., Lin, Y. C., Wang, W., & Lee, W. J. (2008). The application of artificial neural networks and decision tree model in predicting post-operative complication for gastric cancer patients. *Hepato-Gastroenterology*, *55*(84), 1140–1145. PMID:18705347

Cochand-Priollet, B., Koutroumbas, K., Megalopoulou, T. M., Pouliakis, A., Sivolapenko, G., & Karakitsos, P. (2006). Discriminating benign from malignant thyroid lesions using artificial intelligence and statistical selection of morphometric features. *Oncology Reports*, *15*, 1023–1026. PMID:16525694

Davies, K. (2010). *The the revolution in DNA sequencing and the new era of personalized medicine*. New York, NY: Free Press.

Demichelis, F., Della Mea, V., Forti, S., Dalla Palma, P., & Beltrami, C. A. (2002). Digital storage of glass slides for quality assurance in histopathology and cytopathology. *Journal of Telemedicine and Telecare*, *8*(3), 138–142. doi:10.1258/135763302320118979 PMID:12097174

Dey, P., Logasundaram, R., & Joshi, K. (2013). Artificial neural network in diagnosis of lobular carcinoma of breast in fine-needle aspiration cytology. *Diagnostic Cytopathology, 41*(2), 102–106. doi:10.1002/dc.21773 PMID:21987420

Drozdov, I., Ouzounis, C. A., Shah, A. M., & Tsoka, S. (2011). Functional Genomics Assistant (FUGA), a toolbox for the analysis of complex biological networks. *BMC Research Notes, 4*, 462. doi:10.1186/1756-0500-4-462 PMID:22035155

Eugster, M. J., Schmid, M., Binder, H., & Schmidberger, M. (2013). Grid and cloud computing methods in biomedical research. *Methods of Information in Medicine, 52*(1), 62–64. PMID:23318694

Fowsantear, W., Argo, E., Pattinson, C., & Cash, P. (2013). Comparative proteomics of Helicobacter species: The discrimination of gastric and enterohepatic Helicobacter species. *Journal of Proteomics.* PMID:23899588

Fung, K. M., Hassell, L. A., Talbert, M. L., Wiechmann, A. F., Chaser, B. E., & Ramey, J. (2012). Whole slide images and digital media in pathology education, testing, and practice: The Oklahoma experience. *Analytical Cellular Pathology (Amsterdam), 35*(1), 37–40. PMID:21965282

Gagnon, M., Inhorn, S., Hancock, J., Keller, B., Carpenter, D., & Merlin, T. et al. (2004). Comparison of cytology proficiency testing: Glass slides vs. virtual slides. *Acta Cytologica, 48*(6), 788–794. doi:10.1159/000326447 PMID:15581163

Garrison, J. A., Schardt, C., & Kochi, J. K. (2000). Web-based distance continuing education: A new way of thinking for students and instructors. *Bulletin of the Medical Library Association, 88*(3), 211–217. PMID:10928706

Ghaznavi, F., Evans, A., Madabhushi, A., & Feldman, M. (2013). Digital imaging in pathology: Whole-slide imaging and beyond. *Annual Review of Pathology, 8*, 331–359. doi:10.1146/annurev-pathol-011811-120902 PMID:23157334

Giovagnoli, M. R., Cenci, M., Olla, S. V., & Vecchione, A. (2002). Cervical false negative cases detected by neural network-based technology: Critical review of cytologic errors. *Acta Cytologica, 46*(6), 1105–1109. doi:10.1159/000327115 PMID:12462090

Glaser, J. (2011). Cloud computing can simplify HIT infrastructure management. *Healthcare Financial Management, 65*(8), 52–55. PMID:21866720

GlobalData. (2012). *Snapshot: The US cloud computing market for medical imaging.* Retrieved 22/08/2013, from http://www.medicaldevice-network.com/features/featuresnapshot-the-us-cloud-computing-market-for-medical-imaging

Greenbaum, D., & Gerstein, M. (2011). The role of cloud computing in managing the deluge of potentially private genetic data. *The American Journal of Bioethics, 11*(11), 39–41. doi:10.1080/15265161.2011.608242 PMID:22047125

Gutman, D. A., Cobb, J., Somanna, D., Park, Y., Wang, F., & Kurc, T. et al. (2013). Cancer Digital Slide Archive: An informatics resource to support integrated in silico analysis of TCGA pathology data. *Journal of the American Medical Informatics Association.* doi:10.1136/amiajnl-2012-001469 PMID:23893318

Halligan, B. D., Geiger, J. F., Vallejos, A. K., Greene, A. S., & Twigger, S. N. (2009). Low cost, scalable proteomics data analysis using Amazon's cloud computing services and open source search algorithms. *Journal of Proteome Research, 8*(6), 3148–3153. doi:10.1021/pr800970z PMID:19358578

Haymart, M. R., Cayo, M., & Chen, H. (2009). Papillary thyroid microcarcinomas: Big decisions for a small tumor. *Annals of Surgical Oncology, 16*(11), 3132–3139. doi:10.1245/s10434-009-0647-6 PMID:19653044

Hipp, J. D., Lucas, D. R., Emmert-Buck, M. R., Compton, C. C., & Balis, U. J. (2011). Digital slide repositories for publications: lessons learned from the microarray community. *The American Journal of Surgical Pathology, 35*(6), 783–786. doi:10.1097/PAS.0b013e31821946b6 PMID:21552111

Izadi-Mood, N., Sarmadi, S., & Sanii, S. (2013). Quality control in cervicovaginal cytology by cytohistological correlation. *Cytopathology, 24*(1), 33–38. doi:10.1111/j.1365-2303.2011.00926.x PMID:21929578

Jemal, A., Bray, F., Center, M. M., Ferlay, J., Ward, E., & Forman, D. (2011). Global cancer statistics. *CA: a Cancer Journal for Clinicians, 61*(2), 69–90. doi:10.3322/caac.20107 PMID:21296855

Karakitsos, P., Cochand-Priollet, B., Guillausseau, P. J., & Pouliakis, A. (1996). Potential of the back propagation neural network in the morphologic examination of thyroid lesions. *Analytical and Quantitative Cytology and Histology, 18*(6), 494–500. PMID:8978873

Karakitsos, P., Cochand-Priollet, B., Pouliakis, A., Guillausseau, P. J., & Ioakim-Liossi, A. (1999). Learning vector quantizer in the investigation of thyroid lesions. *Analytical and Quantitative Cytology and Histology, 21*(3), 201–208. PMID:10560492

Karakitsos, P., Kyroudes, A., Pouliakis, A., Stergiou, E. B., Voulgaris, Z., & Kittas, C. (2002). Potential of the learning vector quantizer in the cell classification of endometrial lesions in postmenopausal women. *Analytical and Quantitative Cytology and Histology, 24*(1), 30–38. PMID:11865947

Karakitsos, P., Megalopoulou, T. M., Pouliakis, A., Tzivras, M., Archimandritis, A., & Kyroudes, A. (2004). Application of discriminant analysis and quantitative cytologic examination to gastric lesions. *Analytical and Quantitative Cytology and Histology, 26*(6), 314–322. PMID:15678613

Karakitsos, P., Pouliakis, A., Kordalis, G., Georgoulakis, J., Kittas, C., & Kyroudes, A. (2005). Potential of radial basis function neural networks in discriminating benign from malignant lesions of the lower urinary tract. *Analytical and Quantitative Cytology and Histology, 27*(1), 35–42. PMID:15794450

Karakitsos, P., Pouliakis, A., Meristoudis, C., Margari, N., Kassanos, D., & Kyrgiou, M. et al. (2011). A preliminary study of the potential of tree classifiers in triage of high-grade squamous intraepithelial lesions. *Analytical and Quantitative Cytology and Histology, 33*(3), 132–140. PMID:21980616

Karakitsos, P., Stergiou, E. B., Pouliakis, A., Tzivras, M., Archimandritis, A., Liossi, A. I., & Kyrkou, K. (1996). Potential of the back propagation neural network in the discrimination of benign from malignant gastric cells. *Analytical and Quantitative Cytology and Histology, 18*(3), 245–250. PMID:8790840

Khurana, K. K. (2012). Telecytology and its evolving role in cytopathology. *Diagnostic Cytopathology, 40*(6), 498–502. doi:10.1002/dc.22822 PMID:22619124

Kok, M. R., Habers, M. A., Schreiner-Kok, P. G., & Boon, M. E. (1998). New paradigm for ASCUS diagnosis using neural networks. *Diagnostic Cytopathology, 19*(5), 361–366. doi:10.1002/(SICI)1097-0339(199811)19:5<361::AID-DC10>3.0.CO;2-9 PMID:9812231

Kok, M. R., van Der Schouw, Y. T., Boon, M. E., Grobbee, D. E., Kok, L. P., & Schreiner-Kok, P. G. et al. (2001). Neural network-based screening (NNS) in cervical cytology: No need for the light microscope? *Diagnostic Cytopathology, 24*(6), 426–434. doi:10.1002/dc.1093 PMID:11391826

Kondoh, H., Teramoto, K., Kawai, T., Mochida, M., & Nishimura, M. (2013). Development of the Regional EPR and PACS Sharing System on the Infrastructure of Cloud Computing Technology Controlled by Patient Identifier Cross Reference Manager. *Studies in Health Technology and Informatics*, *192*, 1073. PMID:23920847

Konganti, K., Wang, G., Yang, E., & Cai, J. J. (2013). SBEToolbox: A Matlab Toolbox for Biological Network Analysis. *Evolutionary Bioinformatics*, *9*, 355–362. doi:10.4137/EBO. S12012 PMID:24027418

Krishnamurthy, S., Mathews, K., McClure, S., Murray, M., Gilcrease, M., & Albarracin, C. et al. (2013). Multi-Institutional Comparison of Whole Slide Digital Imaging and Optical Microscopy for Interpretation of Hematoxylin-Eosin-Stained Breast Tissue Sections. *Archives of Pathology & Laboratory Medicine*. doi:10.5858/arpa.2012-0437-OA PMID:23947655

Kuo, A. M. (2011). Opportunities and challenges of cloud computing to improve health care services. *Journal of Medical Internet Research*, *13*(3), e67. doi:10.2196/jmir.1867 PMID:21937354

Lee, J., Kim, S., Kim, P., Liu, X., Lee, T., & Kim, K. M. et al. (2013). A novel proteomics-based clinical diagnostics technology identifies heterogeneity in activated signaling pathways in gastric cancers. *PLoS ONE*, *8*(1), e54644. doi:10.1371/journal.pone.0054644 PMID:23372746

Leprevost, F. V., Lima, D. B., Crestani, J., Perez-Riverol, Y., Zanchin, N., Barbosa, V. C., & Carvalho, P. C. (2013). Pinpointing differentially expressed domains in complex protein mixtures with the cloud service of PatternLab for Proteomics. *Journal of Proteomics*, *89*, 179–182. doi:10.1016/j.jprot.2013.06.013 PMID:23796493

Li, G., Zhao, F., & Cui, Y. (2013). Proteomics using mammospheres as a model system to identify proteins deregulated in breast cancer stem cells. *Current Molecular Medicine*, *13*(3), 459–463. PMID:23331018

Ljung, B. M., Chew, K. L., Moore, D. H. II, & King, E. B. (2004). Cytology of ductal lavage fluid of the breast. *Diagnostic Cytopathology*, *30*(3), 143–150. doi:10.1002/dc.20003 PMID:14986293

Lupse, O. S., Vida, M., & Stoicu-Tivadar, L. (2012). Cloud computing technology applied in healthcare for developing large scale flexible solutions. *Studies in Health Technology and Informatics*, *174*, 94–99. PMID:22491119

Madden, K., Flowers, L., Salani, R., Horowitz, I., Logan, S., & Kowalski, K. et al. (2009). Proteomics-based approach to elucidate the mechanism of antitumor effect of curcumin in cervical cancer. *Prostaglandins, Leukotrienes, and Essential Fatty Acids*, *80*(1), 9–18. doi:10.1016/j.plefa.2008.10.003 PMID:19058955

Marchevsky, A. M., Tsou, J. A., & Laird-Offringa, I. A. (2004). Classification of individual lung cancer cell lines based on DNA methylation markers: use of linear discriminant analysis and artificial neural networks. *The Journal of Molecular Diagnostics*, *6*(1), 28–36. doi:10.1016/S1525-1578(10)60488-6 PMID:14736824

Markopoulos, C., Karakitsos, P., Botsoli-Stergiou, E., Pouliakis, A., Gogas, J., Ioakim-Liossi, A., & Kyrkou, K. (1997). Application of back propagation to the diagnosis of breast lesions by fine needle aspiration. *The Breast*, *6*(5), 293–298. doi:10.1016/S0960-9776(97)90008-4

Markopoulos, C., Karakitsos, P., Botsoli-Stergiou, E., Pouliakis, A., Ioakim-Liossi, A., Kyrkou, K., & Gogas, J. (1997). Application of the learning vector quantizer to the classification of breast lesions. *Analytical and Quantitative Cytology and Histology, 19*(5), 453–460. PMID:9349906

Mirza, H., & El-Masri, S. (2013). National Electronic Medical Records integration on Cloud Computing System. *Studies in Health Technology and Informatics, 192*, 1219. PMID:23920993

Mohammed, Y., Mostovenko, E., Henneman, A. A., Marissen, R. J., Deelder, A. M., & Palmblad, M. (2012). Cloud parallel processing of tandem mass spectrometry based proteomics data. *Journal of Proteome Research, 11*(10), 5101–5108. doi:10.1021/pr300561q PMID:22916831

Mouli, K. C., & Sesadri, U. (2013). Single to Multi Clouds for Security in Cloud Computing by using Secret Key Sharing. *Internatioonal Journal of Computers and Technology, 10*(4), 1539–1545.

Muth, T., Peters, J., Blackburn, J., Rapp, E., & Martens, L. (2013). ProteoCloud: A full-featured open source proteomics cloud computing pipeline. *Journal of Proteomics, 88*, 104–108. doi:10.1016/j.jprot.2012.12.026 PMID:23305951

O'Brien, M. J., Takahashi, M., Brugal, G., Christen, H., Gahm, T., & Goodell, R. M. … Winkler, C. (1998). Digital imagery/telecytology. International Academy of Cytology Task Force summary: Diagnostic Cytology Towards the 21st Century: An International Expert Conference and Tutorial. *Acta Cytologica, 42*(1), 148-164.

Pantazopoulos, D., Karakitsos, P., Iokim-Liossi, A., Pouliakis, A., Botsoli-Stergiou, E., & Dimopoulos, C. (1998). Back propagation neural network in the discrimination of benign from malignant lower urinary tract lesions. *The Journal of Urology, 159*(5), 1619–1623. doi:10.1097/00005392-199805000-00057 PMID:9554366

Patel, R. P. (2012). Cloud computing and virtualization technology in radiology. *Clinical Radiology, 67*(11), 1095–1100. doi:10.1016/j.crad.2012.03.010 PMID:22607956

Pouliakis, A., Iliopoulou, D., & Karakitsou, E. (2012). Design and Implementation Issues of an Information System Supporting Cervical Cancer Screening Programs. *Journal of Applied Medical Sciences, 1*(1), 61–91.

Pouliakis, A., & Karakitsos, P. (2011). *Concepts of software design for population based cervical cencer screening.* Paper presented at the 36th European Congress of Cytology. Istanbul, Turkey.

Pouliakis, A., Margari, C., Margari, N., Chrelias, C., Zygouris, D., & Meristoudis, C. et al. (2013). Using classification and regression trees, liquid-based cytology and nuclear morphometry for the discrimination of endometrial lesions. *Diagnostic Cytopathology.* http://dx.doi.org/10.1002/dc.23077 doi:10.1002/dc.23077 PMID:24273089

Renshaw, A. A. (2011). Quality improvement in cytology: Where do we go from here? *Archives of Pathology & Laboratory Medicine, 135*(11), 1387–1390. doi:10.5858/arpa.2010-0606-RA PMID:22032562

Rorive, S. N. D. H., Fossion, C., Delpierre, I., Arbaguia, N., Avni, F., Decaestecker, C., & Salmon, I. (2010). Ultrasound-guided fine-needle aspiration of thyroid nodules: Stratification of malignancy risk using follicular proliferation grading, clinical and ultrasonographic features. *European Journal of Endocrinology.* doi:10.1530/EJE-09-1103 PMID:20219856

Rosenthal, A., Mork, P., Li, M. H., Stanford, J., Koester, D., & Reynolds, P. (2010). Cloud computing: A new business paradigm for biomedical information sharing. *Journal of Biomedical Informatics, 43*(2), 342–353. doi:10.1016/j.jbi.2009.08.014 PMID:19715773

Rudnisky, C. J., Tennant, M. T., Weis, E., Ting, A., Hinz, B. J., & Greve, M. D. (2007). Web-based grading of compressed stereoscopic digital photography versus standard slide film photography for the diagnosis of diabetic retinopathy. *Ophthalmology*, *114*(9), 1748–1754. doi:10.1016/j.ophtha.2006.12.010 PMID:17368543

Schaffer, A. A., Simon, R., Desper, R., Richter, J., & Sauter, G. (2001). Tree models for dependent copy number changes in bladder cancer. *International Journal of Oncology*, *18*(2), 349–354. PMID:11172603

Shannon, P., Markiel, A., Ozier, O., Baliga, N. S., Wang, J. T., & Ramage, D. et al. (2003). Cytoscape: A software environment for integrated models of biomolecular interaction networks. *Genome Research*, *13*(11), 2498–2504. doi:10.1101/gr.1239303 PMID:14597658

Sherman, M. E., Dasgupta, A., Schiffman, M., Nayar, R., & Solomon, D. (2007). The Bethesda Interobserver Reproducibility Study (BIRST), a Web-based assessment of the Bethesda 2001 System for classifying cervical cytology. *Cancer*, *111*(1), 15–25. doi:10.1002/cncr.22423 PMID:17186503

Sohn, J., Do, K. A., Liu, S., Chen, H., Mills, G. B., & Hortobagyi, G. N. et al. (2013). Functional proteomics characterization of residual triple-negative breast cancer after standard neoadjuvant chemotherapy. *Annals of Oncology*. doi:10.1093/annonc/mdt248 PMID:23925999

Solomon, D., Davey, D., Kurman, R., Moriarty, A., O'Connor, D., & Prey, M. et al. (2002). The 2001 Bethesda System: Terminology for reporting results of cervical cytology. *Journal of the American Medical Association*, *287*(16), 2114–2119. doi:10.1001/jama.287.16.2114 PMID:11966386

Stergiou, N., Georgoulakis, G., Margari, N., Aninos, D., Stamataki, M., & Stergiou, E. et al. (2009). Using a web-based system for the continuous distance education in cytopathology. *International Journal of Medical Informatics*, *78*(12), 827–838. doi:10.1016/j.ijmedinf.2009.08.007 PMID:19775933

Stewart, J. III, Miyazaki, K., Bevans-Wilkins, K., Ye, C., Kurtycz, D. F., & Selvaggi, S. M. (2007). Virtual microscopy for cytology proficiency testing: Are we there yet? *Cancer*, *111*(4), 203–209. doi:10.1002/cncr.22766 PMID:17580360

Taylor, C. R. (2011). From microscopy to whole slide digital images: A century and a half of image analysis. *Applied Immunohistochemistry & Molecular Morphology*, *19*(6), 491–493. doi:10.1097/PAI.0b013e318229ffd6 PMID:22089486

Thrall, M., Pantanowitz, L., & Khalbuss, W. (2011). Telecytology: Clinical applications, current challenges, and future benefits. *Journal of Pathology Informatics*, *2*, 51. doi:10.4103/2153-3539.91129 PMID:22276242

Torres-Cabala, C., Bibbo, M., Panizo-Santos, A., Barazi, H., Krutzsch, H., Roberts, D. D., & Merino, M. J. (2006). Proteomic identification of new biomarkers and application in thyroid cytology. *Acta Cytologica*, *50*(5), 518–528. doi:10.1159/000326006 PMID:17017437

Tsilalis, T., Archondakis, S., Meristoudis, C., Margari, N., Pouliakis, A., & Skagias, L. et al. (2012). Assessment of static telecytological diagnoses' reproducibility in cervical smears prepared by means of liquid-based cytology. *Telemedicine Journal and e-Health*, *18*(7), 516–520. doi:10.1089/tmj.2011.0167 PMID:22856666

Uppal, D. S., & Powell, S. M. (2013). Genetics/genomics/proteomics of gastric adenocarcinoma. *Gastroenterology Clinics of North America*, *42*(2), 241–260. doi:10.1016/j.gtc.2013.01.005 PMID:23639639

Varlatzidou, A., Pouliakis, A., Stamataki, M., Meristoudis, C., Margari, N., & Peros, G. et al. (2011). Cascaded learning vector quantizer neural networks for the discrimination of thyroid lesions. *Analytical and Quantitative Cytology and Histology*, *33*(6), 323–334. PMID:22590810

Vooijs, G. P., Davey, D. D., Somrak, T. M., Goodell, R. M., Grohs, D. H., & Knesel, E. A., Jr. … Wilbur, D. C. (1998). Computerized training and proficiency testing. International Academy of Cytology Task Force summary: Diagnostic Cytology Towards the 21st Century: An International Expert Conference and Tutorial. *Acta Cytologica*, *42*(1), 141-147.

Vriesema, J. L., van der Poel, H. G., Debruyne, F. M., Schalken, J. A., Kok, L. P., & Boon, M. E. (2000). Neural network-based digitized cell image diagnosis of bladder wash cytology. *Diagnostic Cytopathology*, *23*(3), 171–179. doi:10.1002/1097-0339(200009)23:3<171::AID-DC6>3.0.CO;2-F PMID:10945904

Wall, D. P., Kudtarkar, P., Fusaro, V. A., Pivovarov, R., Patil, P., & Tonellato, P. J. (2010). Cloud computing for comparative genomics. *BMC Bioinformatics*, *11*, 259. doi:10.1186/1471-2105-11-259 PMID:20482786

Waxer, N., Ninan, D., Ma, A., & Dominguez, N. (2013). How cloud computing and social media are changing the face of health care. *The Physician Executive Journal*, *39*(2), 58-60, 62.

Webb, G. (2012). Making the cloud work for healthcare: Cloud computing offers incredible opportunities to improve healthcare, reduce costs and accelerate ability to adopt new IT services. *Health Management Technology*, *33*(2), 8–9. PMID:22397112

Wolberg, W. H., Tanner, M. A., Loh, W. Y., & Vanichsetakul, N. (1987). Statistical approach to fine needle aspiration diagnosis of breast masses. *Acta Cytologica*, *31*(6), 737–741. PMID:3425134

Wright, A. M., Smith, D., Dhurandhar, B., Fairley, T., Scheiber-Pacht, M., & Chakraborty, S. et al. (2013). Digital slide imaging in cervicovaginal cytology: A pilot study. *Archives of Pathology & Laboratory Medicine*, *137*(5), 618–624. doi:10.5858/arpa.2012-0430-OA PMID:22970841

Yamamura, Y., Nakajima, T., Ohta, K., Nashimoto, A., Arai, K., & Hiratsuka, M. et al. (2002). Determining prognostic factors for gastric cancer using the regression tree method. *Gastric Cancer*, *5*(4), 201–207. doi:10.1007/s101200200035 PMID:12491077

Yim, E. K., & Park, J. S. (2006). Role of proteomics in translational research in cervical cancer. *Expert Review of Proteomics*, *3*(1), 21–36. doi:10.1586/14789450.3.1.21 PMID:16445348

KEY TERMS AND DEFINITIONS

Cloud Computing: A large number of computers connected through a network, capable to run an application on many computers and to configure virtual servers, virtual servers do not have physical presence and can be moved around and scaled up or down without to be noticed by end users, like a cloud.

Cytopathology: A specialty of medicine related to the study and diagnosis of diseases by the examination of cells.

E-Health: Is the healthcare supported by electronics, informatics and tele-communications

E-Learning: Is a broad concept referring to the application of information and communication technologies (ICT) for learning purposes.

Laboratory Information System (LIS): Or Laboratory Information Management System (LIMS) is a software-based system for the support of operations in a modern laboratory, such as workflow, sample tracking, data exchange interfaces, LIS systems are often capable to be connected with medical analyzers for automated extraction and storage of measurements.

Quality Assurance (QA): The set of processes applied in quality systems in order to assure that the characteristics of a product, service or activity will be fulfilled, QA attempts to improve and stabilize products, services or activities.

Quality Control (QC): The set of processes by which entities review the quality of all factors involved in product, service or activity, during QC processes, the products, services and activities are tested or validated in order to reveal defects and problems, before their release.

Screening: In the medical world is the examination of a group of persons in order to identify healthy persons from those who have an undiagnosed disease or have high risk to get sick.

Telecytology: The application of cytopathology from distance.

Telediagnosis: Is the determination of a disease at a site remote from the patient based on transmitted data.

Chapter 14
A Case Study of the Health Cloud

Roma Chauhan
IILM Graduate School of Management, India

ABSTRACT

Initiatives have recently been taken to facilitate effective sharing and collaboration of healthcare information. The process undertaken to manage healthcare data is always in debate. The healthcare industry is encouraged to leverage technology solution for providing improved services to patients and doctors. The chapter explains the need of the healthcare process re-engineering through the implementation of Software as a Service (SaaS). It also highlights the potential and challenges of integrating SaaS-based health cloud in the healthcare industry. This chapter explores the exciting journey of the Indian healthcare transformation through technology implementation. Moreover, the chapter discusses the different healthcare clouds and deployment models. It illustrates SaaS-based solutions for the healthcare segment and argues that cloud-based healthcare and mobile healthcare by use of portable devices can make health consultation convenient for patients across the world.

INTRODUCTION

With the ascending health care expenditure, healthcare service providers are steadily seeking mechanisms to stay competitive and provide quality service to the customers. However, not much research has been done on the implementation of the Business Process Re-engineering (BPR) for the healthcare systems. Healthcare industry has conventionally focused on breakthroughs in operating procedures and technology to stay competitive. However, healthcare service providers have started to understand that BPR initiatives could be a better solution to achieve competitive advantage.

Reengineering modus operandi enable healthcare service providers to take a precise look at the processes involved within the organization, identifying redundancy and inefficiency that can be removed from the system. The process reengineering methods are used by managers to discover the best processes for performing work, and these processes can be reengineered for optimized output (Weicher et al., 1995). A core business process

DOI: 10.4018/978-1-4666-6118-9.ch014

usually creates value by the capabilities it gives the company for competitiveness. A finite number of such vital business processes can be determined in a company, and improving those processes can lead to business enhancement.

The advantage of reinventing hospitals holds the tangible and realistic promise of profoundly cutting on cost and dramatically enhancing the quality of care provided (Harmon, 1996). The recognized reasons for the emergence of BPR are identified as consumers, global competition, technological development and IT (Francis & McIntosh, 1997). For re-engineered processes, IT is an enabler and, for any reengineering program, it is necessary to consider the enormous benefits achieved by using technologies such as document image processing and expert systems (Morris & Brandon, 1993).

With the globalized fierce competition in healthcare arena, it has become absolutely necessary for the healthcare service providers to trans-

form and execute technology enabled processes for healthcare record management. The improved process enhances patient doctor collaboration and efficient management of patient records.

A health cloud is the interconnection of a large number of computers and servers dedicated to cater for the needs of the healthcare industry. The healthcare service is delivered to the user who can be a doctor or patient through the internet connection. The cloud service allows users to access the hardware and software managed by the third parties at remote locations (Figure1). As a result, Cloud computing has brought major transformation in how information is stored and accessed. The entire scenario, today, has drifted from desktop centric to document the centric context, while the cloud computing framework encourages re-use of IT capabilities.

The primary value proposition of cloud computing is to pay only for the services a user consumes. As an example, organizations can

Figure 1. Health Cloud infrastructure
Data Source: Image by Author

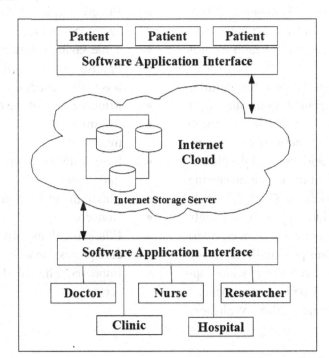

run multiple applications in the cloud and pay for only what they use based on the number of virtual CPU's, storage and network utilization. The cloud model can be useful to run software, handle testing, expand storage and simplify collaboration. It enables computing infrastructure to be considered as a service and leads to enhanced agility and scalability.

BACKGROUND

Cloud Computing is an interesting methodology enabled by delivering software, infrastructure and the entire computation platform as a service. Contrary to traditional Web hosting providers, cloud computing, delivers pay-per-click services. It means users only have to pay for the resources they use over time (Dawoud, Takouna & Meinel, 2010). These services are offered over the Internet by large data and computing centers (Feng, Chen & Liu, 2010).

The cloud computing is a service oriented and not application oriented. It offers on-demand virtualized resources as an assessable and chargeable service (Buyya, Yeo & Venugopal, 2008). It can also make convenient for the patients to find and keep track of their own health records (Grogan, 2006).

The healthcare applications for cellular network had gradually gained momentum over the last few years (Blake, 2008). The escalation in the invasion of mobile networks in remote rural villages in India and the mobile phones have become an important device for enhancing doctor-patient communication (Bali & Singh, 2007). The mobile technology is increasingly augmenting functions of handheld devices, smart phones and PDAs that are potentially replacing the use of computer based substitutes while supporting mobility needs of patients and medical practitioners (Ikhu-Omoregbe, 2008). With these

benefits, it is increasingly becoming possible to create innovative applications for developing countries that can shift the paradigm of delivering services and resolving problems nurtured by the healthcare systems (Perera, 2009).

Recent trends include accessing information any time across the globe which can be achieved by shifting towards the healthcare cloud. This delivery model can make healthcare more efficient and effective and at a comparatively technology budgets of less cost (Horowitz, 2011). In spite of rising security and privacy risks, the healthcare organizations can certainly take benefits of cloud computing solutions and bring immense benefits to improve the quality of service to the patients and reduce overall healthcare costs (Muir, 2011).

SOCIAL TRANSFORMATION DRIVE AND THE CLOUD

The electronic healthcare has brought transformation to the society. It has emerged as a promising field with the following benefits for the society:

- Effective channel for creating the health awareness among citizens.
- Time saving solution.
- Precise information about doctors' and hospitals' schedule.
- Minimization of the cost of medicine.
- Minimization of the cost of health treatment.
- Save with hospitals with interference of middlemen.
- Maximum utilization of hospital resources.
- Convenience for doctor patient interaction.
- Efficient collaborative platform for healthcare professionals.
- Improved clinical data management and access.

CLOUD DEPLOYMENT MODELS

The deployment model describes where the physical server is deployed and how it is managed. The following cloud deployment models can be classified into different categories on the basis of their functionality:

Private Cloud

The private computing service is dedicatedly owned and used by the enterprise. The private cloud service is deployed within the organization datacenter and behind the firewall that makes it highly secure. The pool of resources on the cloud is only accessible to a single organization leading to a higher level of control.

Public Cloud

The public cloud provides access to computing resources over the Internet. The infrastructure cost is shared among end users making it affordable. It offers superior scalability and sharing of resources. The organizations can use this service without being aware of where the data is located and stored.

Hybrid Cloud

A hybrid cloud is a combination of public and the private cloud. It enables shared Application Program Interface (API) to enable hybrid operation. The hybrid cloud allows cost benefit of public cloud and security feature of private cloud.

Community Cloud

It is shared cloud service environment limited to set of organization or people. They are built to meet the needs of specific market segments such like healthcare. The community that has to share common concerns will preferably select the option of community cloud for effective collaboration.

CLOUD COMPUTING MODELS

The cloud computing technology is flourishing paradigm, and it will evolve in coming years. The cloud service archetypal models can be described as:

Issues, Controversies Software as a Service (SaaS)

The on-demand software is accessed as a Web based service through the cloud infrastructure. The Web based application has data and software centralized that can be accessed through Web browser. The cloud service provider maintains storage, application and network for the consumer. The end user does not require managing any software upgrade, storage, server and network infrastructure (Peter et al., 2009).

Platform as a Service (PaaS)

By using PaaS, the geographically distributed development teams can collaboratively work on software development projects. The service allows software developers to build Web applications without any complexity of installing tools on their workstation. The PaaS offering includes application design, development, test and deployment.

Infrastructure as a Service (IaaS)

The service delivery model enables with the assistance to lease hardware, operating system, storage and network capacity in a virtualized manner. The end user need is not required to manage the underlying cloud infrastructure and has control over operating systems, storage and deployed applications (Mell & Grance (2011). The IaaS offering includes virtual server space, bandwidth and IP address.

THE KEY PLAYERS

There are multiple companies offering cloud based healthcare service; a few to name are Practo Technologies, Healcon Labs, Helping Doc, Doc-Suggest, MocDoc and Insta Health. Refer Table 1 to check Website ranking of key SaaS based health players.

With the rising demand of digitization, the healthcare digitization is at peak with the leading competitors such like: Practo (allow doctor patient connectivity, digitized records, billing and reminders), DocSuggest (Helps find suitable doctors, schedule appointments via Website or call), Mocdoc (Books appointment, offers SMS reminders, follow up calls and digitized records), SmartRx (Book appointment, offer access to patient records, alert on diagnostics and e-consultation) (Adarsh, 2013).

Practo Technologies leading competitors are mentioned in the Table 1. The stat given above indicates change is user preferences. The key drivers of SaaS healthcare are Practo, HelpingDoc, Healcon

Labs and SmartRx, users are comparatively spending between 11 to 25 minutes average on these Websites. The ranking of Practo Technologies is the highest for Indian and Global scenario. The company is able to make a remarkable position is the fierce competition using creative strategy, which are discussed later in the chapter.

CLOUD BASED HEALTH CARE: A CASE STUDY

Practo Technologies[1] was formed in year 2008. The vision of the company was to make medical information digitally accessible to patients and doctors. With all these features at pleasing price, solutions providers like Practo aimed to create the most efficient healthcare experience for people in India and gradually around the world. The aim was to improve the patient experience for finding and meeting a doctor.

Traditionally the healthcare records were created manually and stored on shelves. Managing of records stored in files traditionally was of not much use. With the evolution of technology, there has been a paradigm shift in the manner the healthcare industry functions. The medical records are electronically stored and managed. With the

Table 1. Website ranking

No	Company Name	Website	Global Rank	Indian Rank	Daily Time on Site (min)	Bounce Rate on Site (%)
1	Practo Technologies	practo.com	29,692	2,263	11:33	29.60
2	HelpingDoc	helpingdoc.com	73,739	8,509	13:34	32.40
3	DocSuggest	docsuggest.com	89,185	9,289	2:20	55.40
4	NamasteDoc	namastedoc.com	450,357	57,963	2:47	43.90
5	Insta Health Solution	instahealthsolutions.com	1,198,332	78,573	3:12	44.80
6	Healcon Labs	healcon.com	65,532	6,045	25:45	23.40
7	MocDoc	mocdoc.in	548,675	70,421	1:45	61.50
8	SmartRx	Smartrx.in	438,264	44,881	23.07	21.10

Source: www.Alexa.com

acceptance of cloud computing the healthcare patient data is stored at a remote server location on the internet.

The Cloud Software

The cloud based software is developed to meet the needs of doctors and patients can be classified as:

Practo Ray

Practo Ray is a cloud based flagship product that allows patients to search for doctors and book their appointment online. The dedicated online platform for health professionals and intelligent system that lets users know when the doctor is available. The user friendly and effective practice management software supports online appointment booking, electronic medical records (EMR) and enables effective clinic-patient communication.

Practo Hello

It is the first automated call based software that enables patients to call and book their appointment instantly. The automated voice service responds to the calls made by the patients to book an appointment. The Interactive Voice Response System (IVRS) solution for doctors lets them manage the phone calls made to their clinics and access call recordings while ensuring that no call goes unanswered.

Practo Group

It is an online collaborative platform dedicated to healthcare community. The online forum enables healthcare professionals to share views, meet other members and promote their health events. The group service enabled collaboration among like-minded healthcare fraternity.

The Cloud Service

The cloud software service has a number of benefits and challenges. Below are discussion point of benefits and challenges and the key selling strategies opted by Practo Technologies for selling their services to the clients:

Benefits

Bringing cloud into use in businesses, it will not just save the cost of staff required to manage servers, but will also require lesser servers and with that less power consumption (Padhy, Patra & Satapathy, 2012). E-health cloud data may be used by decision makers for planning and budgeting for healthcare services (AbuKhousa, Mohamed & Al-Jaroodi, 2012). Moreover, Cloud computing has the potential to significantly reduce IT costs and complexities. It improves resources utilization and service delivery (Maria, Fenu & Surcis, 2009) while providing on-demand self-service to users that come as a package with pay per use. The organizations offering a cloud service can expect rapid and elastic provisioning with minimal service provider interaction. The advantages of having a SaaS base cloud system include:

- The health cloud provides the opportunity of improved patient care since the unified patient records can be shared effectively with other medical specialists if required. Moreover, the digital records are available anytime anywhere to view the patient's medical history comprehensively.
- The internet based health cloud offers the service opportunity at a reduced price, as a collaborative environment brings shared cost among participants with the flexibility to pay for actual resource utilization.

- The health cloud solves the issue of scarce IT infrastructure and healthcare professionals enabling rural and remote communities to use the healthcare service.
- The cloud based health service strengthens the ability to monitor spread out of diseases. It can be used as an alert system for diseases outbreak or can be used to identify the infectious regions, the disease spreading patterns and the probable reasons of the outbreaks.
- The strategic decision makers can use the health loud for planning and budgeting health services while the integrated approach can help in predicting future healthcare needs.

Challenges

It is convenient for healthcare providers and patients to have electronic health record applications and services over the cloud. This adoption may lead to enormous security challenges related with user authentication, access control, policy integration and trust management (Wu et al., 2010). The challenges leaded to lot of difficulties in the idea being accepted. Doctors were very apprehensive about buying the software online. The challenges of a SaaS based system can be classified as:

- The user acceptance to cloud emerged as a vital issue. The doctors are not very open to the idea of technology to manage their operations and other healthcare practices.
- The cloud based healthcare service should be continuously available on-demand, with no interruptions. The cloud based service should not be compromised due to hardware, software or network failure.
- The cloud services do offer security measures, but there is a challenge about data security. Data security and privacy are the primary concerns for the healthcare in-

dustry. As the service becomes distributed in nature, the chances of erroneous data increases.
- The cloud should have the potential of scalability (an exponential increase of the healthcare records over a period of time).
- High security concerns are the prime concerns for open environments. It is necessary to provide cloud service with adequate access control and authentication mechanisms to ensure secure data transfer between the client and the service provider.
- With the rise in the numbers of users and the complexity of the cloud based healthcare network, the cloud based resources should be maintained in a reliable manner to avoid any future disruption of the service.

Key Selling Strategy

Selling software to SME appeared as a challenge for Practo Technologies. They creatively designed their strategies to reach a large number of customers. After rigorous follow up with the doctors and the clinics, it came as a surprise that most of the doctors were not online. Selling of internet based software to that segment appeared difficult. Following listed are strategies developed and implemented by Practo team to sell the SaaS based health care service:

- Don't focus on the number of registered users for the software but try to add value to the software product and enhance its lifetime value.
- The advantage of selling SaaS was that you can push the customer to buy the software service at an affordable price. A user can pay for a month, six months, annually and further stretching up to five years of time.
- Diversify the product line. Sell many products not one.

- Broaden geographical reach to connect with the customers. Practo headquartered at Bangalore decided to move beyond the capital, reaching out more places.
- Practo followed aggressive pricing policy. No negotiation on the registration and usage price. They steadily followed the policy for a long time. Zero discounts were offered to the customers. The product was priced uniformly irrespective of different geographic locations and financial status.
- The IT in the healthcare market may a niche, but it's a world-wide territory with global internet connectivity. Use Internet to sell the service.
- Spreading awareness about the product through trade shows and discussion forums.
- Strategically planned short duration reporting sales cycle to analyze and monitor the sales figures across the country.
- Initially, the company focused on developing a high-end value based product.

The SWOT Analysis

Practo Technologies is currently in a highly lucrative and rapidly dynamic market. They foresee their strengths as the ability to respond apprehensively to the market dictates and provide custom designed software and services to clients including patients and doctors. In addition, through aggressive marketing and quality management strategies creatively designed Practo intends to become a well-respected leader in the list of software providers for the healthcare industry. SWOT analysis showcases comprehensive competencies of Practo and enormous opportunities to capture the potential market.

Strengths

- Unsatisfied clients of the competitors.

- Dedicated sales team with short term sales cycle monitoring.
- Customized software to meet patient and doctor needs.
- Innovation with software service diversification.
- Strategically planned sales cycle.
- Cloud based easy to use software interface.

Weaknesses

- Lack of a concrete well established network.
- Weak brand and software service awareness .

Opportunities

- The IT healthcare market is niche.
- Need of superior quality, precise and relevant on-time information availability.
- Improvement in mobile technology and rise of m-healthcare.
- After sales service on monthly basis.
- Limited features offered by HelpingDoc, Healcon and SARAL software.
- An aggressive and focused marketing campaign.
- Participation in health care Expo and other community building platforms.

Threats

- New marketing strategies and tactics by established companies.
- Neutral or no brand image.
- Current IT Infrastructure.
- Hesitation of healthcare professionals to leverage technology in current systems.
- Unawareness about SaaS models and the payment options.

PORTABLE HEALTHCARE

With the advancement, in the mobile technology ample opportunities to improve patient's health and well-being have emerged in recent years. Mobile and other PDA devices are increasingly being accepted by large volume of users due to its rising affordability. Mobile technology is extensively used to support mobile driver healthcare known as mHealth. mHealth technologies provide real time monitoring and detection of transition in health status, support the acceptance and maintenance of a healthy lifestyle, offer expeditious diagnosis of health conditions and promote the implementation of interventions ranging from promoting patient self-care to provide remote healthcare services.

With the dynamic changes in the standards, high-quality, user-friendly wireless consumer devices, such as mobile phones, have gained popularity. The mobile devices are available with the user for most of the time and not only provides mobile communication, but also sensing, analytic, and visual capabilities and the access to the cloud. The problems of computer based health care is charged with infrastructure issues like lack of electricity, maintenance issues in heat and dust of tropical climate, moral and ethical issues in providing quality care, knowledge gaps of users, supply of medicines and other healthcare and ambiguous clinical competence (Wootton, 2001). The cloud based light weight applications can be utilized to support healthcare practices to a major extent.

The semi literate people in rural areas are now becoming efficient mobile users and innovation have diffused into arena of m-commerce, m-health, m-learning and m-governance projects across the developing world (Donner, 2008). It is observed that user friendliness and low start up cost make m-health emerge as an interesting option in the developing world. The applications can be customized to fit the complexities of local healthcare delivery networks and appropriate financial models can be figured out (Kaplan, 2006).

With the support from the mobile technology, the SaaS based healthcare software can reach larger chunk of the population.

FUTURE RESEARCH DIRECTIONS

Research on cloud based healthcare is an emerging area of interest and can be the solution to various healthcare industry collaboration issues. . Though the technologies related to healthcare cloud have been in existence for quite some time, the knowledge and experience about their business use is quite limited. Further research work is suggested to be conducted in the form of empirical analysis of data gathered from healthcare professionals and patients to understand the acceptability of healthcare cloud. In addition, I would like to investigate region wise cloud penetration and identify usage patterns of users from different geographic locations.

CONCLUSION

With the advancement of the mobile technology, ample opportunities to improve patient's health and well-being have emerged in recent years. mHealth technologies provide real time monitoring and detection of transition of health status, support the acceptance and maintenance of a healthy lifestyle, offer expeditious diagnosis of health conditions and promote the implementation of interventions ranging from promoting patient self-care to providing remote healthcare services.

With the dynamic changes in the standards, high-quality, user-friendly wireless consumer devices, such as mobile phones, have gained popularity. The mobile devices are available with the user for most of the time and not only provide mobile communication, but also sensing, analytic, and visual capabilities and the access to the cloud. The problems of computer based health care include infrastructure issues like lack of electricity, maintenance issues in heat and dust of tropical climate, moral and ethical issues in providing quality care, knowledge gaps of users, supply of medicines and other healthcare and ambiguous clinical competence (Wootton, 2001).

The semi-literate people in rural areas are now becoming efficient mobile users and innovation has diffused into the arena of m-commerce, m-health, m-learning and m-governance projects across the developing world (Donner, 2008). It is observed that user friendliness and low startup cost make m-health emerge as an interesting option in the developing world. The applications can be customized to fit the complexities of local healthcare delivery networks and appropriate financial models can be figured out (Kaplan, 2006).

Finally, the recent trend of accepting cloud computing in the healthcare can improve and solve considerable collaborative information concerns in healthcare organizations including the cost optimization factor. The accepted cloud based applications will bring obvious benefits to patients, physicians, insurance companies, pharmacies, imaging centers and many more when sharing information across medical organizations.

The e-Health Cloud showcases an enabling technology solution for many healthcare providers encountering various concerns of rising healthcare delivery costs, information sharing, and scarcity of healthcare professionals. The benefits gained are suppressed by issues of trust, privacy, and security, in addition to many technical issues, that must be addressed before healthcare providers can fully adopt and trust the-Health Cloud. With improvements in standards of mobile technologies, the access to healthcare records and information has become convenient for patients and healthcare practitioners.

However, challenges of security and interoperability will elevate leading to slow adoption of the cloud computing model. But the implementation of best practices in the design, deployment and use will hopefully generate a future growth of the cloud based systems, despite all the obstacles. It is not uncommon for emerging technologies to have associated challenges. However, if the challenges are mismanaged or ignored, technology adoption can be a risky affair.

REFERENCES

AbuKhousa, E., Mohamed, N., & Al-Jaroodi, J. (2012). E-Health Cloud: Opportunities and Challenges. *Future Internet, 4*, 621–645. doi:10.3390/fi4030621

Adarsh, V. (2013). Hospitals & doctors gain from health startups as online healthcare brings a windfall for companies. *Economc Times*. Retrieved August 18, 2013, from http://articles.economictimes.indiatimes.com/2013-06-20/news/40093911_1_doctors-digitisation-practo-technologies

Bali, S., & Singh, A. J. (2007). Mobile phone consultation for community health care in rural north India. *Journal of Telemedicine and Telecare, 13*(8), 421–424. doi:10.1258/135763307783064421 PMID:18078555

Blake, H. (2008). Innovation in practice: mobile phone technology in patient care. *British Journal of Community Nursing, 13*(4), 160. doi:10.12968/bjcn.2008.13.4.29024 PMID:18595303

Buyya, R., Yeo, C. S., & Venugopal, S. (2008). Market-oriented Cloud computing: Vision, hype, and reality for delivering IT services as computing utilities. *Future Generation Computer Systems, 25*(6), 599–616. doi:10.1016/j.future.2008.12.001

Dawoud, W., Takouna, I., & Meinel, C. (2010). Infrastructure as a service security: Challenges and solutions. In *Proceedings of Informatics and Systems (I*FOS), The 7th International Conference. I*FOS.

Donner, J. (2008). Research approaches to mobile use in the developing world: A review of the literature. *The Information Society, 24*(3), 140–159. doi:10.1080/01972240802019970

Feng, J., Chen, Y., & Liu, P. (2010). Bridging the Missing Link of Cloud Data Storage Security in AWS. In *Proceedings of Consumer Communications and networking Conference (CC*C)*. IEEE.

Francis, A., & McIntosh, R. (1997). The market, technological and industry context of business process re-engineering in the UK. *International Journal of Operations & Production Management, 17*(4), 344–364. doi:10.1108/01443579710159941

Grogan, J. (2006). EHRs and information availability: Are you at risk? *Health Management Technology, 27*(5), 16. PMID:16739432

Harmon, R. L. (1996). *Reinventing the business: Preparing today's enterprise for tomorrow's technology*. New York: Free Press.

Horowitz, B. (2011). *Cloud computing brings challenges for health care data storage, privacy*. Retrieved July 23, 2013 from http://www.eweek.com/c/a/Health-Care-IT/Cloud-Computing-Brings-Challenges-for-Health-Care-Data-Storage-Privacy-851608/

Ikhu-Omoregbe. (2008). Formal modeling and design of mobile prescription applications. *Journal of Health Informatics in Developing Countries, 2*(2).

Kaplan, W. A. (2006). Can the ubiquitous power of mobile phones be used to improve health outcomes in developing countries? *Globalization and Health, 2*(1), 9. doi:10.1186/1744-8603-2-9 PMID:16719925

Maria, A. F., Fenu, G., & Surcis, S. (2009). An Approach to Cloud Computing Network. In *Proceedings of the 3rd International Conference on Theory and Practice of Electronic Governance*. Bogota, Colombia: Academic Press.

Mell, P., & Grance, T. (2011). The NIST Definition of Cloud Computing. *NIST Special Publication*, 800-145.

Morris, D., & Brandon, J. (1993). *Reengineering your Business*. New York: McGraw-Hill.

Muir, E. (2011). *Challenges of cloud computing in healthcare integration*. Retrieved from http://www.zdnet.com/news/challenges-of-cloud-computing-in-healthcare-integration/6266971

Padhy, P. R., Patra, M. R., & Satapathy, S. C. (2012). Design and Implementation of a Cloud based Rural Healthcare Information System Model. *Universal Journal of Applied Computer Science & Technology, 2*(1), 149–157.

Perera, I. (2009). Implementing Healthcare Information in Rural Communities in Sri Lanka: A Novel Approach with Mobile Communication. *Journal of Health Informatics in Developing Countries, 3*(2). PMID:21822397

Peter, M., & Tim, G. (2009). *The NIST definition of Cloud Computing* (Version 15). Information Technology Laboratory. Retrieved August 20, 2013, from http://www.hexistor.com/blog/bid/36511/The-NIST-Definition-of-Cloud-Computing

Weicher, M., Chu, W., Lin, W. C., Le, V., & Yu, D. (1995). *Business Process Reengineering Analysis and Recommendations*. Baruch College. Retrieved from http://www.netlib.com/bpr1.htm

Wootton, R. (2001). Telemedicine and developing countries & successful implementation will require. *Journal of Telemedicine and Telecare*, *7*(1), 1–6. doi:10.1258/1357633011936589 PMID:11576471

Wu, R., Ahn, G. J., Hu, H., & Singhal, M. (2010). Information flow control in cloud computing. In *Proceedings of 6th International Conference on Collaborative Computing: Networking, Applications and Worksharing* (CollaborateCom) (pp. 1-7). IEEE.

KEY TERMS AND DEFINITIONS

Business Process Re-engineering (BPR): Business strategies crafted to design and analyze the workflow within an organization. The business transformation leads to process improvement by defining better mechanisms on how people should work and processes to be conducted.

Cloud Computing: In the phrase cloud computing, cloud is a metaphor used for 'internet'. It is a contemporary computer based internet technique where different services of storage, server and application are delivered to the user, online through internet connection. It reduces the cost, simplifies data management and improves the imparted service in a secure manner.

Health Cloud: The cloud designed specifically for imparting healthcare services to the users. It improves collaboration between doctors and patients in a secure environment and provides access to data irrespective of time and location.

Interactive Voice Response (IVR): A technology that allows a computer to interact with humans through voice. It does not require human interventions and voice messages are pre-recorded to deliver updated information to the users.

Software as a Service (SaaS): In the SaaS cloud model, software is sold to a client in the form of service. The service is available on-demand to users, and the user only pays for the resources used. The application service providers host application and data on the cloud.

ENDNOTES

[1] www.practo.com accessed 10 June 2013

Chapter 15
Demystifying Quality of Healthcare in the Cloud

Anastasius Moumtzoglou
Hellenic Society for Quality and Safety in Healthcare, Greece & P. & A. Kyriakou Children's Hospital, Greece

ABSTRACT

Healthcare services have experienced a sharp increase in demand while the shortages in licensed healthcare professionals have formed one of the toughest challenges that healthcare providers face. In addition, illness has become more complex while advancement in technology and research have expedited the rise of modern and more effective diagnoses and treatment techniques. Cloud computing allows healthcare professionals to share medical records, including all sorts of image and accuracy while new applications or workloads can be started much faster, without going through the entire procurement process or testing the interoperability of the entire infrastructure. Moreover, although the notion of organizational culture is now routinely invoked in organizations and management literature, it remains an elusive concept. However, it is clear that managing the culture is one path towards improving healthcare, and cloud computing introduces a dynamic system adaptation, affecting the quality of care. This is explored in this chapter.

INTRODUCTION

Healthcare services experience a sharp increase in the demand while the shortages in licensed healthcare professionals form one of the toughest challenges, which healthcare providers confront. In addition, illness becomes more complex while advancement in technology and research have expedited the rise of contemporary and more effective diagnoses and treatment techniques (Singh et al., 2008). Furthermore, contention among the

healthcare industry has become apparent (Douglas & Ryman, 2003). Different healthcare arrangements specify differing models of services to suit the needs of various budget categories and disease levels. The marketplace is intensely competitive while the guidance from supervising authorities obligates vulnerable and non-performing hospitals out of business.

In this context, the healthcare industry is transformed to an information centric model, characterized by collaborative workflows, infor-

DOI: 10.4018/978-1-4666-6118-9.ch015

mation sharing, and open standards that support cooperation. Information is harvested and repurposed for more appropriate referrals and medical research to keep the promise of personalized health and care. This availability ensures that the most current, complete insights and clinical expertise are available to deliver comprehensive, integrated and coordinated care focused on value creation rather than consumption.

Health information technology has evolved over the years from departmental solutions to incorporate larger solutions at the venture level, and from stand-alone systems that accommodate bounded and local solutions to more complementary ones that support inclusive and unified solutions (Lenz & Reichert, 2006). The complexity of health information technology has also evolved from passive and reactive to more interactive and proactive systems with more focus on the quality of care (Saranummi, 2008; Saranummi, 2009; Saranummi, 2011; Vasilakos & Lisetti, 2010).

Overall, an ecosystem evolves that continually generates and exchanges insights and brings relevant insights into health and care decisions. It is efficient, with the flexibility to respond dynamically to changing needs and the latest medical breakthroughs. Cloud computing, information management, and business analytics are the key enablers of these capabilities.

Cloud computing allows healthcare professionals to share medical records, including all sorts of image and accuracy. Moreover, healthcare providers pay per use; with no long-term costs; hardware installation is not required, and the software set-up takes only a short period. Finally, the recipient may securely check results without downloading any software while records can be uploaded, viewed or forwarded from any DICOM source.

In general, cloud computing provides three additional aspects from a hardware provisioning and pricing point of view:

- The appearance of infinite computing resources available on demand.
- The elimination of an up-front commitment by cloud users.
- The ability to pay for use of computing resources on a short-term basis.

By the same token, cloud computing results in shifting costs from capital expenditures to operational expense, which helps cash flow, and consolidates different management systems permitting all elements of the data center to be controlled by a single management system. Additionally, rapid provisioning allows administrators to commission or decommission computing resources with a few mouse clicks. Finally, new applications or workloads can be started much faster, without going through the entire procurement process or testing the interoperability of the entire infrastructure. However, cloud latency is adequate for many common applications, but it may not be suitable for applications that must be hyper-responsive. Beyond any doubt, unwinding the sound integrations of the healthcare system could cause the entire system to fail if the wrong component is removed. Moreover, data could be disseminated across time zones and continents, revealing a whole assortment of latent issues for organizations dealing with privacy laws.

Cloud computing has made tremendous strides forward while experts predict a profuse number of firms joining the cloud or developing their own; new services arising to lead the clouds and the data within them, and the clouds' expansion transforming information technology and work life worldwide. There are many explanations why businesses and organizations are flocking to the clouds. Cloud services can be deployed in much less time than usual ones, so information technology undertakings are completed and delivered to market much sooner. Those activities will also be affordable, and potentially of higher-quality while, at the same time, staff members absolve for other creative activities. Cloud services make it easier to innovate and thereby open up new revenue streams.

The businesses and organizations that utilize cloud services recognize yet another advantage. Labor, to a greater extent, moves out of the old limits of a timetable in a physical place of business. Productivity happens at all hours of the day and night, off-site, as well as on-site. Computer software can unquestionably move toward far greater use if it liberates itself from space and time. In that respect, the promise of cloud computing is located at computational power that is boundlessly broad and ubiquitous. Reflective organizations and enterprises have begun exploring cloud computing and many more appear poised to join them. They and we can hope for exciting things to understand.

Thus, the objective of the chapter is to analyze the features and types of cloud services, describe cloud technologies and cloud-based systems for healthcare information technology, and demystify the quality of healthcare in the Cloud.

BACKGROUND

The Internet, which has its origin in telephony applications of the early 1990s, is often referred to as 'The Cloud'. By entering the new millennium, the Internet was referred as broadband, and the term "in the cloud" was highly trusted. Telephone services were committed to 'The Cloud' to route phone call, faxes, and live feed connections. Then, around the middle of the decade, Computational Cloud Services, called "Cloud Computing" was firmly in the vocabulary as a way to describe what the user was doing: accessing computing services in the cloud.

At the beginning of the decade, companies began building their Websites in such a way that users could utilize their services exclusively through the use of a browser. Shortly, through the use of more powerful technologies, "in the cloud" applications became commonplace. By the middle of the decade, most leading corporations with a strong Web presence had reasonable and reliable operation of their services exclusively 'in the cloud'.

The 'Cloud' represents a fundamental change in the use of IT services, which involves a shift from owning and managing the IT system to accessing IT systems as a service. The term Cloud Services, a distinct terminology from outsourced IT hosting comes from the fact that the Internet has often been depicted as a 'Cloud'. Cloud Services have been defined as the services that meet the following criteria (Soman, 2011):

- Consumers neither own the hardware on which data processing and storage happen, nor the software that performs the data processing.
- Consumers have the ability to access and use the service at any time over the Internet.

As a result, the definition of Cloud Services is twofold. The first part pertains to the ownership of the actual hardware and software that is used to perform data storage and data processing while the second part refers to the client's ability to access the service remotely when it needs to use it.

On the other hand, as definitions evolved, Cloud Computing denoted the influence of cloud, and implied the user experience moving away from personal computers to a "cloud" of computers. In this context, the National Institute of Standards and Technology (NIST) defined Cloud Computing as 'a model for enabling ubiquitous, convenient, on-demand network access to a shared pool of configurable computing resources (e.g., networks, servers, storage, applications, and services) that can be rapidly provisioned and released with minimal management effort or service provider interaction'. This cloud model is composed of five essential characteristics, three service models, and four deployment models (Mell & Grance, 2011). Essential characteristics, according to NIST, include on-demand self-service, broad network access, resource pooling, rapid elasticity, and measured service. Service Models include Software as a Service (SaaS), Platform as a Service (PaaS), and Infrastructure as a Service (IaaS) while deployment models include the Private cloud, the Community cloud, the Public cloud, and the Hybrid cloud.

Moreover, research firm IDC (Gens, 2008) described Cloud Computing as 'an emerging IT development, deployment and distribution model, enabling real-time delivery of products, services and solutions over the Internet'. It also defined Cloud Services as 'Consumer and Business products, services and solutions that are delivered and consumed in real-time over the Internet'.

Finally, analyst firm Gartner (Gartner, 2009) defined Cloud Computing as 'a model of computing in which scalable and flexible IT-enabled capabilities are delivered as a service to external customers using Internet technologies'.

Overall, the definition of cloud computing is based on two meanings: on one hand, it describes the infrastructure used to construct the application; on the other hand it describes the establishment of such infrastructure on cloud computing applications.

As far as health care is concerned, the trend appears to be irreversible. Software applications and information once in the realm of a local computer or a local server are now in the sphere of the public Internet. Private health information once confined to local networks is migrating onto the Internet. Patients voluntarily grant access to their health records while the collection and management of this data is entirely legal.

FEATURES AND TYPES OF CLOUD SERVICES

Remote access over the Internet is the predominant feature of Cloud Services. Moreover, we use Cloud Services on demand, that is, when we want them, to the extent we need to. Utilization is typically measured in terms of metrics such as Data Storage space used, CPU usage, period for which we have subscribed to the service, number of concurrent user accounts we have, or any other such metric. Cloud Service vendors build their infrastructure assuming that the demand for using it is likely to be elastic. They also develop Cloud Services assuming platform-independence and shared usage. Platform independence means that the services are accessed through any standard Internet Browser while shared usage implies that the host infrastructure is shared between different subscribers. It is this shared use of resources that allow Cloud providers to offer a 'pay-as-you-go' payment type.

On the other hand, there are several different types of IT requirements that can be fulfilled by Cloud Services (Soman, 2011):

- Software Cloud Services (also called SaaS i.e., Software as a Service).

These are Cloud Services wherein subscribers access and use a software application over Internet. These applications are also called "Web-based applications" and they run from within Internet Browsers on the user's computer. When talking of Cloud Services in the context of Healthcare IT, one is typically referring to this category of Cloud Services.

- Computational Cloud Services (also called Cloud Computing).

This refers to a class of Cloud services that allow access and use of computational resources and data storage resources over the Internet. These services essentially make available a computer of customizable capacity to a subscriber who is interested in developing and running his own software programs.

- Cloud Web Services (also called Application Programming Interface (API) Services).

These Cloud Services encompass a variety of services which allow users to access and integrate data manipulation or storage functionality over the Internet.

- Platform Cloud Services.

These refer to a class of Cloud services that enable software developers to access and utilize a proprietary platform on the Internet for building and deploying third party applications.

CLOUD TECHNOLOGIES

There are three fundamental aspects pertaining to Cloud-based services (Soman, 2011):

1. Browser-based applications.

Browser-based applications are different from native applications, which run on personal computers. Native Applications are those that run entirely on the computer on which they are invoked. A native application uses only the computing resources and storage of the computer which was used to launch the application. Conversely, browser based applications are applications that run from within Internet Browsers. They are conceptually similar to Client Server applications, which require a powerful central computer, but there are two distinct characteristics:

a. Browser based applications can only be invoked from inside a standard browser.
b. The Client and the Server are not (necessarily) a part of a Local Area Network.

2. Optimal utilization of server resources.

Cloud Service Providers see variable levels of utilization of their services. This variability has two components. Firstly, the number of concurrent users accessing the service is different at different times. Secondly, the processing and storage of resources required by any particular user are never constant.

Technologies for scaling and resource partitioning are at the heart of Cloud Services because without these technologies, the Cloud business model would not be feasible. Load Balancing denotes a mechanism for balanced or even distribution of load across multiple physical resources, such as servers, storage devices or communication links.

A server load balancer is responsible for balancing the load of incoming requests among an array of physical servers. Virtualization allows a single physical resource to be used like many resources or multiple physical resources to be used like a single resource. There are several types of virtualization, depending on the nature of the physical resource that is 'virtualized'. In this context, server virtualization implies that a single physical server is converted into several logical servers, storage virtualization a single storage device that is converted into multiple logical storage devices, or vice-versa, and network virtualization allows the user to split a single communication link into separate channels assigned to different processes.

Finally, multi-tenancy is the principal of architecting applications such that a single instance of the application running on the server is visible as separate instances of the same application for each of the clients connected to it.

3. Datacenters

Datacenter is where the user's data is processed and stored. Some of the design considerations for Datacenters are as below (Soman, 2011):

a. Datacenters are typically located in places where the risk of natural disasters and man-made disasters.
b. Buildings used to house Datacenters typically do not accommodate other offices and businesses. The area around the Datacenter is generally well lit and easy to monitor. It is easy to control access into the premises where the Datacenter is housed.
c. Datacenters have areas with raised flooring.
d. Datacenters have air-conditioning.
e. Datacenters have different levels of physical security.
f. Datacenters have assured solid electric supply.
g. Datacenters have state of the art fire prevention and fire protection systems.

From a networking perspective (Soman, 2011):

a. Datacenters have high-bandwidth data pipes with various levels of redundancy.
b. Datacenters have all the elements installed that are required to continually run Intranet services.
c. Datacenters achieve the most advanced Network security tools including intrusion detection, firewalls, antivirus systems, and systems that guard against spamming, Denial of Service Attacks, and all known malware.

Lastly (Soman, 2011):

a. Datacenters employ qualified system administrators.

b. Datacenters support systems and processes in place to keep smooth functioning 24x7 and throughout the year.
c. Datacenters have a disaster recovery plan.

Moreover, 'Private Cloud' is the terminology used to describe a Cloud Service type of infrastructure put in place for the use of a single organization. The 'Datacenter' for the private cloud could be located physically within the organization itself, or in rented space at a regular Datacenter. On the other hand, the benefit of the Private Cloud is the security it offers. An infrastructure that has elements in the Public Cloud and the Private Cloud is referred to as a Hybrid Cloud. Finally, the traditional SaaS (Software as a Service) model is used by several vendors of healthcare IT solutions to deliver services to their customers. In this model, the solution is installed and hosted on servers which are housed at a Datacenter, rather than on-premise. It can be accessed by the practice remotely over the Internet, using technologies such as Virtual Private Networks (VPN) or similar remote-access technologies (rather than a browser) while the billing model is 'pay-as-you go'.

A VPN (virtual private network) is a computer network that is layered on top of other underlying computer networks. It allows for transfer of data between two private networks in such a way that the data travelling over the VPN is not visible to or accessible to the underlying computer networks.

CLOUD-BASED SYSTEMS FOR HEALTHCARE IT

The healthcare industry is different from most other industries. It is highly sensitive, and there are several entities that have to deal with healthcare data. This includes care providers, hospital administration staff, payers, labs, and patients themselves. The key differences between the healthcare industry and other industries, in which Cloud-based systems have been used, include (Soman, 2011):

- **High Risk Industry:** The healthcare industry impacts individuals to a greater extent than any other industry.
- **Highly Regulated:** Numerous regulations govern the provision of healthcare.
- **Multiple Stakeholders:** There is a large number of stakeholders in the healthcare industry. This includes the patients, the physicians, the nurse practitioners, the hospitals/clinics, their administrative staff members, the payers/ insurance companies, employers, pharmaceutical companies, technology vendors, device manufacturers, government bodies, and so on.
- **Slow Pace of Adoption:** The healthcare industry has traditionally been slow to adopt IT, especially the smaller clinics and individual physician practices.
- **Small and Large Providers:** The small providers typically do not have the resources to evaluate or experiment with advanced IT systems. On the other hand, there are several large multi-specialty hospitals whose IT requirements are distinctly different from those of office practitioners.
- **Long Term Relationships:** Changing IT systems often is not easy and there is, therefore, an assumption that any product adopted would be advantageous to use for several years.

Given all of these differences, it is not clear that Cloud-based systems would work as well in the healthcare industry as they have in other industry verticals, unless Cloud-based healthcare solutions address these specific attributes of the industry.

From a clinical perspective, an EMR (electronic medical record) leads to improvement in the quality of care provided to patients. Cloud-based EMRs are, therefore, a key component of any Cloud-based healthcare offering. An EMR is a computer-based documentation of a patient's medical history including illnesses, examinations, reports, diagnosis and the care administered. Electronic Medical Records are created and maintained by care providers when a patient avails service from the provider.

The following key pieces of medical information are a part of virtually all EMR systems (Soman, 2011):

- Patient Identification Information.
- Information about Patient Allergies and Habits.
- Immunization Record.
- Medical History.
- Benefits of EMR.

There are significant advantages to using EMR when compared to the traditional paper-based records and charts (Soman, 2011):

- Storage,
- Usage in Emergency,
- Duplication and Transportation Costs,
- Uniformity,
- Risks,
- Audit/Reporting,
- Integration,
- Efficiency.

Cloud-based EMR systems have all the features and capabilities of in house-EMR systems. Many Cloud-based systems have rich and especially easy-to-use interfaces along with the ability to customize the fields in the records. Cloud-based EMR systems make it even easier to access or transfer medical information to any point, for example, to the point of care in an emergency. Cloud-based EMR systems also make it easier to provide access to the records of the patient via patient portals.

A Cloud-based medical practice management application enables a healthcare provider to manage and streamline business management tasks and workflows. A 'workflow' is a series of steps followed in order to achieve a specific purpose. Provision of healthcare involves implementation of various workflows within the practice, mirroring the movement of the patient within the system. Medical Practice Management relates to the operation of various workflows within the practice. Medical Practice Management Systems are, therefore, the key to ensuring that all operations within the practice run smoothly and efficiently.

Cloud-based Practice Management software generally supports features such as (Soman, 2011):

- Appointment scheduling of patients.
- Eligibility and authorization.
- Physician scheduling, scheduling surgery or other procedures for patients.
- Tracking patient referrals.
- Patient account management.
- Managing patients as they move from admission to discharge including information on hospital rounds.
- Managing patient recall.
- Claims submission and processing, automated follow-ups, collections and remittance advice.
- Managing the schedules of employees of the clinic.
- Managing the inventory of medical supplies and office materials.
- Inter and intra clinic/location communication.
- HIPAA compliance.
- Patient portal.

In a Cloud-based Practice Management solution, the software is accessed in a browser over the Internet, which is why continuous Internet availability is crucial. Cloud-based Practice Management solutions can be customized, although admittedly to a limited extent when compared to on-site solutions. However, Cloud-based solutions can effectively compete with the on-site solutions in terms of functionality and features.

A patient portal is essentially a Website on which patients can log in and access most portions of their medical records. In a patient portal, the information is presented in a manner which makes it easy for the patient to understand the nature of his conditions and his treatment. Most Patient Portals also provide for some level of interactivity with the healthcare provider.

Patient Portals represent one of the key advantages of Cloud-based systems over in-house systems. A Patient Portal interfaces with sensitive, private information of individuals, which should be securely available and Web-accessible at all times. It is, therefore, best if the responsibility of managing the patient portal is assigned to an entity that has the expertise, the infrastructure, the resources and experience to develop and achieve high availability, high security information systems. Most clinics or physician practices do not have this capability, nor is it practically feasible to invest in infrastructure and human resources in order to undertake such capability. It is, therefore, best to opt for a Patient Portal that is Cloud-based.

Many Practice Management systems and EMR systems include ePrescription capability as a part of their overall functionality. An ePrescription system is a computerized system in which the prescription is either entered by the physician/nurse practitioner or generated on the basis of information available to the system. The prescription can be automatically communicated to pharmacies associated with the healthcare provider. Further, ePrescription systems also have inbuilt rules/databases pertaining to drug-drug allergies and appropriateness of each drug in the context of various health conditions.

An ePrescription system brings several benefits (Soman, 2011):

- It eliminates the possibility of a prescription being incorrectly interpreted due to poor handwriting, thereby reducing medical errors.
- It reduces the occurrence of drug-drug allergies and the possibility of inappropriate drug being administered in the view of the patients' comprehensive medical history.
- It makes ordering refills easier since prior prescriptions can be easily accessed electronically.
- ePrescriptions are also found to increase compliance by patients simply because they are more convenient.

A Cloud-based ePrescription system is likely to be much more highly available and secure and thus be able to communicate prescriptions to pharmacies with a higher reliability than an in-house system. Secondly, a Cloud-based system is more likely to cooperate with more and more pharmacy chains over time, enhancing the number of pharmacies the ePrescriptions can be sent to.

Even if a clinic does not use Cloud-based systems for practice management, it is a brilliant idea to consider Cloud-based systems for data backup and secondary storage. The way most Cloud-based backup systems work is as follows (Soman, 2011).

There is software installed on one or more of the computers within the facility (called the backup client) connected to the primary storage. The backup client tracks the changes to the data stored on the primary storage at regular intervals and communicates the changes to the Cloud-based storage space of the service provider.

The backup client encrypts all information before it is communicated to Cloud storage. Secondly, bandwidth requirements are significantly reduced because the client only communicates the changes that have occurred in the data since the last backup run, rather than transmitting all the details again.

A notable special case of a data backup system is the Picture Archival and Communication System ('PACS'). In the process of administering healthcare, numerous images, graphs, pictures and scans are generated. This includes images from X-Rays, ultrasound machines, MRI and CT scans, endoscopy, mammograms, computed radiography, etc. Even scanned images of paper documents are often required to be stored, when legacy paper-based data is digitized via scanning. In order to ensure uniformity, a standard format used to store and communicate pictorial information has been defined—the Digital Imaging and Communications in Medicine ('DICOM').

Cloud-based Laboratory solutions are available for various functions such as Microbiology, histology and cytology processes, Synoptic/Antibiogram reporting, Image/Document capture, Inventory Management, Voice recording, Blood bank. They have all the functionality of on-site solutions. Cloud-based Radiology systems are similar to PACS systems. These systems support basic Radiology workflows where physicians can register examination requests for existing or new patients, and select appropriate billing rules. It is also possible to interface laboratory devices directly to Cloud-based systems. This means that the readings from instruments or captured images are directly uploaded to the cloud.

Overall, cloud-based healthcare IT systems are easier to get started; distinctly cost effective when compared to on-site solutions; more convenient, especially for smaller clinics and private physician practices, while allow physicians to collaborate on any medical data easily, and work on the system from anywhere, including from home.

DEMYSTIFYING QUALITY OF HEALTH CARE IN THE CLOUD

Although the notion of organizational culture is now routinely invoked in organizations and management literature, it remains an elusive concept, fraught with competing interpretations and eluding a consensual definition. Firstly, there is the family of approaches that see culture as something that an organization *is* (here culture serves as a metaphor for describing an organization rather than being seen as something easily identifiable or separable from the organization itself). Indeed, post-modern perspectives on organizational culture challenge the notion of organizations and their cultures as concrete entities. In contrast, there is the collection of approaches that picture of culture as something that an organization *has* aspects or variables of the organization that can be isolated, described, and manipulated.

Organizational culture emerges from that which is shared between colleagues in an organization, including shared beliefs, attitudes, values, and norms of behavior. Rivalry and competition between groups may come out as a key feature of the overall organizational culture. Nonetheless, organizational culture appears to be a deciding factor in understanding the potential of any organization to perform and compete, and some work in health care confirms this. Indeed, many organizations—public and private—place great emphasis on shaping their cultures as a means of improving organizational readiness. It is clear that managing the culture is one path towards improving health care.

Organizational culture can also be influenced by factors outside of the organization. The dedicated professional ethic and sense of professional identity seen in the health professions attest to the importance of supraorganizational norms. Firstly, extensive and simultaneous change on all the many different aspects of organizational culture is unfeasible and probably not even desirable. Secondly, the nature of the cultural destination for the health systems and other healthcare organizations is currently far from clearly specified. Thirdly, cultural change cannot easily be wrought from the top down by simple exhortation.

In essence, there are two key policy choices in the management of cultural diversity. The first is whether one partner's culture should prevail as opposed to striving for a balance of contributions from the contributory cultures. The second choice addresses whether to attempt integration of the partners' cultures (with the purpose of deriving synergy from them) versus a preference for segregating the cultures within the organization (with the purpose of avoiding potential conflict and reducing the energy devoted towards cultural management). These policy choices give rise to four possible bases for accommodating cultural diversity: synergy, domination, segregation, and breakdown. The first three provide a basis for establishing cultural fit, whilst the fourth results in apathy or organizational cost.

In any case, it is clear that managing the culture is one path towards improving health care while researchers have asserted that improving the quality of health care involves change. In this context, cloud computing introduces a dynamic system adaptation, affecting the quality of care, which is based on the following characteristics:

- **Agility:** The agile organization values technology that allows it to be quick, resourceful and adaptable, quickly and consistently delivering results in the face of uncertainty and change.
- **Reliability:** Reliability in health care involves regular use of appropriate treatments and processes of care that have been shown to produce more favorable outcomes. However, adoption of a health care reliability culture, such as the one described, has been limited by significant challenges.
- **Virtualization:** In the hospital environment, client virtualization bridges the gap between available resources and end-user satisfaction. Client virtualization allows providers of information technology to

align their services with efficiency, access, and quality goals, providing a valuable tool for achieving them.

In virtualized client environments, the image of a real desktop is replaced by a virtual one running on a server. Each user accesses a single virtual PC while virtual PCs run concurrently on top of the virtualization layer. Moreover, although many virtual PCs run on a single server, the crash of a single virtual PC does not mean the collapse of other virtual PCs on the same server. Overall, Client virtualization can facilitate:

- Greater investment in customer-facing capabilities.
- Regulatory compliance.
- Customer service.

- **Scalability:** The ability to scale for future growth.
- **Resilience:** Resilience is the inherent ability of a system to improve its functioning during all stages of changes and disturbances so that it can sustain required operations. Resilience engineering enables an organization to cope with unexpected developments, and maintain the ability to adapt when demand goes beyond the organization's standard operating margins.

Resilience focuses on how and what we can learn from successes and error avoidance rather than just a reactive search for 'causes' and superficial remedies. However, from a human factors perspective, resilience refers to the ability, within complex and high-risk organizations, to understand how failure is avoided and how success is obtained.

Resilience has three interconnected levels: (1) the individual or cognitive/knowledge-based; (2) micro-organizational or team/intergroup dynamics and (3) macro-organizational or entire organization. This means that resilience can be described as a property of individuals as well as teams within their workplace.

There are three stages of resilience which describe different standards of functioning. These include:

- Reactive (or brittle) represents the most critical point and is characterized by a mere response to failure that means an individual, group or organization is easily overwhelmed by even minor disruptions and deviations from standard practice. It can stem from the belief that the absence of failure indicates that hazards are not available and/or that countermeasures are adequate to handle unexpected occurrences
- Interactive (or partial resilience), which represents an intermediate stage where there is attention to failure but not anticipation of it
- Proactive (or full resilience), which represents the mature stage where deviations are worthy of more attention, but also there is an unwavering commitment to proactively seek out proof testing assumptions about risk and the overall 'health' of the system

- **Advanced Analytics- New Data Visualisation Techniques:** Advanced analytics and new data visualization techniques help unlock the power of data to make an informed decision making and, ultimately, higher quality, lower cost care.
- **Usability:** Usability constitutes one of the key features of every system and is primarily concerned with making a system easy to understand and use.

Finally, Mobile Cloud Computing, which refers to an infrastructure where data storage and processing occur outside of the mobile device, introduces the concept of personalized care since mobile cloud applications affect the computing power and data storage away from mobile phones and into the cloud. As a result, they move applications and mobile computing to a much broader range of mobile subscribers.

ISSUES, CONTROVERSIES, PROBLEMS

Cloud services amount to three developments that are relevant to an ethical analysis (Timmermans et al., 2010):

1. The shifting of control from technology users to the third parties servicing the cloud.
2. The storage of data in different physical locations across multiple servers around the world.
3. The interconnection of various services across the cloud.

These developments complement with the limitations of current e-health systems (AbuKhousa & Najati, 2012):

- High cost of implementing and maintaining health information technology as it requires investments in software, hardware, technical infrastructure, IT professionals, and training.
- Fragmentation of health information technology and poor exchange of patient data since health information technology, in most cases, exists as separate small clinical or administrative systems within different departments of the healthcare provider's organization.
- Lack of regulations mandating the use and protection of electronic health care data capture and dissemination.
- Lack of a Health Cloud model and development standards.

These developments play a vital role in the analysis of the following ethical issues of cloud services (Timmermans et al., 2010).

1. **Control:** Customers or users of a cloud service relinquish control over computation and data (Haeberlen, 2010; Kandukuri & Rakshit, 2009; Grimes, Jaeger, and Lin (2009). The loss of control can become problematic if something goes wrong. The risks associated with cloud services are prohibited entry, data corruption, infrastructure failure, or unavailability/outing (Paquette, Jaeger, and Wilson, 2010). As a result, if something goes wrong it can be difficult to determine who has caused the problem (Haeberlen, 2010). Contributing to this is the fact that the boundary between what is part of one's own IT infrastructure and what lies outside it is blurred. Systems can extend the boundaries of various parties and meet the security perimeters that these parties have put in place. This process is called de-perimeterisation.
2. **Problem of Many Hands:** Cloud services typically make sense in 'a service-oriented architecture (SOA), where all functionality consists of services which can be aggregated into larger applications performing functions to end-users' (Soman, 2011).
3. **Self-Determination:** In a world of ubiquitous and unlimited data sharing and storage among organizations, self-determination is challenged. This not only raises privacy issues but also puts at stake the confidence and trust of in today's evolving information society (Cavoukian, 2008).
4. **Accountability:** Accountability requires detailed records of actions by its users in the cloud. It is, therefore, important to consider what is being recorded, and who the record is made available to, as there can be a tension

between privacy and accountability (Pearson & Charlesworth, 2009). Moreover, in a de-parameterized world not only the periphery of the organizations IT infrastructure blurs, also the limits of the organization's accountability become less clear.

5. **Ownership:** Besides data actively stored in the cloud by users, the cloud also generates information to provide accountability, to improve the services provided, or other reasons such as running or security. Although identity-based systems will provide many benefits, unknown risks and threats are emerging. As Cavoukian (2008) states 'identity fraud and theft are the diseases of the Information Age made possible by the surfeit of personal data in circulation, along with new forms of discrimination and social engineering made possible by asymmetries of data, information and knowledge'.

6. **Function Creep:** Data collected for specific purposes, over time might be used for other purposes (function creep).

7. **Monopoly and Lock-in:** If only a handful of companies are able to achieve a dominant position in the market for cloud services, this might lead abuse or could be harmful otherwise to the interests of the users (Nelson, 2010).

8. **Privacy:** Companies providing cloud services save terabytes of sensitive personal information, which is then stored in data centers in countries around the world. As a result, a key factor affecting the development and adoption of cloud services is how these companies, and the countries in which they operate, address privacy issues (Nelson, 2010).

9. **Privacy across (Cultural) Borders:** Cloud services prepare for a dialogue between different cultures by providing the infrastructure to exchange, collaborate and communicate across cultural borders. However, different opinions on privacy are further enhanced by cultural differences.

10. **Cultural Imperialism and Dealing with Diversity:** Cloud services may lead to increasing cultural homogenization, suppressing local cultures, due to the fact that large corporations, which dominate the cloud, implement Western values into cloud applications (Ess, 2008).

On the other hand, healthcare services are delivered by individuals with a variety of beliefs and values. Moreover, patients come from different economic and cultural backgrounds. As a result, the opportunities for misunderstanding are numerous.

In addition, Cloud Computing can significantly reduce IT costs and complexities but enhances resources utilization and faces various technical challenges:

-   Most healthcare providers require high availability of the Health Cloud services.
-   The health cloud requires unfailing reliability for the provided services.
-   Huge numbers of medical records and images related to millions of people will be stored in Health Clouds. The data may be replicated for high reliability and better access at different locations and across large geographic distances.
-   Scalability requires dynamic organization and reconfiguration as well as an automatic resizing of used virtualized hardware resources (Vaquero et al., 2009).
-   Health Cloud services must be flexible to meet individual healthcare requirements; they also must be easily configurable to meet with different needs.
-   Services for the Health Cloud can be provided from various cloud service provid-

ers. As a result, a good level of interoperability facilitates easy migration among different available systems.

- It is crucial to offer cloud services, which underpin appropriate and equitable access control and authentication mechanisms to protect the transfer data to and from clients and service providers.

- Health Cloud services amplify the main concerns in e-health systems (Goldman & Hudson, 2000; Kelly, 2002).

- Health Clouds increase the complexity of network maintainability compared to an individual e-health system.

- Health Clouds require significant changes to clinical and business processes and also to the organizational boundaries in the healthcare industry.

- There are still no clear regulations and guidelines for clinical, technical and business practices of healthcare in the e-context.

- Ownership of data in the health clouds is a place with no clear guidelines.

Among all the challenges listed above, trust, privacy and security emerge as the major concerns for the Cloud. Hence, several efforts in this area strive to provide solutions to address these concerns and improve the security and privacy of the Health Cloud.

Finally, there are open issues in delivering cloud services:

- Policy enforcement within the Health Cloud could prove extremely difficult.

- It may only be possible to verify that data processing takes place somewhere within the cloud, and not the specific places where this takes place.

- It may be difficult to determine the processors of data.

- It may be difficult to know the evolution of the cloud service, as Cloud Computing is subject to a paradigm shift in user requirements from traditional approaches.

SOLUTIONS AND RECOMMENDATIONS

The Health Cloud has the potential to support collaborative work among different healthcare sectors through connecting healthcare applications and integrating their high volume of information sources. Dispersed healthcare professionals and hospitals will be able to build networks, collaborate and exchange information more efficiently. Overall, collecting patients' data in a central location as the Health Cloud results in many benefits:

- The ability to provide a unified patient medical record containing patient data from all patient encounters across all operators results in improving patient care.

- The ability to take advantage of the capabilities of Cloud Computing creates a collaborative economic environment. Moreover, the flexibility to only pay for actual resource utilization shares the overhead costs among the participants resulting in reduced cost.

- The ability to overcome shortage issues in terms of information technology infrastructure and health care professionals ameliorates the issue of resources scarcity.

- The storage of clinical data in the cloud enables health organizations supplying related entities with information on patient safety and the quality of care.

- The Health Cloud provides an integrated platform, which hosts an impressive information repository, which can be uniformly and globally accessed, affecting research.

- The Health Cloud increases the ability to monitor the spread of infectious diseases and/or other disease outbreaks.
- Decision makers can use the Health Cloud data for planning and budgeting for healthcare services.
- The Cloud serves as a broker between healthcare providers and healthcare payers streamlining financial operations.
- The Health Cloud facilitates clinical trials since health organizations could partner with pharmaceutical companies and medical research institutions for clinical trials on new medicines.
- The sharing of data allows for the creation of specialized registries targeted for specific types of patients such as cancer and diabetes registries.

FUTURE RESEARCH DIRECTIONS

Despite all the efforts, the Health Cloud is still in its infancy. However, the models so far proposed indicate the emergence of more comprehensive approaches that will satisfy the requirements of the healthcare professionals. Moreover, although several differences exist between Cloud Computing and multi-agent systems, some common problems can be identified, and various benefits can be obtained by their combined use. Until now, the research activities in the area of Cloud Computing are primarily focused on the efficient use of the computing infrastructure, service delivery, data storage, scalable virtualization techniques, and energy efficiency. Moreover, we could say that the main focus of Cloud Computing research is on the adept use of the infrastructure at reduced cost. On the contrary, research activities in the field of agents are more focused on the intelligent aspects of agents and their use for developing complex applications. In this context, the main

problems are related to issues such as a complex system simulation, adaptive systems, software-intensive applications, distributed computational intelligence, and collective learning.

In spite of these differences, Cloud Computing and multi-agent systems share issues and research topics, and overlap in the need to be investigated. In particular, Cloud Computing can provide a powerful, reliable, predictable and scalable computing infrastructure for the implementation of multi-agent systems. On the other side, software agents can be used as critical components for implementing intelligence in Cloud Computing systems making them more adjusting, adaptable, and self-directing in resource management, service provisioning and in running extensive applications.

In this frame of reference, the Health Cloud will evolve from being a static repository of data into an active resource that health professionals rely on throughout their daily practice. With new capabilities for accessing online expert systems and applications, Cloud Intelligence will allow tapping into information, analysis, and contextual recommendations in more integrated ways. Virtual agents will migrate to personalized support and assistance that provides information and performs useful tasks.

CONCLUSION

Adopting the Health Cloud to provide information technology solutions for the healthcare industry comes with many advantages:

- Reducing the cost of owning and maintaining an information technology infrastructure and support staff within each organization.
- Providing better integration and exchange of medical records across multiple organizations and scattered geographical areas.

- Allowing multiple parties to streamline processes, enhance diagnosis, support medical research activities, and simplify administrative operations.
- Increasing the availability, scalability and flexibility of the health information systems.

Accordingly, it is clear that the Health Cloud presents promising opportunities for the healthcare industry but still faces significant challenges. These challenges include patient care quality and safety, increasing healthcare costs, computing and access speeds, backup capabilities, security, resources scarcity; and most importantly, collaboration and knowledge sharing among healthcare professionals at local and international levels. Nevertheless, the Health Cloud is an appropriate method to provide a solution to the value equation 'high quality services at the lowest cost'.

REFERENCES

AbuKhousa, E., Mohamed, N., & Al-Jaroodi, J. (2012). e-Health Cloud: Opportunities and Challenges. *Future Internet*, *4*, 621–645. doi:10.3390/fi4030621

AbuKhousa, E., & Najati, H. A. (2012). UAE-IHC: Steps towards Integrated E-Health Environment in UAE. In *Proceedings of the 4th e-Health and Environment Conference in the Middle East*. Dubai, UAE: Academic Press.

Beauchamp, T. L., & Childress, J. F. (2001). *Principles of biomedical ethics*. Oxford University Press.

Cavoukian, A. (2008). Privacy in the clouds. *Identity Journal*, 89-108.

Douglas, T. J., & Ryman, J. A. (2003). Understanding competitive advantage in the general hospital industry: Evaluating strategic competencies. *Strategic Management Journal*, *24*, 333–347. doi:10.1002/smj.301

Ess, C. (2008). Culture and Global Networks, Hope for a Global Ethics? In J. van den Hoven, & J. Weckert (Eds.), *Information Technology and Moral Philosophy* (pp. 195–225). New York: Cambridge University Press.

Gartner, Inc. (2009). *Defining Gartner Highlights Five Attributes of Cloud Computing*. Retrieved June 1, 2013, from http://www.gartner.com/it/page.jsp?id=1035013

Gens, F. (2008). *Defining Cloud Services and Cloud Computing*. Retrieved June 1, 2013, from http://blogs.idc.com/ie/?p=190

Goldman, J., & Hudson, Z. (2000). Virtually exposed: Privacy and e-health. *Health Affairs*, *19*, 140–148. doi:10.1377/hlthaff.19.6.140 PMID:11192397

Grimes, J. M., Jaeger, P. T., & Lin, J. (2009). *Weathering the Storm: The Policy Implications of Cloud Computing*. Retrieved June 1, 2013, from http://nora.lis.uiuc.edu/images/iConferences/CloudAbstract13109FINAL.pdf

Haeberlen, A. (2010). A case for the accountable cloud. *SIGOPS Operating Systems Review*, *44*, 52–57. doi:10.1145/1773912.1773926

Kandukuri, R., & Rakshit, A. (2009). Cloud Security Issues. In *Proceedings of the 2009 IEEE international Conference on Services Computing, 2009* (pp. 517-520). Lincoln, NE: University of Nebraska Press.

Kelly, E. P., & Unsal, F. (2002). Health information privacy and e-healthcare. *International Journal of Healthcare Technology and Management, 4,* 41–52. doi:10.1504/IJHTM.2002.001128

Kerridge, I., Lowe, M., & McPhee, J. (2005). *Ethics and law for the health professions.* Sydney: Federation Press.

Lenz, R., & Reichert, M. (2006). IT support for healthcare processes—Premises, challenges, perspectives. *Data and Knowledge Engineering Journal, 61,* 39–58. doi:10.1016/j.datak.2006.04.007

Mell, P., & Grance, T. (2011). *The NIST Definition of Cloud Computing.* Gaithersburg, MD: NIST.

Nelson, M. R. (2010). The Cloud, the Crowd, and Public Policy. *Issues in Science and Technology.* Retrieved June 1, 2013, from http://www.issues.org/25.4/nelson.html

Paquette, S., Jaeger, P. T., & Wilson, S. C. (2010). Identifying the security risks associated with governmental use of cloud computing. *Government Information Quarterly, 27*(3), 245–253. doi:10.1016/j.giq.2010.01.002

Pearson, S., & Charlesworth, A. (2009). Accountability as a Way Forward for Privacy Protection in the Cloud. In M. G. Jaatun, G. Zhao, & C. Rong (Eds.), *Cloud Computing* (pp. 131–144). Berlin: Springer-Verlag. doi:10.1007/978-3-642-10665-1_12

Pieters, W., & Cleeff, A. (2009). The precautionary principle in a world of digital dependencies. *IEEE Computer, 42*(6), 50–56. doi:10.1109/MC.2009.203

Saranummi, N. (2008). In the spotlight: Health information systems. *IEEE Reviews in Biomedical Engineering, 1,* 15–17. doi:10.1109/RBME.2008.2008217 PMID:22274895

Saranummi, N. (2009). In the spotlight: Health information systems—PHR and value based healthcare. *IEEE Reviews in Biomedical Engineering, 2,* 15–17. doi:10.1109/RBME.2009.2034699 PMID:22275039

Saranummi, N. (2011). In the spotlight: Health information systems - Mainstreaming mHealth. *IEEE Reviews in Biomedical Engineering, 4,* 17–19. doi:10.1109/RBME.2011.2176998 PMID:22273787

Singh, H., Naik, A. D., Rao, R., & Petersen, L. A. (2008). Reducing diagnostic errors through effective communication: Harnessing the power of information technology. *Journal of General Internal Medicine, 23,* 489–494. doi:10.1007/s11606-007-0393-z PMID:18373151

Soman, A. K. (2011). *Cloud-based Solutions for Healthcare IT.* Science Publishers. doi:10.1201/b10737

Timmermans, J., Ikonen, V., Stahl, B. C., & Bozdag, E. (2010). The Ethics of Cloud Computing: A Conceptual Review. In *Proceedings of Cloud Computing Technology and Science (CloudCom), 2010 IEEE Second International Conference,* (pp. 614-620). IEEE.

Vasilakos, A. V., & Lisetti, C. (2010). Special section on affective and pervasive computing for healthcare. *IEEE Transactions on Information Technology in Biomedicine, 14,* 183–185. doi:10.1109/TITB.2010.2043299 PMID:20684047

ADDITIONAL READING

Soman, A. K. (2011). *Cloud-based Solutions for Healthcare IT.* Science Publishers. doi:10.1201/b10737

KEY TERMS AND DEFINITIONS

Browser-Based Applications: Different from native applications, which run on personal computers. Native Applications are those that run entirely on the computer on which they are invoked. A native application uses only the computing resources and storage of the computer which was used to launch the application. Conversely, browser based applications are applications that run from within Internet Browsers.

Cloud Computing: A model for enabling ubiquitous, convenient, on-demand network access to a shared pool of configurable computing resources (e.g., networks, servers, storage, applications, and services) that can be rapidly provisioned and released with minimal management effort or service provider interaction.

Cloud Services: The definition of Cloud Services is twofold. The first part pertains to the ownership of the actual hardware and software that is used to perform data storage and data processing while the second part refers to the client's ability to access the service remotely when it needs to use it.

Cloud Web Services: A variety of services which allow users to access and integrate data manipulation or storage functionality over the Internet.

Cloud-Based EMR Systems: Have all the features and capabilities of in house-EMR systems.

Datacenters: Where the user's data is processed and stored.

Platform Cloud Services: A class of Cloud services that enable software developers to access and utilize a proprietary platform on the Internet for building and deploying third party applications.

Scalability: The ability to scale for future growth.

Software Cloud Services: Cloud Services wherein subscribers access and use a software application over Internet. These applications are also called "Web-based applications" and they run from within Internet Browsers on the user's computer. When talking of Cloud Services in the context of Healthcare IT, one is typically referring to this category of Cloud Services.

Virtualization: Allows a single physical resource to be used like many resources or multiple physical resources to be used like a single resource.

Compilation of References

Abadi, D. J., Carney, D., Çetintemel, U., Cherniack, M., Convey, C., Lee, S.,... Zdonik, S. (2003). Aurora: A new model and architecture for data stream management. *The VLDB Journal—The International Journal on Very Large Data Bases, 12*(2), 120-139.

Abbadi, I. M., Namiluko, C., & Martin, A. (2011, December). Insiders analysis in cloud computing focusing on home healthcare system. In Proceedings of Internet Technology and Secured Transactions (ICITST), (pp. 350-357). IEEE.

Abreu, R. M., Froufe, H. J., Queiroz, M. J., & Ferreira, I. C. (2010). MOLA: A bootable, self-configuring system for virtual screening using AutoDock4/Vina on computer clusters. *Journal of Cheminformatics, 2*(1), 10. doi:10.1186/1758-2946-2-10 PMID:21029419

AbuKhousa, E., & Najati, H. A. (2012). UAE-IHC: Steps towards integrated e-health environment in UAE. In *Proceedings of the 4th e-Health and Environment Conference in the Middle East*. Dubai, UAE: Academic Press.

AbuKhousa, E., Mohamed, N., & Al-Jaroodi, J. (2012). E-Health Cloud: Opportunities and Challenges. *Future Internet, 4*, 621–645. doi:10.3390/fi4030621

Act, H. I. T. E. C. H. (n.d.). *HealthIT.gov*. Retrieved November 18, 2013, from http://www.healthit.gov/policy-researchers-implementers/hitech-act-0

aDam LeVenthaL, B. (2008). Flash storage memory. *Communications of the ACM, 51*(7).

Adarsh, V. (2013). Hospitals & doctors gain from health startups as online healthcare brings a windfall for companies. *Economc Times*. Retrieved August 18, 2013, from http://articles.economictimes.indiatimes.com/2013-06-20/news/40093911_1_doctors-digitisation-practo-technologies

Admins, R. (2011). Reddit's May 2010. *State of the Servers Report, 11*.

Afgan, E., Baker, D., Coraor, N., Chapman, B., Nekrutenko, A., & Taylor, J. (2010). Galaxy CloudMan: Delivering cloud compute clusters. *BMC Bioinformatics, 11*(Suppl 12), S4. doi:10.1186/1471-2105-11-S12-S4 PMID:21210983

Ahuja, S. P., Mani, S., & Zambrano, J. (2012). A survey of the state of Cloud computing in healthcare. *Network and Communication Technologies, 1*(2), 12–19.

Akyildiz, I. F., Su, W., Sankarasubramaniam, Y., & Cayirci, E. (2002a). A survey on sensor networks. *IEEE Communications Magazine, 40*(8), 102–114. doi:10.1109/MCOM.2002.1024422

Akyildiz, I. F., Su, W., Sankarasubramaniam, Y., & Cayirci, E. (2002b). Wireless sensor networks: a survey. *Computer Networks, 38*(4), 393–422. doi:10.1016/S1389-1286(01)00302-4

Albino, A., & Jacinto, V. (2009). *Implementação da escala de alerta precoce - EWS*. Portimão.

Al-Enazi, T., & El-Masri, S. (2013). HL7 Engine Module for Healthcare Information Systems. *Journal of Medical Systems*, *37*(6), 9986. doi:10.1007/s10916-013-9986-8 PMID:24154569

Al-Janabi, S., Huisman, A., Willems, S. M., & Van Diest, P. J. (2012). Digital slide images for primary diagnostics in breast pathology: A feasibility study. *Human Pathology*, *43*(12), 2318–2325. doi:10.1016/j.humpath.2012.03.027 PMID:22901465

Alley, D., Ahmed, T., Androvich, J., Archibald, S., Baker, A. S., Fultz, N., ... Wilson, K. (2012). The Cloud computing guide for healthcare. *Focus Research*, 1-22.

Alliance, H. I. T. R. U. S. T. (2013). *Common Security Framework*. Retrieved December 07, 2013, from http://www.hitrustalliance.net/commonsecurityframework/

Almeida, J. S., Gruneberg, A., Maass, W., & Vinga, S. (2012). Fractal MapReduce decomposition of sequence alignment. *Algorithms for Molecular Biology; AMB*, *7*(1), 12. doi:10.1186/1748-7188-7-12 PMID:22551205

Almeida, J. S., & Noble, P. A. (2000). Neural computing in microbiology. *Journal of Microbiological Methods*, *43*(1), 1–2. doi:10.1016/S0167-7012(00)00200-1 PMID:11084224

AlSairafi, S., Emmanouil, F.-S., Ghanem, M., Giannadakis, N., Guo, Y., Kalaitzopoulos, D., & Wendel, P. (2003). The design of discovery net: Towards open grid services for knowledge discovery. *International Journal of High Performance Computing Applications*, *17*(3), 297–315. doi:10.1177/1094342003173003

Amazon Free Usage Tier Website. (2013). *Amazon Free Usage Tier website*. Retrieved September 2, 2013, from http://aws.amazon.com/free

Amazon. (2012). *Amazon S3 - The First Trillion Objects*. Author.

Amazon. (2013a). *1000 Genomes Project and AWS*. Retrieved 22/12/2013, 2013, from http://aws.amazon.com/1000genomes/

Amazon. (2013b). *Amazon Elastic Compute Cloud (Amazon EC2)*. Retrieved 19/12/2013, from http://aws.amazon.com/ec2/

Amazon. (n.d.). *Amazon Simple Storage Service (S3)*. Retrieved from http://aws.amazon.com/s3/

Amqp. (2013). *Official Amqp website*. Retrieved August 23, 2013, from http://www.amqp.org

Ananthanarayanan, R., Gupta, K., Pandey, P., Pucha, H., Sarkar, P., Shah, M., & Tewari, R. (2009). Cloud analytics: Do we really need to reinvent the storage stack. In *Proceedings of the 1st USENIX Workshop on Hot Topics in Cloud Computing (HOTCLOUD'2009)*. San Diego, CA: USENIX.

Angiuoli, S. V., Matalka, M., Gussman, A., Galens, K., Vangala, M., & Riley, D. R. et al. (2011). CloVR: A virtual machine for automated and portable sequence analysis from the desktop using cloud computing. *BMC Bioinformatics*, *12*, 356. doi:10.1186/1471-2105-12-356 PMID:21878105

Angiuoli, S. V., White, J. R., Matalka, M., White, O., & Fricke, W. F. (2011). Resources and costs for microbial sequence analysis evaluated using virtual machines and cloud computing. *PLoS ONE*, *6*(10), e26624. doi:10.1371/journal.pone.0026624 PMID:22028928

Annas, G. J. (2003). HIPAA regulations-a new era of medical-record privacy? *The New England Journal of Medicine*, *348*(15), 1486–1490. doi:10.1056/NEJMlim035027 PMID:12686707

Apache Software Foundation. (2013). *Hadoop—Apache Software Foundation project home page*. Retrieved 23/12/2013, 2013, from http://hadoop.apache.org/

Apache UIMA. (n.d.). Retrieved September 19, 2013, from http://uima.apache.org/

Arah, O. A., Westery, G. P., Hurst, J., & Klazinga, N. S. (2006). A conceptual framework for the OECD Health Care Quality Indicators Project. *International Journal for Quality in Health Care*, (18): 5–13. doi:10.1093/intqhc/mzl024 PMID:16954510

Armbrust, M., Fox, A., Griffith, R., Joseph, A. D., & Katz, R. (2009). *Above the Clouds: A Berkeley View of Cloud Computing*. Reliable Adaptive Distributed Systems Laboratory White Paper. Berkeley, CA: University of California.

Armbrust, M., Fox, A., Griffith, R., Joseph, A. D., Katz, R., & Konwinski, A. et al. (2010). A view of cloud computing. *Communications of the ACM, 53*(4), 50–58. doi:10.1145/1721654.1721672

Arns, M., de Ridder, S., Strehl, U., Breteler, M., & Coenen, A. (2009). Efficacy of neurofeedback treatment in ADHD: The effects on inattention, impulsivity and hyperactivity: A meta-analysis. *Clinical EEG and Neuroscience, 40*(3), 180–189. doi:10.1177/155005940904000311 PMID:19715181

ARRA. (2009). *American Recovery and Reinvestment Act of 2009.* Retrieved December 07, 2013, from http://www.gpo.gov/fdsys/pkg/BILLS-111hr1enr/pdf/BILLS-111hr1enr.pdf

Ashdown, L., & Kyte, T. (2011). *Oracle Database Concepts, 11g Release 2 (11.2).* Oracle.

Astion, M. L., & Wilding, P. (1992). Application of neural networks to the interpretation of laboratory data in cancer diagnosis. *Clinical Chemistry, 38*(1), 34–38. PMID:1733603

AT&T. (2012). *Medical Imaging in the Cloud.* Retrieved 26/08/2013, 2012, from https://www.corp.att.com/healthcare/docs/medical_imaging_cloud.pdf

Avorn, J., & Schneeweiss, S. (2009). Managing drug-risk information—What to do with all those new numbers. *The New England Journal of Medicine, 361*(7), 647–649. doi:10.1056/NEJMp0905466 PMID:19635948

Aylward, S. (2010). *Cloud computing in healthcare – Private, public, or somewhere in between.* The Official Microsoft Blog, New & Perspectives. Retrieved from http://blogs.technet.com/b/microsoft_blog/archive/2010/06/28/cloud-computing-in-healthcare-private-public-or-somewhere-in-between.aspx

Baden-Powell, R. (1908). Scouting for Boys. London: Windsor House, Bream's Buildings, E.C. (First published ed.), C.A. Pearson.

Bahga, A., & Madisetti, V. (2013). A cloud-based approach for interoperable electronic health records (EHRS). *IEEE Journal of Biomedical and Health Informatics, 17*(5), 894–906. doi:10.1109/JBHI.2013.2257818

Bajikar, S. (2002, June 20). *Trusted platform module (tpm) based security on notebook pcs-white paper.* Mobile Platforms Group, Intel Corporation.

Bakhouya, M., & Gaber, J. (2008). *Ubiquitous and pervasive application design.* Paper presented in IEEE International Conference on Pervasive Services, Proceedings of the 2nd Workshop on Agent-Oriented Software Engineering Challenges for Ubiquitous and Pervasive Computing (AUPC). Rome, Italy.

Bali, S., & Singh, A. J. (2007). Mobile phone consultation for community health care in rural north India. *Journal of Telemedicine and Telecare, 13*(8), 421–424. doi:10.1258/135763307783064421 PMID:18078555

Barham, P., Dragovic, B., Fraser, K., Hand, S., Harris, T., & Ho, A. et al. (2003). Xen and the art of virtualization. *ACM SIGOPS Operating Systems Review, 37*(5), 164–177. doi:10.1145/1165389.945462

Barkley, R. A. (1997). Behavioral inhibition, sustained attention, and executive functions: Constructing a unifying theory of ADHD. *Psychological Bulletin, 121*(1), 65. doi:10.1037/0033-2909.121.1.65 PMID:9000892

Beauchamp, T. L., & Childress, J. F. (2001). *Principles of biomedical ethics.* Oxford University Press.

Bellare, M., Goldreich, O., & Goldwasser, S. (1994). Incremental cryptography: The case of hashing and signing. In Advances in Cryptology—CRYPTO'94 (pp. 216-233). Springer.

Bellare, M., Goldreich, O., & Goldwasser, S. (1995). Incremental cryptography and application to virus protection. In *Proceedings of the Twenty-Seventh Annual ACM Symposium on Theory of Computing* (pp. 45-56). ACM.

Bellare, M., Guérin, R., & Rogaway, P. (1995). *XOR MACs: New methods for message authentication using finite pseudorandom functions.* Springer.

Bellare, M., Pointcheval, D., & Rogaway, P. (2000). Authenticated key exchange secure against dictionary attacks. In *Proceedings of Advances in Cryptology—Eurocrypt 2000* (pp. 139–155). Bruges, Belgium: Springer. doi:10.1007/3-540-45539-6_11

Berger, B. (2005). Trusted computing group history. *Information Security Technical Report, 10*(2), 59–62. doi:10.1016/j.istr.2005.05.007

Berkelaar, M., Eikland, K., & Notebaert, P. (2004). *lpsolve: Open source (mixed-integer) linear programming system.* Eindhoven University of Technology.

Bertino, E., & Sandhu, R. (2005). Database security - Concepts, approaches, and challenges. *IEEE Transactions on Dependable and Secure Computing, 2*(1), 2–19. doi:10.1109/TDSC.2005.9

Best, R. M. (1980). Preventing software piracy with crypto-microprocessors.[). IEEE.]. *Proceedings of IEEE Spring COMPCON, 80,* 466–469.

Bethencourt, J., Sahai, A., & Waters, B. (2007). Ciphertext-policy attribute-based encryption. In *Proceedings of Security and Privacy* (pp. 321–334). IEEE.

Bhattacharya, I. (2012). Healthcare Data Analytics on the Cloud. *Online Journal of Health and Allied Sciences, 11*(1).

Blaisdell, R. (2013). *Cloud computing advantages for the healthcare industry.* Retrieved from http://webcache.googleusercontent.com/search?q=cache:http://www.rickscloud.com/5-cloud-computing-advantages-for-the-healthcare-industry/

Blake, H. (2008). Innovation in practice: mobile phone technology in patient care. *British Journal of Community Nursing, 13*(4), 160. doi:10.12968/bjcn.2008.13.4.29024 PMID:18595303

Bluetooth, S. I. G. (BSIG). (2013). Health Device Profile. *Health Device Profile - Bluetooth Technology Special Interest Group.* Retrieved October 23, 2013, from https://www.bluetooth.org/en-us/specification/assigned-numbers/health-device-profile

Bollineni, P. K., & Neupane, K. (2011). *Implications for adopting cloud computing in e-Health.* (Unpublished Master's Thesis). School of Computing, Blekinge Institute of Technology.

Boon, M. E., & Kok, L. P. (1993). Neural network processing can provide means to catch errors that slip through human screening of pap smears. *Diagnostic Cytopathology, 9*(4), 411–416. doi:10.1002/dc.2840090408 PMID:8261846

Boshier, A. (2000). Windows Management Instrumentation: A Simple, Powerful Tool for Scripting Windows Management. *MSDN Magazine, 4.*

Botts, N., Thoms, B., Noamani, A., & Horan, T. A. (2010). Cloud Computing Architectures for the Underserved: Public Health Cyberinfrastructures through a Network of HealthATMs. In R. H. Sprague, Jr. (Ed.), *43rd Hawaii International Conference on System Sciences* (HICSS) (pp. 1-10). Honolulu, HI: IEEE.

Bouckaert, J., Van Dijk, T., & Verboven, F. (2010). Access regulation, competition, and broadband penetration: An international study. *Telecommunications Policy, 34*(11), 661–671. doi:10.1016/j.telpol.2010.09.001

Bouwman, H., & MacInnes, I. (2006). Dynamic business model framework for value webs.[). IEEE.]. *Proceedings of System Sciences, 2,* 43–43.

Bracci, F., Corradi, A., & Foschini, L. (2012). Database security management for healthcare SaaS in the Amazon AWS Cloud. In Proceedings of Computers and Communications (ISCC), (pp. 812-819). IEEE.

Brust, C., & Sarnikar, S. (2011). Decision Modeling for Healthcare Enterprise IT Architecture Utilizing Cloud Computing. In *Proceedings of 17th Americas Conference on Information Systems* (AMCIS). Association for Information Systems.

Buxmann, P., Weitzel, T., von Westarp, F., & König, W. (1999). The standardization problem: An economic analysis of standards in information systems. In *Proceedings of the 1st IEEE Conference on Standardisation and Innovation in Information Technology SIIT '99* (pp. 57-162). IEEE.

Buyya, R., Yeo, C. S., Venugopal, S., Broberg, J., & Brandic, I. (2009). Cloud computing and emerging IT platforms: Vision, hype, and reality for delivering computing as the 5th utility. *Future Generation Computer Systems, 25*(6), 599–616. doi:10.1016/j.future.2008.12.001

Carolan, C. C. A. J., Gaede, S., Baty, J., Brunette, G., Licht, A., Remmell, J., … Weise, J. (2009). *Introduction to cloud computing architecture* (White Paper). Academic Press.

Carr, C. D., & Moore, S. M. (2003). IHE: A model for driving adoption of standards. *Computerized Medical Imaging and Graphics, 27*(2-3), 137–146. doi:10.1016/S0895-6111(02)00087-3 PMID:12620304

Carr-Hill, R. A. (1992). The measurement of patient satisfaction. *Journal of Public Health Medicine, 14*(3), 236–249. PMID:1419201

Carstoiu, D., Cernian, A., & Olteanu, A. (2010). *Hadoop Hbase-0.20.2 performance evaluation.* Paper presented at the New Trends in Information Science and Service Science (NISS). New York, NY.

Carter, G. M., Newhouse, J. P., & Relles, D. A. (1990). *How Much Change in the Case Mix Index Is DRG Creep? (RAND Report #3826)*. Santa Barbara, CA: RAND.

Casebeer, L. L., Strasser, S. M., Spettell, C. M., Wall, T. C., Weissman, N., Ray, M. N., & Allison, J. J. (2003). Designing tailored Web-based instruction to improve practicing physicians' preventive practices. *Journal of Medical Internet Research, 5*(3), e20. doi:10.2196/jmir.5.3.e20 PMID:14517111

Cattell, R. (2011). Scalable SQL and NoSQL data stores. *SIGMOD Record, 39*(4), 12–27. doi:10.1145/1978915.1978919

Cavoukian, A. (2008). Privacy in the clouds. *Identity Journal,* 89-108.

CDC CHF. (2013). *Center of disease control chronic heart failure factsheet.* Retrieved September 2, 2013, from http://www.cdc.gov/dhdsp/data_statistics/fact_sheets/fs_heart_failure.htm

Centers for Medicare & Medicaid Services. (2008). Retrieved July 20, 2013 from http://downloads.cms.gov/cmsgov/archived-downloads/SMDL/downloads/SMD073108.pdf

Chan, I. (2008). *Oracle Database Performance Tuning Guide, 10g Release 2 (10.2).* Oracle.

Chen, J. L., Tsai, C. W., Chiang, M. C., & Yang, C. S. (2013). A high performance cloud-based protein-ligand docking prediction algorithm. *BioMed Research International,* 909717.

Chen, J., Qian, F., Yan, W., & Shen, B. (2013). Translational biomedical informatics in the cloud: present and future. *BioMed Research International,* 658925.

Chen, L., & Hoang, D. B. (2011). Towards Scalable, Fine-Grained, Intrusion-Tolerant Data Protection Models for Healthcare Cloud. In Proceedings of Trust, Security and Privacy in Computing and Communications (TrustCom), (pp. 126-133). IEEE.

Chiang, F., Braun, R., & Hughes, J. (2006). A biologically-inspired multi-agent framework for autonomic service management. *International Journal of Pervasive Computing and Communications, 2*(3), 261–276. doi:10.1108/17427370780000155

Chien, C. W., Lee, Y. C., Ma, T., Lee, T. S., Lin, Y. C., Wang, W., & Lee, W. J. (2008). The application of artificial neural networks and decision tree model in predicting post-operative complication for gastric cancer patients. *Hepato-Gastroenterology, 55*(84), 1140–1145. PMID:18705347

Chih-Jen, H. (2008). Telemedicine information monitoring system. In Proceedings of e-health Networking, Applications and Services, (pp. 48-50). IEEE.

Chodorow, K. (2013). *MongoDB: the definitive guide.* Sebastopol, CA: O'Reilly.

Chronaki, C., Pakarinen, V., Jalonen, M., Porrasmaa, J., Berler, A., & Tarhonen, T. (2012). HL7 CDA in the national ePrescription efforts of Finland & Greece: A comparison. *Studies in Health Technology and Informatics*, *174*, 38–43. PMID:22491107

Cochand-Priollet, B., Koutroumbas, K., Megalopoulou, T. M., Pouliakis, A., Sivolapenko, G., & Karakitsos, P. (2006). Discriminating benign from malignant thyroid lesions using artificial intelligence and statistical selection of morphometric features. *Oncology Reports*, *15*, 1023–1026. PMID:16525694

Coleman, E. A., Parry, C., Chalmers, S., & Min, S. J. (2006). The care transitions intervention: Results of a randomized controlled trial. *Archives of Internal Medicine*, *166*(17), 1822–1828. doi:10.1001/archinte.166.17.1822 PMID:17000937

Continua Health Alliance (CHA). (2013). About the Alliance. *About the Alliance - Continua Health Alliance*. Retrieved October 23, 2013, from http://www.continuaalliance.org/about-the-alliance

Contreras, M., Germán, E., Chi, M., & Sheremetov, L. (2004). Design and implementation of a FIPA compliant Agent Platform in.NET. *Journal of Object Technology*, *3*(9), 5–28. doi:10.5381/jot.2004.3.9.a1

CORDIS. (n.d.). Big data at your service. In *Digital agenda for Europe*. European Commission. Retrieved November 26, 2013, from http://ec.europa.eu/digital-agenda/en/news/big-data-your-service

Costa, L., & Silva, F. (2010). Um Software de gerenciamento baseado no padrão WBEM-WMI. *Sistemas de Informação & Gestão de Tecnologia*, *5*.

Craciunas, S. S., Haas, A., Kirsch, C. M., Payer, H., Röck, H., Rottmann, A., et al. (2010). Information-acquisition-as-a-service for cyber-physical cloud computing. In *Proceedings of the 2nd USENIX conference on Hot topics in cloud computing* (pp. 14-14). USENIX Association.

Cumberlidge, M. (2007). *Business Process Management with JBoss JBPM: A Practical Guide for Business Analysts, Develop Business Process Models for Implementation in a Business Process Management Sytem*. Packt Publishing.

D'Agostino, D., Clematis, A., Quarati, A., Cesini, D., Chiappori, F., Milanesi, L., & Merelli, I. (2013). Cloud infrastructures for in silico drug discovery: Economic and practical aspects. *BioMed Research International*, 138012.

Davies, K. (2010). *The the revolution in DNA sequencing and the new era of personalized medicine*. New York, NY: Free Press.

Dawoud, W., Takouna, I., & Meinel, C. (2010). Infrastructure as a service security: Challenges and solutions. In *Proceedings of Informatics and Systems (I*FOS), The 7th International Conference*. I*FOS.

De Paris, R., Frantz, F. A., de Souza, O. N., & Ruiz, D. D. (2013). wFReDoW: A cloud-based Web environment to handle molecular docking simulations of a fully flexible receptor model. *BioMed Research International*, 469363.

Dean, J., & Ghemawat, S. (2008). MapReduce: Simplified data processing on large clusters. *Communications of the ACM*, *51*(1), 107–113. doi:10.1145/1327452.1327492

Delgado, M. (2011). The evolution of health care it: Are current us privacy policies ready for the clouds? In *Proceedings of Services (SERVICES)*, (pp. 371-378). IEEE.

Della Valle, E., Cerizza, D., Bicer, V., Kabak, Y., Laleci, G., Lausen, H., & DERI-Innsbruck, S. M. S. M. (2005). The need for semantic web service in the eHealth. In *Proceedings of W3C workshop on Frameworks for Semantics in Web Services*. Academic Press.

Demichelis, F., Della Mea, V., Forti, S., Dalla Palma, P., & Beltrami, C. A. (2002). Digital storage of glass slides for quality assurance in histopathology and cytopathology. *Journal of Telemedicine and Telecare*, *8*(3), 138–142. doi:10.1258/135763302320118979 PMID:12097174

Deng, M., Petkovic, M., Nalin, M., & Baroni, I. (2011). A Home Healthcare System in the Cloud--Addressing Security and Privacy Challenges. In *Proceedings of IEEE International Conference on Cloud Computing* (CLOUD) (pp. 549 - 556). IEEE Computer Society.

Department of Economic and Social Affairs. Population Division. (2001). World Population Ageing: 1950-2050. New York: United Nations.

Department of Economic and Social Affairs. Population Division. (2007). *World Population Ageing 2007*. New York: United Nations.

Deshpande, S. U. (1982). ILIS--An integrated laboratory information system: Biochemistry and hematology. *Clinical Chemistry*, *28*(2), 271–276. PMID:7055947

Devanbu, P., Gertz, M., Martel, C., & Stubblebine, S. G. (2002). Authentic third-party data publication. In *Data and Application Security* (pp. 101–112). Schoorl, The Netherlands: Springer US. doi:10.1007/0-306-47008-X_9

Devaney, G., & Lead, W. (2011). *Guideline for the use of the modified early warning score (MEWS)*. Academic Press.

Dey, P., Logasundaram, R., & Joshi, K. (2013). Artificial neural network in diagnosis of lobular carcinoma of breast in fine-needle aspiration cytology. *Diagnostic Cytopathology*, *41*(2), 102–106. doi:10.1002/dc.21773 PMID:21987420

Di Tommaso, P., Orobitg, M., Guirado, F., Cores, F., Espinosa, T., & Notredame, C. (2010). Cloud-Coffee: Implementation of a parallel consistency-based multiple alignment algorithm in the T-Coffee package and its benchmarking on the Amazon Elastic-Cloud. *Bioinformatics (Oxford, England)*, *26*(15), 1903–1904. doi:10.1093/bioinformatics/btq304 PMID:20605929

Dias, K., Ramacher, M., Shaft, U., Venkataramani, V., & Wood, G. (2005). Automatic performance diagnosis and tuning in Oracle. In *Proceedings of the 2005 CIDR Conf*. CIDR.

DICOM. (2006). *Digital Imaging and Communication in Medicine*. Retrieved December 07, 2013, from http://medical.nema.org/dicom/

Diffie, W., Van Oorschot, P. C., & Wiener, M. J. (1992). Authentication and authenticated key exchanges. *Designs, Codes and Cryptography*, *2*(2), 107–125. doi:10.1007/BF00124891

Dijkstra, E. W. (1959). A note on two problems in connection with graphs. *Numeriche Mathematic*, *1*(1), 269–271. doi:10.1007/BF01386390

Dimitrova, M., Lozanova, S., Lahtchev, L., & Roumenin, C. (2012). A framework for design of cloud compatible medical. In *Proceedings of the 13th ACM International Conference on Computer Systems and Technologies (CompSysTech)* (pp. 195-200). Ruse, Bulgaria: ACM.

Dimopoulou, E. (2006). *Implementation of an advanced spatial technological system for emergency situations*. Paper presented at FIG Workshop on eGovernance Knowledge Management and eLearning. Budapest, Hungary.

Domiter, V. (2004). Constraint Delaunay triangulation using plane subdivision. In *Proceedings of the 8th Central European Seminar on Computer Graphics*. Retrieved August 13, 2014, from http://www.cescg.org/CESCG-2004/web/Domiter-Vid/

Donabedian, A. (1980). *Exploration in Quality Assessment and Monitoring: The Definition of Quality and Approaches to its Management* (Vol. 1). Ann Arbor, MI: Health Administration Press.

Donner, J. (2008). Research approaches to mobile use in the developing world: A review of the literature. *The Information Society*, *24*(3), 140–159. doi:10.1080/01972240802019970

dotNetRdf library. (n.d.). Retrieved from http://www.dotnetrdf.org

Douglas, T. J., & Ryman, J. A. (2003). Understanding competitive advantage in the general hospital industry: Evaluating strategic competencies. *Strategic Management Journal*, *24*, 333–347. doi:10.1002/smj.301

Drake, S., Hu, W., McInnis, D., Sköld, M., Srivastava, A., & Thalmann, L. … Wolski, A. (2005). Architecture of Highly Available Databases. In M. Malek, M. Reitenspieß, & J. Kaiser (Eds.), Service Availability (Vol. 3335, pp. 1–16). Springer.

DROOL. (n.d.). Retrieved from http://www.jboss.org/drools/

Drozdov, I., Ouzounis, C. A., Shah, A. M., & Tsoka, S. (2011). Functional Genomics Assistant (FUGA), a toolbox for the analysis of complex biological networks. *BMC Research Notes*, *4*, 462. doi:10.1186/1756-0500-4-462 PMID:22035155

Duarte, J., Salazar, M., Quintas, C., Santos, M., Neves, J., Abelha, A., & Machado, J. (2010). Data Quality Evaluation of Electronic Health Records in the Hospital Admission Process. In *Proceedings of International Conference on Computer and Information Science*, (pp. 201–206). Academic Press.

Duda, R. O., Hart, P. E., & Stork, D. G. (2001). *Pattern classification* (2nd ed.). New York: Wiley.

Dudley, J. T., & Butte, A. J. (2010). In silico research in the era of cloud computing. *Nature Biotechnology*, *28*(11), 1181–1185. doi:10.1038/nbt1110-1181 PMID:21057489

Dudley, J. T., Pouliot, Y., Chen, R., Morgan, A. A., & Butte, A. J. (2010). Translational bioinformatics in the cloud: an affordable alternative. *Genome Medicine*, *2*(8), 51. doi:10.1186/gm172 PMID:20691073

Dyer, J. G., Lindemann, M., Perez, R., Sailer, R., Van Doorn, L., & Smith, S. W. (2001). Building the IBM 4758 secure coprocessor. *Computer*, *34*(10), 57–66. doi:10.1109/2.955100

Dynastream Innovations Inc. (DII). (2013). ANT+. *ANT+ Vision*. Retrieved October 24, 2013, from http://www.thisisant.com/company/

Dyson, R. G. (2004). Strategic development and SWOT analysis at the University of Warwick. *European Journal of Operational Research*, *152*(3), 631–640. doi:10.1016/S0377-2217(03)00062-6

Edworthy, S. M. (2001). Telemedicine in developing countries: May have more impact than in developed countries. *British Medical Journal*, *323*(7312), 524. doi:10.1136/bmj.323.7312.524 PMID:11546681

Ekonomou, E., Fan, L., Buchanan, W., & Thuemmler, C. (2011). An Integrated Cloud-based Healthcare Infrastructure. In *Proceedings of IEEE Third International Conference on Cloud Computing Technology and Science* (CloudCom) (pp. 532-536). Athens, Greece: IEEE.

ElephantDrive. (n.d.). Retrieved from http://aws.amazon.com/solutions/case-studies/elephantdrive/

Elstein, A. S. (2004). On the origins and development of evidence-based medicine and medical decision making. *Inflammation Research*, *53*(Suppl 2), S184–S189. doi:10.1007/s00011-004-0357-2 PMID:15338074

Endomondo. (n.d.). Retrieved from http://www.endomondo.com/

Ess, C. (2008). Culture and global networks, hope for a global ethics? In J. van den Hoven, & J. Weckert (Eds.), *Information Technology and Moral Philosophy* (pp. 195–225). New York: Cambridge University Press.

Eugster, M. J., Schmid, M., Binder, H., & Schmidberger, M. (2013). Grid and cloud computing methods in biomedical research. *Methods of Information in Medicine*, *52*(1), 62–64. PMID:23318694

European Commission (EU). (2013). Living Healthy, Ageing Well. *Digital Agenda for Europe*. Retrieved October 24, 2013, from http://ec.europa.eu/digital-agenda/en/life-and-work/living-healthy-ageing-well

European Commission. (2013a). ESFRI. *Research & Innovation Infrastructures*. Retrieved December 1, 2013, from http://ec.europa.eu/research/infrastructures/index_en.cfm?pg=esfri

European Commission. (2013b). Improving health reporting mechanisms. *Public Health*. Retrieved December 22, 2013, from http://ec.europa.eu/health/data_collection/tools/mechanisms/index_en.htm

Evidence-Based Medicine Working Group. (1992). Evidence-based medicine: A new approach to teaching the practice of medicine. *Journal of the American Medical Association*, *268*(17), 2420–2425. doi:10.1001/jama.1992.03490170092032 PMID:1404801

ExtremeTech. (2013). *Just how big are porn sites?* Retrieved September 2, 2013, from http://www.extremetech.com/computing/123929-just-how-big-are-porn-sites

Feng, F., & Watanabe, T. (2004). Search of continuous nearest target objects along route on large hierarchical road network. In *Proceedings of the 14th Data Engineering Workshop* (DEWS). Kaga City, Japan: DEWS.

Feng, J., Chen, Y., & Liu, P. (2010). Bridging the Missing Link of Cloud Data Storage Security in AWS. In *Proceedings of Consumer Communications and networking Conference (CC*C)*. IEEE.

Feng, X., Grossman, R., & Stein, L. (2011). PeakRanger: A cloud-enabled peak caller for ChIP-seq data. *BMC Bioinformatics*, *12*, 139. doi:10.1186/1471-2105-12-139 PMID:21554709

Fernando, N., Loke, S. W., & Rahayu, W. (2013). Mobile cloud computing: A survey. *Future Generation Computer Systems*, *29*, 84–106. doi:10.1016/j.future.2012.05.023

Fitbit. (n.d.). Retrieved from http://www.fitbit.com/

Forschungscampus Connected Technologies (FCT). (2013). Forschnungscampus Connected Technologies. In *Connected Living e.v.: Forschnungscampus*. Retrieved October 23, 2013, from http://www.connected-living.org/projekte/forschnungscampus

Foursquare. (n.d.). Retrieved from https://foursquare.com

Fowsantear, W., Argo, E., Pattinson, C., & Cash, P. (2013). Comparative proteomics of Helicobacter species: The discrimination of gastric and enterohepatic Helicobacter species. *Journal of Proteomics*. PMID:23899588

Fox, G., Balsoy, O., Pallickara, S., Uyar, A., Gannon, D., & Slominski, A. (2002). Community Grids. In Proceedings of Computational Science—ICCS 2002 (pp. 22-38). Springer.

Francis, A., & McIntosh, R. (1997). The market, technological and industry context of business process re-engineering in the UK. *International Journal of Operations & Production Management*, *17*(4), 344–364. doi:10.1108/01443579710159941

Frost & Sullivan. (2012). *U.S. Hospital Health Data Analytics Market: Growing EHR Adoption Fuels A New Era in Analytics*. Retrieved November 18, 2013, from http://www.frost.com/c/10046/sublib/display-report.do?id=NA03-01-00-00-00

Fuchs, T., Birbaumer, N., Lutzenberger, W., Gruzelier, J. H., & Kaiser, J. (2003). Neurofeedback treatment for attention-deficit/hyperactivity disorder in children: A comparison with methylphenidate. *Applied Psychophysiology and Biofeedback*, *28*(1), 1–12. doi:10.1023/A:1022353731579 PMID:12737092

Fulmer, J. (n.d.). *Siege HTTP regression testing and benchmarking utility*. Retrieved from http://www.joedog.org/JoeDog/Siege

Fung, K. M., Hassell, L. A., Talbert, M. L., Wiechmann, A. F., Chaser, B. E., & Ramey, J. (2012). Whole slide images and digital media in pathology education, testing, and practice: The Oklahoma experience. *Analytical Cellular Pathology (Amsterdam)*, *35*(1), 37–40. PMID:21965282

Gaber, J. (2006). New paradigms for ubiquitous and pervasive applications. In *Proceedings of First Workshop on Software Engineering Challenges for Ubiquitous Computing*. Lancaster, UK: Academic Press.

Gagnon, M., Inhorn, S., Hancock, J., Keller, B., Carpenter, D., & Merlin, T. et al. (2004). Comparison of cytology proficiency testing: Glass slides vs. virtual slides. *Acta Cytologica*, *48*(6), 788–794. doi:10.1159/000326447 PMID:15581163

Gardner-Thorpe, J., Love, N., Wrightson, J., Walsh, S., & Keeling, N. (2006). The value of Modified Early Warning Score (MEWS) in surgical in-patients: a prospective observational study. *Annals of the Royal College of Surgeons of England*, *88*(6), 571–575. doi:10.1308/003588406X130615 PMID:17059720

Garets, D., & Davis, M. (2006). *Electronic medical records vs. electronic health records: Yes, there is a difference* (policy white paper). Chicago: HIMSS Analytics.

Garrison, J. A., Schardt, C., & Kochi, J. K. (2000). Web-based distance continuing education: A new way of thinking for students and instructors. *Bulletin of the Medical Library Association*, 88(3), 211–217. PMID:10928706

Gartner, Inc. (2009). *Defining Gartner Highlights Five Attributes of Cloud Computing*. Retrieved June 1, 2013, from http://www.gartner.com/it/page.jsp?id=1035013

Gavan, T. L., & King, J. W. (1970). An evaluation of the microbiology portions of the 1969 basic, comprehensive, and special College of American Pathologists proficiency testing surveys. *American Journal of Clinical Pathology*, 54(3), 514–520. PMID:4918179

GÉANT. (n.d.). Retrieved December 5, 2013, from http://www.geant.net

Gens, F. (2008). *Defining Cloud Services and Cloud Computing*. Retrieved June 1, 2013, from http://blogs.idc.com/ie/?p=190

Gens, F. (2011). Top 10 Predictions. In IDC Predictions 2012: Competing for 2020. IDC.

Gentleman, R. (2008). *R programming for bioinformatics*. Boca Raton, FL: CRC Press. doi:10.1201/9781420063684

Georgiou, A., Callen, J., Westbrook, J., Prgomet, M., & Toouli, G. (2007). Information and communication processes in the microbiology laboratory--Implications for computerised provider order entry. *Studies in Health Technology and Informatics*, 129(2), 943–947. PMID:17911854

Georgiou, A., Prgomet, M., Toouli, G., Callen, J., & Westbrook, J. (2011). What do physicians tell laboratories when requesting tests? A multi-method examination of information supplied to the microbiology laboratory before and after the introduction of electronic ordering. *International Journal of Medical Informatics*, 80(9), 646–654. doi:10.1016/j.ijmedinf.2011.06.003 PMID:21757400

Gerla, M. (2012). Vehicular Cloud Computing. In *Proceedings of Ad Hoc Networking Workshop (Med-Hoc-Net)*, (pp. 152-155). IEEE.

Ghaznavi, F., Evans, A., Madabhushi, A., & Feldman, M. (2013). Digital imaging in pathology: Whole-slide imaging and beyond. *Annual Review of Pathology*, 8, 331–359. doi:10.1146/annurev-pathol-011811-120902 PMID:23157334

Ghosh, R., Longo, F., Naik, V. K., & Trivedi, K. S. (2010). Quantifying resiliency of IaaS cloud. In *Proceedings of Reliable Distributed Systems* (pp. 343–347). IEEE.

Giacomelli, P. (2012). *HornetQ messaging developers' guide*. Packt Publishing.

Giacomini, M., Ruggiero, C., Calegari, L., & Bertone, S. (2000). Artificial neural network based identification of environmental bacteria by gas-chromatographic and electrophoretic data. *Journal of Microbiological Methods*, 43(1), 45–54. doi:10.1016/S0167-7012(00)00203-7 PMID:11084227

Giovagnoli, M. R., Cenci, M., Olla, S. V., & Vecchione, A. (2002). Cervical false negative cases detected by neural network-based technology: Critical review of cytologic errors. *Acta Cytologica*, 46(6), 1105–1109. doi:10.1159/000327115 PMID:12462090

Giuffre, G. (2006). Topical dorzolamide for the treatment of cystoid macular edema in patients with retinitis pigmentosa. *American Journal of Ophthalmology*, 142(4), 707–708. doi:10.1016/j.ajo.2006.06.042 PMID:17011883

Glaser, J. (2011). Cloud computing can simplify HIT infrastructure management. *Healthcare Financial Management*, 65(8), 52–55. PMID:21866720

GlobalData. (2012). *Snapshot: The US cloud computing market for medical imaging*. Retrieved 22/08/2013, from http://www.medicaldevice-network.com/features/featuresnapshot-the-us-cloud-computing-market-for-medical-imaging

Godinho, R. (2011). *Availability, Reliability and Scalability in Database Architecture*. Universidade do Minho.

Goldman, J., & Hudson, Z. (2000). Virtually exposed: Privacy and e-health. *Health Affairs*, 19, 140–148. doi:10.1377/hlthaff.19.6.140 PMID:11192397

Goncalves, A., Tikhonov, A., Brazma, A., & Kapushesky, M. (2011). A pipeline for RNA-seq data processing and quality assessment. *Bioinformatics (Oxford, England)*, 27(6), 867–869. doi:10.1093/bioinformatics/btr012 PMID:21233166

Goodgame, J. C., Pottage, J. C. Jr, Jablonowski, H., Hardy, W. D., Stein, A., & Fischl, M. et al. (2000). Amprenavir in combination with lamivudine and zidovudine versus lamivudine and zidovudine alone in HIV-1-infected antiretroviral-naive adults: Amprenavir PROAB3001 International Study Team. *Antiviral Therapy*, 5(3), 215–225. PMID:11075942

Google Charts. (n.d.). Retrieved from https://developers. google.com/chart/

Google. (n.d.). *Google Cloud Storage Service*. Retrieved from http://code.google.com/apis/storage/

Greenbaum, D., & Gerstein, M. (2011). The role of cloud computing in managing the deluge of potentially private genetic data. *The American Journal of Bioethics*, 11(11), 39–41. doi:10.1080/15265161.2011.60824 2 PMID:22047125

Grimes, J. M., Jaeger, P. T., & Lin, J. (2009). *Weathering the storm: The policy implications of cloud computing*. Retrieved June 1, 2013, from http://nora.lis.uiuc.edu/ images/iConferences/CloudAbstract13109FINAL.pdf

Grogan, J. (2006). EHRs and information availability: Are you at risk? *Health Management Technology*, 27(5), 16. PMID:16739432

Groves, P., Kayyali, B., Knott, D., & Van Kuiken, S. (2013). *The 'big data' revolution in healthcare: Accelerating value and innovation*. McKinsey & Company.

Gunter, T. D., & Terry, N. P. (2005). The emergence of national electronic health record architectures in the United States and Australia: models, costs, and questions. *Journal of Medical Internet Research*, 7(1). doi:10.2196/ jmir.7.1.e3 PMID:15829475

Guo, L., Guo, Y., & Tian, X. (2010). *IC cloud: A design space for composable cloud computing*. Paper presented at the Cloud Computing (CLOUD). New York, NY.

Guo, Y., Kuo, M., & Sahama, T. (2012). Cloud computing for healthcare research information sharing. In *Proceedings of the 4th IEEE International Conference on Cloud Computing Technology and Science* (CloudCom) (pp. 889-894). Taipei, Taiwan: IEEE.

Guo, Y.-K., & Guo, L. (2011). IC cloud: Enabling compositional cloud. *International Journal of Automation and Computing*, 8(3), 269–279. doi:10.1007/s11633-011-0582-4

Gutman, D. A., Cobb, J., Somanna, D., Park, Y., Wang, F., & Kurc, T. et al. (2013). Cancer Digital Slide Archive: An informatics resource to support integrated in silico analysis of TCGA pathology data. *Journal of the American Medical Informatics Association*. doi:10.1136/ amiajnl-2012-001469 PMID:23893318

Haeberlen, A. (2010). A case for the accountable cloud. *SIGOPS Operating Systems Review*, 44, 52–57. doi:10.1145/1773912.1773926

Hajmeer, M. N., Basheer, I. A., & Najjar, Y. M. (1997). Computational neural networks for predictive microbiology: Application to microbial growth. *International Journal of Food Microbiology*, 34(1), 51–66. doi:10.1016/ S0168-1605(96)01169-5 PMID:9029255

Halligan, B. D., Geiger, J. F., Vallejos, A. K., Greene, A. S., & Twigger, S. N. (2009). Low cost, scalable proteomics data analysis using Amazon's cloud computing services and open source search algorithms. *Journal of Proteome Research*, 8(6), 3148–3153. doi:10.1021/pr800970z PMID:19358578

Hanna, E. M., Mohamed, N., & Al-Jaroodi, J. (2012). The Cloud: Requirements for a Better Service. In Proceedings of Cluster, Cloud and Grid Computing (CCGrid), (pp. 787-792). IEEE.

HAPI. (2013). *Official HAPI website*. Retrieved September 2, 2013, from http://hl7api.sourceforge.net

Harding, H. B. (1965a). Quality control in microbiology. *Hospital Topics*, 43(10), 77–80. doi:10.1080/00185868. 1965.9954565 PMID:5831293

Harding, H. B. (1965b). Quality control in microbiology: II. *Hospital Topics*, *43*(11), 79–85. doi:10.1080/00185868.1965.9954597 PMID:5843067

Harmon, R. L. (1996). *Reinventing the business: Preparing today's enterprise for tomorrow's technology*. New York: Free Press.

Harris, B. (2012). 5 ways cloud computing will transform healthcare. *Healthcare IT News*. Retrieved from http://www.healthcareitnews.com/news/5-ways-cloud-computing-will-transform-healthcare

Haykin, S. S. (1994). *Neural networks: A comprehensive foundation*. Toronto: Macmillan.

Haymart, M. R., Cayo, M., & Chen, H. (2009). Papillary thyroid microcarcinomas: Big decisions for a small tumor. *Annals of Surgical Oncology*, *16*(11), 3132–3139. doi:10.1245/s10434-009-0647-6 PMID:19653044

HBase. (n.d.). Retrieved from http://hbase.apache.org/

Health Level Seven International (HL7). (2013). About HL7. *About Health Level Seven International*. Retrieved October 23, 2013, from http://www.hl7.org/about/index.cfm?ref=nav

Healthcare & Life Sciences. (n.d.). Retrieved November 28, 2013, from http://www.cloudera.com/content/cloudera/en/solutions/industries/healthcare-life-sciences.html

Healthcare IT Q1 2013 Funding and M&A Report. (n.d.). MERCOM Capital Group.

He, C., Fan, X., & Li, Y. (2013). Toward Ubiquitous Healthcare Services with a Novel Efficient Cloud Platform. *IEEE Transactions on Bio-Medical Engineering*, *60*(1), 230–234. doi:10.1109/TBME.2012.2222404 PMID:23060318

Heiler, S. (1995). Semantic interoperability. *ACM Computing Surveys*, *27*(2), 271–273. doi:10.1145/210376.210392

Held, M., Wolfe, P., & Crowder, H. P. (1974). Validation of subgradient optimization. *Mathematical Programming*, *6*(1), 62–88. doi:10.1007/BF01580223

Heymans, S., McKennirey, M., & Phillips, J. (2011). Semantic validation of the use of SNOMED CT in HL7 clinical documents. *Journal of Biomedical Semantics*, *2*(1), 2. doi:10.1186/2041-1480-2-2 PMID:21762489

HighCharts JS. (n.d.). Retrieved from http://www.highcharts.com/

HIPAA. (1996). *Health Insurance Portability and Accountability Act of 1996*. Retrieved from http://www.gpo.gov/fdsys/pkg/PLAW-104publ191/html/PLAW-104publ191.htm

Hipp, J. D., Lucas, D. R., Emmert-Buck, M. R., Compton, C. C., & Balis, U. J. (2011). Digital slide repositories for publications: lessons learned from the microarray community. *The American Journal of Surgical Pathology*, *35*(6), 783–786. doi:10.1097/PAS.0b013e31821946b6 PMID:21552111

HL7. (2012). *HL7 Website*. Retrieved from http://www.hl7.org/

HL7. (2013). *Official HL7 website*. Retrieved August 23, 2013, from http://www.hl7.org

Hofmarcher, M. M., Oxley, H., & Rusticelli, E. (2007). *Improved Health System Performance through better Care Coordination* (OECD Health Working Papers, No. 30). OECD Publishing.

Holland, J. (1975). *Adaptation in natural and artificial systems*. Ann Arbor, MI: The University of Michigan Press.

Hommes, F. A., Brewster, M. A., Burton, B. K., Buist, N. R., Elsas, L. J., & Goldsmith, B. M. et al. (1990). Proficiency testing for biochemical genetics laboratories: The first 10 rounds of testing. *American Journal of Human Genetics*, *46*(5), 1001–1004. PMID:2339686

Hong, D., Rhie, A., Park, S. S., Lee, J., Ju, Y. S., & Kim, S. et al. (2012). FX: An RNA-Seq analysis tool on the cloud. *Bioinformatics (Oxford, England)*, *28*(5), 721–723. doi:10.1093/bioinformatics/bts023 PMID:22257667

Hood, M. N., & Scott, H. (2006). Introduction to picture archive and communication systems. *Journal of Radiology Nursing*, *25*(3), 69–74. doi:10.1016/j.jradnu.2006.06.003

Hornet, Q. (2013). *Official HornetQ website*. Retrieved August 13, 2013, from http://www.jboss.org/hornet

Horowitz, B. (2011). *Cloud computing brings challenges for health care data storage, privacy*. Retrieved July 23, 2013 from http://www.eweek.com/c/a/Health-Care-IT/Cloud-Computing-Brings-Challenges-for-Health-Care-Data-Storage-Privacy-851608/

Hsu, C. H., Lin, C. Y., Ouyang, M., & Guo, Y. K. (2013). Biocloud: Cloud computing for biological, genomics, and drug design. *BioMed Research International, 909470.*

Hu, Y., Lu, F., Khan, I., & Bai, G. (2012). A cloud computing solution for sharing healthcare information. In *Proceedings of the 7th International Conference for Internet Technology and Secured Transactions* (ICITST) (pp. 465-470). London, UK: ICITST.

Huang, C. C., Lin, C. Y., Chang, C. W., & Tang, C. Y. (2013). Enzyme reaction annotation using cloud techniques. *BioMed Research International, 140237.*

Huffaker, B., Fomenkov, M., & Claffy, K. (2011). Geocompare: a comparison of public and commercial geolocation databases. In *Proceedings of Network Mapping and Measurement Conference (NMMC).* NMMC.

Hung, C. L., & Hua, G. J. (2013). Cloud computing for protein-ligand binding site comparison. *BioMed Research International, 170356.*

Hunt, J. (2013). *The Silent Scandal of Patient Safety.* UK Government Speeches. Retrieved July 17, 2013 from https://www.gov.uk/government/speeches/the-silent-scandal-of-patient-safety

IBM. (n.d.). *InfoSphere Platform.* Retrieved December 4, 2013, from http://www-01.ibm.com/software/data/infosphere/

IDC. (2008). *IDC market analysis: IT spend on cloud services to grow to $42 billion / 25% of spend by 2012.* Retrieved June 1, 2013 from http://blogs.idc.com/ie/?p=190

Ikhu-Omoregbe. (2008). Formal modeling and design of mobile prescription applications. *Journal of Health Informatics in Developing Countries, 2*(2).

International, I. H. E. (IHE). (2013a). Integrating the Healthcare Enterprise. *IHE - Integrating the Healthcare Enterprise* Retrieved October 23, 2013, from http://www.ihe.net/

International, I. H. E. (IHE). (2013b). PCD Profile Rosetta Terminology Mapping. *PCD Profile Rosetta Terminology Mapping - IHE wiki.* Retrieved October 23, 2013, from http://http://wiki.ihe.net/index.php?title=PCD_Profile_Rosetta_Terminology_Mapping

Ioannidis, J. P., Tarone, R., & McLaughlin, J. K. (2011). The false-positive to false-negative ratio in epidemiologic studies. *Epidemiology (Cambridge, Mass.), 22*(4), 450–456. doi:10.1097/EDE.0b013e31821b506e PMID:21490505

ISO/IEC. (1994). Information technology - Open Systems Interconnection - Basic Reference Model: The Basic Model. In *ISO/IEC 7498.1:1994(E)* (pp. 1-68). ISO/IEC.

ISO/IEC/IEEE. (2010). ISO/IEC/IEEE Health Informatics–Personal Health Device Communication–Part 20601: Application Profile–Optimized Exchange Protocol. In ISO/IEEE 11073-20601:2010(E) (pp. 1-208). IEEE.

ISO/IEEE. (2004). ISO/IEEE Health Informatics–Point-Of-Care Medical Device Communication–Part 10101. In ISO/IEEE 11073-10101:2004(E) (pp. 0-492). IEEE.

IT Union. (2008). *Implementing e-health in developing countries.* ITU Tech Report.

Ivanov, D., Kliem, A., & Kao, O. (2013). Transformation Middleware for Heterogeneous Healthcare Data in Mobile E-health Environments. In *Proceedings of the 2013 IEEE Second International Conference on Mobile Services* (pp. 39-46). IEEE Computer Society.

Izadi-Mood, N., Sarmadi, S., & Sanii, S. (2013). Quality control in cervicovaginal cytology by cytohistological correlation. *Cytopathology, 24*(1), 33–38. doi:10.1111/j.1365-2303.2011.00926.x PMID:21929578

Jemal, A., Bray, F., Center, M. M., Ferlay, J., Ward, E., & Forman, D. (2011). Global cancer statistics. *CA: a Cancer Journal for Clinicians, 61*(2), 69–90. doi:10.3322/caac.20107 PMID:21296855

Jha, S., Katz, D. S., Luckow, A., Merzky, A., & Stamou, K. (2011). Understanding Scientific Applications for Cloud Environments. In R. Buyya, J. Nroberg, & A. Goscinski (Eds.), *Cloud Computing: Principles and Paradigms* (pp. 345–371). Wiley. doi:10.1002/9780470940105.ch13

JMS. (2013). *Official JMS specification.* Retrieved August 13, 2013, from http://www.oracle.com/technetwork/java/docs-136352.html

Jo, H., Jeong, J., Lee, M., & Choi, D. H. (2013). Exploiting GPUs in virtual machine for BioCloud. *BioMed Research International, 939460.*

Jourdren, L., Bernard, M., Dillies, M. A., & Le Crom, S. (2012). Eoulsan: A cloud computing-based framework facilitating high throughput sequencing analyses. *Bioinformatics (Oxford, England)*, 28(11), 1542–1543. doi:10.1093/bioinformatics/bts165 PMID:22492314

Kaelber, D. C., Foster, W., Gilder, J., Love, T. E., & Jain, A. K. (2012). Patient characteristics associated with venous thromboembolic events: a cohort study using pooled electronic health record data. *Journal of the American Medical Informatics Association*, 19(6), 965–972. doi:10.1136/amiajnl-2011-000782 PMID:22759621

Kajan, L., Yachdav, G., Vicedo, E., Steinegger, M., Mirdita, M., Angermuller, C., … Rost, B. (2013). Cloud prediction of protein structure and function with PredictProtein for Debian. *BioMed Research International*, 398968.

Kandukuri, R., & Rakshit, A. (2009). Cloud Security Issues. In *Proceedings of the 2009 IEEE international Conference on Services Computing*, (pp. 517-520). Lincoln. NE: University of Nebraska Press.

Kanungo, R. (2012). Are clinical microbiology laboratories missing out quality control and quality assurance in laboratory management? *Indian Journal of Medical Microbiology*, 30(1), 1–2. doi:10.4103/0255-0857.93012 PMID:22361752

Kaplan, W. A. (2006). Can the ubiquitous power of mobile phones be used to improve health outcomes in developing countries? *Globalization and Health*, 2(1), 9. doi:10.1186/1744-8603-2-9 PMID:16719925

Karakitsos, P., Cochand-Priollet, B., Guillausseau, P. J., & Pouliakis, A. (1996). Potential of the back propagation neural network in the morphologic examination of thyroid lesions. *Analytical and Quantitative Cytology and Histology*, 18(6), 494–500. PMID:8978873

Karakitsos, P., Cochand-Priollet, B., Pouliakis, A., Guillausseau, P. J., & Ioakim-Liossi, A. (1999). Learning vector quantizer in the investigation of thyroid lesions. *Analytical and Quantitative Cytology and Histology*, 21(3), 201–208. PMID:10560492

Karakitsos, P., Kyroudes, A., Pouliakis, A., Stergiou, E. B., Voulgaris, Z., & Kittas, C. (2002). Potential of the learning vector quantizer in the cell classification of endometrial lesions in postmenopausal women. *Analytical and Quantitative Cytology and Histology*, 24(1), 30–38. PMID:11865947

Karakitsos, P., Megalopoulou, T. M., Pouliakis, A., Tzivras, M., Archimandritis, A., & Kyroudes, A. (2004). Application of discriminant analysis and quantitative cytologic examination to gastric lesions. *Analytical and Quantitative Cytology and Histology*, 26(6), 314–322. PMID:15678613

Karakitsos, P., Pouliakis, A., Kordalis, G., Georgoulakis, J., Kittas, C., & Kyroudes, A. (2005). Potential of radial basis function neural networks in discriminating benign from malignant lesions of the lower urinary tract. *Analytical and Quantitative Cytology and Histology*, 27(1), 35–42. PMID:15794450

Karakitsos, P., Pouliakis, A., Meristoudis, C., Margari, N., Kassanos, D., & Kyrgiou, M. et al. (2011). A preliminary study of the potential of tree classifiers in triage of high-grade squamous intraepithelial lesions. *Analytical and Quantitative Cytology and Histology*, 33(3), 132–140. PMID:21980616

Karakitsos, P., Stergiou, E. B., Pouliakis, A., Tzivras, M., Archimandritis, A., Liossi, A. I., & Kyrkou, K. (1996). Potential of the back propagation neural network in the discrimination of benign from malignant gastric cells. *Analytical and Quantitative Cytology and Histology*, 18(3), 245–250. PMID:8790840

Kasson, P. M. (2013). Computational biology in the cloud: Methods and new insights from computing at scale. In *Proceedings of Pacific Symposium on Biocomputing*, (pp. 451-453). Academic Press.

Kazandjian, V. A. (1991). Performance Indicators: Pointer-dogs in disguise- A commentary. *Journal of the American Medical Record Association*, 62(9), 34–36. PMID:10112933

Kazandjian, V. A. (2002). *Accountability through Measurement: A Global Healthcare Imperative.* Milwaukee, WI: ASQ Quality Press.

Kazandjian, V. A. (2012). Quality is Not an Accident: The Planning for a Safe Journey through the Healthcare System. *International Journal of Reliable and Quality E-Healthcare, 1*(2), 1–11. doi:10.4018/ijrqeh.2012040101

Kazandjian, V. A., & Lied, T. (1999). *Healthcare Performance Measurement: Systems Design and Evaluation.* ASQC Quality Press.

Kazandjian, V. A., & Lipitz-Snyderman, A. (2010). HIT or Miss: The application of health care information technology to managing uncertainty in clinical decision making. *Journal of Evaluation in Clinical Practice, 17*(6), 1108–1113. PMID:20630010

Kelley, D. R., Schatz, M. C., & Salzberg, S. L. (2010). Quake: Quality-aware detection and correction of sequencing errors. *Genome Biology, 11*(11), R116. doi:10.1186/gb-2010-11-11-r116 PMID:21114842

Kelly, E. P., & Unsal, F. (2002). Health information privacy and e-healthcare. *International Journal of Healthcare Technology and Management, 4*, 41–52. doi:10.1504/IJHTM.2002.001128

Kerridge, I., Lowe, M., & McPhee, J. (2005). *Ethics and law for the health professions.* Sydney: Federation Press.

Khansa, L., Forcade, J., Nambari, G., Parasuraman, S., & Cox, P. (2012). Proposing an intelligent cloud-based electronic health record system. *International Journal of Business Data Communications and Networking, 8*(3), 57–71. doi:10.4018/jbdcn.2012070104

Khayati, M., & Akaichi, J. (2008). Incremental approach for continuous k-nearest neighbors queries on road. *International Journal of Intelligent Information and Database Systems, 2*(2), 204–221. doi:10.1504/IJIIDS.2008.018255

Khetrapal, A., & Ganesh, V. (2006). *HBase and Hypertable for large scale distributed storage systems.* Dept. of Computer Science, Purdue University.

Khurana, K. K. (2012). Telecytology and its evolving role in cytopathology. *Diagnostic Cytopathology, 40*(6), 498–502. doi:10.1002/dc.22822 PMID:22619124

Kifor, T., Varga, L., Álvarez, S., Vázquez-Salceda, J., & Willmott, S. (2006). Privacy issues of provenance in electronic healthcare record systems. In *Proceedings of the 1st Int. Workshop on Privacy and Security in Agent-Based Collaborative Environments (PSACE 2006).* PSACE.

Kijl, B., Bouwman, H., Haaker, T., & Faber, E. (2005). *Dynamic Business Models in Mobile Service Value Networks: A Theoretical and Conceptual Framework.* FRUX Deliverable.

Kim, Y., Gurumurthi, S., & Sivasubramaniam, A. (2006). *Understanding the performance-temperature interactions in disk I/O of server workloads.* Paper presented at the High-Performance Computer Architecture. New York, NY.

Kim, S., Cho, N., Lee, Y., Kang, S.-H., Kim, T., Hwang, H., & Mun, D. (2010). Application of density-based outlier detection to database activity monitoring. *Information Systems Frontiers*, 1–11.

Kirsch, C., Pereira, E., Sengupta, R., Chen, H., Hansen, R., Huang, J., et al. (2012). Cyber-physical cloud computing: The binding and migration problem. In *Proceedings of the Conference on Design, Automation and Test in Europe* (pp. 1425-1428). EDA Consortium.

Kliem, A., Hovestadt, M., & Kao, O. (2012). Security and Communication Architecture for Networked Medical Devices in Mobility-Aware eHealth Environments. In *Proceedings of the 2012 IEEE First International Conference on Mobile Services* (pp. 112-114). IEEE.

Koenig, J. (2004). *JBoss jBPM white paper.* JBoss Labs.

Koh, H. C., & Tan, G. (2011). Data mining applications in healthcare. *Journal of Healthcare Information Management, 19*(2), 64. PMID:15869215

Kohn, L. T., Corrigan, J. M., & Donaldson, M. S. (2000). *To err is human: building a safer health system.* Washington, DC: National Academy Press.

Kohonen, T. (1982). Self-Organized Formation of Topologically Correct Feature Maps. *Biological Cybernetics, 43*, 59–69. doi:10.1007/BF00337288

Kohonen, T. (1984). *Self-Organization and Associative Memory.* Berlin: SpringerVerlag.

Kohonen, T. (2001). *Self-organizing maps* (3rd ed.). Berlin: Springer. doi:10.1007/978-3-642-56927-2

Ko, J., Lu, C., Srivastava, M. B., Stankovic, J. A., Terzis, A., & Welsh, M. (2010). Wireless sensor networks for healthcare. *Proceedings of the IEEE*, *98*(11), 1947–1960. doi:10.1109/JPROC.2010.2065210

Kok, M. R., Habers, M. A., Schreiner-Kok, P. G., & Boon, M. E. (1998). New paradigm for ASCUS diagnosis using neural networks. *Diagnostic Cytopathology*, *19*(5), 361–366. doi:10.1002/(SICI)1097-0339(199811)19:5<361::AID-DC10>3.0.CO;2-9 PMID:9812231

Kok, M. R., van Der Schouw, Y. T., Boon, M. E., Grobbee, D. E., Kok, L. P., & Schreiner-Kok, P. G. et al. (2001). Neural network-based screening (NNS) in cervical cytology: No need for the light microscope? *Diagnostic Cytopathology*, *24*(6), 426–434. doi:10.1002/dc.1093 PMID:11391826

Kolahdouzan, M., & Shahabi, C. (2004). *Vornoi-based K nearest neighbor search for spatial network databases.* Paper presented at the 30th VLDB Conference. Toronto, Canada.

Kolahdouzan, M., & Shahabi, C. (2005). Alternative solutions for continuous K-nearest neighbor queries in spatial network databases. *Springer Science*, *9*(4), 321–341.

Kondoh, H., Teramoto, K., Kawai, T., Mochida, M., & Nishimura, M. (2013). Development of the Regional EPR and PACS Sharing System on the Infrastructure of Cloud Computing Technology Controlled by Patient Identifier Cross Reference Manager. *Studies in Health Technology and Informatics*, *192*, 1073. PMID:23920847

Konganti, K., Wang, G., Yang, E., & Cai, J. J. (2013). SBEToolbox: A Matlab Toolbox for Biological Network Analysis. *Evolutionary Bioinformatics*, *9*, 355–362. doi:10.4137/EBO.S12012 PMID:24027418

Koumpouros, I. (2012). *Information and Communication Technologies & Society.* Athens, Greece: New Technologies Publications.

Krampis, K., Booth, T., Chapman, B., Tiwari, B., Bicak, M., Field, D., & Nelson, K. E. (2012). Cloud BioLinux: Pre-configured and on-demand bioinformatics computing for the genomics community. *BMC Bioinformatics*, *13*, 42. doi:10.1186/1471-2105-13-42 PMID:22429538

Krishnamurthy, S., Mathews, K., McClure, S., Murray, M., Gilcrease, M., & Albarracin, C. et al. (2013). Multi-Institutional Comparison of Whole Slide Digital Imaging and Optical Microscopy for Interpretation of Hematoxylin-Eosin-Stained Breast Tissue Sections. *Archives of Pathology & Laboratory Medicine.* doi:10.5858/arpa.2012-0437-OA PMID:23947655

Kuntz, I. D. (1992). Structure-based strategies for drug design and discovery. *Science*, *257*(5073), 1078–1082. doi:10.1126/science.257.5073.1078 PMID:1509259

Kuo, M. H., Kushniruk, A., Borycki, E., Lai, F., & Dorjgochoo, S. Altangerel, & Jigjidsuren, C. (2012). A cloud computing based platform for sharing healthcare research information. In *Proceedings of the 13th International Conference on Collaboration Technologies and Systems* (CTS) (pp. 504-508). Denver, CO: CTS.

Kuo, A. M. (2011). Opportunities and Challenges of Cloud Computing to Improve Health Care Services. *Journal of Medical Internet Research*, *13*(3), e67. doi:10.2196/jmir.1867 PMID:21937354

Lakshman, A., & Malik, P. (2010). Cassandra: A decentralized structured storage system. *SIGOPS Oper. Syst. Rev.*, *44*(2), 35–40. doi:10.1145/1773912.1773922

Langmead, B., Hansen, K. D., & Leek, J. T. (2010). Cloud-scale RNA-sequencing differential expression analysis with Myrna. *Genome Biology*, *11*(8), R83. doi:10.1186/gb-2010-11-8-r83 PMID:20701754

Langmead, B., Schatz, M. C., Lin, J., Pop, M., & Salzberg, S. L. (2009). Searching for SNPs with cloud computing. *Genome Biology*, *10*(11), R134. doi:10.1186/gb-2009-10-11-r134 PMID:19930550

Laprie, J. C. (2008). From dependability to resilience. In *Proceedings of 38th IEEE/IFIP Int. Conf. on Dependable Systems and Networks.* IEEE.

Lavy, M. M., & Meggitt, A. J. (2001). *Windows Management Instrumentation (WMI)*. New Riders. Retrieved from http://www.google.pt/books?id=DD1jA3RgFEMC

Leavitt, N. (2010). Will NoSQL databases live up to their promise? *Computer*, *43*(2), 12–14. doi:10.1109/MC.2010.58

Lee, S. T., Lin, C. Y., & Hung, C. L. (2013). GPU-based cloud service for Smith-Waterman algorithm using frequency distance filtration scheme. *BioMed Research International*, 721738.

Lee, C. H., Birch, D., Wu, C., Silva, D., Tsinalis, O., Li, Y., & Guo, Y. (2013). Building a generic platform for big sensor data application. In *Proceedings of Big Data* (pp. 94–102). IEEE. doi:10.1109/BigData.2013.6691559

Lee, H., Yang, Y., Chae, H., Nam, S., Choi, D., & Tangchaisin, P. et al. (2012). BioVLAB-MMIA: A cloud environment for microRNA and mRNA integrated analysis (MMIA) on Amazon EC2. *IEEE Transactions on Nanobioscience*, *11*(3), 266–272. doi:10.1109/TNB.2012.2212030 PMID:22987133

Lee, J., Kim, S., Kim, P., Liu, X., Lee, T., & Kim, K. M. et al. (2013). A novel proteomics-based clinical diagnostics technology identifies heterogeneity in activated signaling pathways in gastric cancers. *PLoS ONE*, *8*(1), e54644. doi:10.1371/journal.pone.0054644 PMID:23372746

Lenz, R., & Reichert, M. (2006). IT support for healthcare processes—Premises, challenges, perspectives. *Data and Knowledge Engineering Journal*, *61*, 39–58. doi:10.1016/j.datak.2006.04.007

Leprevost, F. V., Lima, D. B., Crestani, J., Perez-Riverol, Y., Zanchin, N., Barbosa, V. C., & Carvalho, P. C. (2013). Pinpointing differentially expressed domains in complex protein mixtures with the cloud service of PatternLab for Proteomics. *Journal of Proteomics*, *89*, 179–182. doi:10.1016/j.jprot.2013.06.013 PMID:23796493

Li, N., Hou, J., & Sha, L. (2003). Design and analysis of MST-based topology control algorithm. In *Proceedings of the 22th Annual Joint Conference on the IEEE INFOCOM*. San Francisco, CA: IEEE.

Li, W., Yan, J., Yan, Y., & Zhang, J. (2010). Xbase: Cloud-enabled information appliance for healthcare. In I. Manolescu, S. Spaccapietra, J. Teubner, M. Kitsuregawa, A. Leger, F. Naumann, A. Ailamaki, & F. Ozcan (Eds.), *13th International Conference on Extending Database Technology (EDBT 2010)*, (vol. 426, pp. 675-680). ACM.

Li, Y., Guo, L., & Guo, Y. (2012). *CACSS: Towards a Generic Cloud Storage Service*. Paper presented at the CLOSER. New York, NY. Retrieved from http://dblp.uni-trier.de/db/conf/closer/closer2012.html#LiGG12

Li, G., Zhao, F., & Cui, Y. (2013). Proteomics using mammospheres as a model system to identify proteins deregulated in breast cancer stem cells. *Current Molecular Medicine*, *13*(3), 459–463. PMID:23331018

Lilford, R., Mohammed, M. A., Spiegelhalter, D., & Thomson, R. (2004). Use and misuse of process and outcome data in managing performance of acute medical care: Avoiding institutional stigma. *Lancet*, *363*, 1147–1154. doi:10.1016/S0140-6736(04)15901-1 PMID:15064036

Li, M., Yu, S., Ren, K., & Lou, W. (2010). Securing personal health records in cloud computing: Patient-centric and fine-grained data access control in multi-owner settings. In *Proceedings of Security and Privacy in Communication Networks* (pp. 89–106). Springer. doi:10.1007/978-3-642-16161-2_6

Lindner, M. A., McDonald, F., Conway, G., & Curry, E. (2011). Understanding Cloud Requirements-A Supply Chain Lifecycle Approach. In *Proceedings of Cloud Computing 2011, The Second International Conference on Cloud Computing, GRIDs, and Virtualization* (pp. 20-25). Academic Press.

Lindner, M., Galán, F., Chapman, C., Clayman, S., Henriksson, D., & Elmroth, E. (2010). The cloud supply chain: A framework for information, monitoring, accounting and billing. In *Proceedings of 2nd International ICST Conference on Cloud Computing (CloudComp 2010)*. ICST.

Lindner, M., McDonald, F., McLarnon, B., & Robinson, P. (2011). Towards automated business-driven indication and mitigation of VM sprawl in Cloud supply chains. In *Proceedings of Integrated Network Management (IM)* (pp. 1062–1065). IEEE. doi:10.1109/INM.2011.5990505

Liu, X., Han, J., Zhong, Y., Han, C., & He, X. (2009). *Implementing WebGIS on Hadoop: A case study of improving small file I/O performance on HDFS*. Paper presented at the Cluster Computing and Workshops. New York, NY.

Liu, F., Tong, J., Mao, J., Bohn, R., Messina, J., Badger, L., & Leaf, D. (2011). NIST cloud computing reference architecture. *NIST Special Publication, 500*, 292.

Li, Y., Guo, L., & Guo, Y. (2013). An Efficient and Performance-Aware Big Data Storage System. In *Cloud Computing and Services Science* (pp. 102–116). Springer. doi:10.1007/978-3-319-04519-1_7

Ljung, B. M., Chew, K. L., Moore, D. H. II, & King, E. B. (2004). Cytology of ductal lavage fluid of the breast. *Diagnostic Cytopathology, 30*(3), 143–150. doi:10.1002/dc.20003 PMID:14986293

Löhr, H., Sadeghi, A. R., & Winandy, M. (2010). Securing the e-health cloud. In *Proceedings of the 1st ACM International Health Informatics Symposium* (pp. 220-229). ACM.

Loke, S. (2007). *Context-Aware Pervasive Systems: Architectures for a New Breed of Applications*. Boca Raton, FL: Auerbach Publications.

Lomotey, R. K., Jamal, S., & Deters, R. (2012). SOPHRA: A Mobile Web Services Hosting Infrastructure in mHealth. In Proceedings of Mobile Services (MS), (pp. 88-95). IEEE.

Lounis, A., Hadjidj, A., Bouabdallah, A., & Challal, Y. (2012). Secure and Scalable Cloud-based Architecture for e-Health Wireless sensor networks. In Proceedings of Computer Communications and Networks (ICCCN), (pp. 1-7). IEEE.

Lubar, J. F., Swartwood, M. O., Swartwood, J. N., & O'Donnell, P. H. (1995). Evaluation of the effectiveness of EEG neurofeedback training for ADHD in a clinical setting as measured by changes in TOVA scores, behavioral ratings, and WISC-R performance. *Biofeedback and Self-Regulation, 20*(1), 83–99. doi:10.1007/BF01712768 PMID:7786929

Luck, M., McBurney, P., & Preist, C. (2003). *Agent technology: Enabling next generation computing (a roadmap for agent based computing)*. AgentLink/University of Southampton.

Lupşe, O. S., Vida, M. M., & Stoicu-Tivadar, L. (2012). Cloud Computing and Interoperability in Healthcare Information Systems. In P. Lorenz & P. Dini (Eds.), *The First International Conference on Intelligent Systems and Applications (INTELLI 2012)* (pp. 81-85). IARIA.

Lupse, O. S., Vida, M., & Stoicu-Tivadar, L. (2012). Cloud computing technology applied in healthcare for developing large scale flexible solutions. *Studies in Health Technology and Informatics, 174*, 94–99. PMID:22491119

Machado, J., Abelha, A., Novais, P., Neves, J., & Neves, J. (2010). Quality of service in healthcare units. *International Journal of Computer Aided Engineering and Technology, 2*(4), 436–449. doi:10.1504/IJCAET.2010.035396

Machado, J., Miranda, M., Gonçalves, P., Abelha, A., Neves, J., & Marques, J. A. (2010). *AIDATrace: Interoperation platform for active monitoring in healthcare environments*. Academic Press.

Mack, R., Mukherjea, S., Soffer, A., Uramoto, N., Brown, E., & Coden, A. et al. (2004). Text analytics for life science using the unstructured information management architecture. *IBM Systems Journal, 43*(3), 490–515. doi:10.1147/sj.433.0490

Madden, K., Flowers, L., Salani, R., Horowitz, I., Logan, S., & Kowalski, K. et al. (2009). Proteomics-based approach to elucidate the mechanism of antitumor effect of curcumin in cervical cancer. *Prostaglandins, Leukotrienes, and Essential Fatty Acids, 80*(1), 9–18. doi:10.1016/j.plefa.2008.10.003 PMID:19058955

Manyika, J., Chui, M., Brown, B., Bughin, J., Dobbs, R., & Roxburgh, C. et al. (2011). *Big data: The next frontier for innovation, competition, and productivity*. McKinsey Global Institute.

Marchevsky, A. M., Tsou, J. A., & Laird-Offringa, I. A. (2004). Classification of individual lung cancer cell lines based on DNA methylation markers: use of linear discriminant analysis and artificial neural networks. *The Journal of Molecular Diagnostics*, *6*(1), 28–36. doi:10.1016/S1525-1578(10)60488-6 PMID:14736824

Maria, A. F., Fenu, G., & Surcis, S. (2009). An Approach to Cloud Computing Network. In *Proceedings of the 3rd International Conference on Theory and Practice of Electronic Governance*. Bogota, Colombia: Academic Press.

MarketsAndMarkets. (2011). *World Healthcare IT (Provider and Payor) Market - Clinical (EMR, PACS, RIS, CPOE, LIS) & Non-Clinical (RCM, Billing, Claims) Information systems Trends, opportunities & Forecast till 2015*. Retrieved November 28, 2013, from http://www.marketsandmarkets.com/Market-Reports/healthcare-information-technology-market-136.html

MarketsAndMarkets. (2012). *Healthcare Cloud Computing (Clinical, EMR, SaaS, Private, Public, Hybrid) Market – Global Trends, Challenges, Opportunities & Forecasts (2012–2017)*. Retrieved November 28, 2013, from http://www.marketsandmarkets.com/Market-Reports/cloud-computing-healthcare-market-347.html

Markopoulos, C., Karakitsos, P., Botsoli-Stergiou, E., Pouliakis, A., Gogas, J., Ioakim-Liossi, A., & Kyrkou, K. (1997). Application of back propagation to the diagnosis of breast lesions by fine needle aspiration. *The Breast*, *6*(5), 293–298. doi:10.1016/S0960-9776(97)90008-4

Markopoulos, C., Karakitsos, P., Botsoli-Stergiou, E., Pouliakis, A., Ioakim-Liossi, A., Kyrkou, K., & Gogas, J. (1997). Application of the learning vector quantizer to the classification of breast lesions. *Analytical and Quantitative Cytology and Histology*, *19*(5), 453–460. PMID:9349906

Martí, R., Delgado, J., & Perramon, X. (2004). Security specification and implementation for mobile e-health services. In *Proceedings of e-Technology, e-Commerce and e-Service* (pp. 241–248). IEEE. doi:10.1109/EEE.2004.1287316

McGregor, C. (2011). A cloud computing framework for real-time rural and remote service of critical care. In *Proceedings of the 24th International Symposium on Computer-Based Medical Systems (CBMS)* (pp. 1-6). Bristol, UK: IEEE.

McKenna, A., Hanna, M., Banks, E., Sivachenko, A., Cibulskis, K., & Kernytsky, A. et al. (2010). The Genome Analysis Toolkit: A MapReduce framework for analyzing next-generation DNA sequencing data. *Genome Research*, *20*(9), 1297–1303. doi:10.1101/gr.107524.110 PMID:20644199

McKnight, J., Babineau, B., & Gahm, J. (2011). *North American Health Care Provider Information Market Size & Forecast*. ESG-Enterprise Strategy Group.

MediaWiki. (n.d.). Retrieved from http://www.mediawiki.org

Meersman, D., Hadzic, F., Hughes, J., Razo-Zapata, I., & De Leenheer, P. (2013). Health Service Discovery and Composition in Ambient Assisted Living: The Australian Type 2 Diabetes Case Study. In Proceedings of System Sciences (HICSS), (pp. 1337-1346). IEEE.

Mell, P., & Grance, T. (2011). The NIST Definition of Cloud Computing. *NIST Special Publication*, 800-145.

Mell, P., & Grance, T. (2009). The NIST Definition of Cloud Computing. *National Institute of Standards and Technology*, *53*(6), 50.

Mell, P., & Grance, T. (2011). The NIST definition of cloud computing (draft). *NIST Special Publication*, *800*(145), 7.

Mell, P., & Grance, T. (2011). *The NIST definition of cloud computing*. Gaithersburg, MD: NIST.

Mersenne. (2013). *Great Internet Mersenne Prime Search 2012*. Retrieved September 15, 2013, from http://www.mersenne.org/

Metropolis, N., Rosenbluth, A. W., Rosenbluth, M. N., Teller, A. H., & Teller, E. (1953). Equations of state calculations by fast computing machines. *The Journal of Chemical Physics*, *21*(6), 1087–1091. doi:10.1063/1.1699114

Microsoft Corporation (MS). (2013). Explore HealthVault. *HealthVault - Overview*. Retrieved October 23, 2013, from http://www.healthvault.com/us/en/overview

Microsoft. (2013a). *WMI Overview*. Retrieved August 16, 2013, from http://technet.microsoft.com/en-us/library/cc753534.aspx

Microsoft. (2013b). *Win32_PerfFormattedData_PerfProc_Process class*. Retrieved August 16, 2013, from http://msdn.microsoft.com/en-us/library/windows/desktop/aa394277(v=vs.85).aspx

Microsoft. (2013c). *Win32_PerfFormattedData_PerfOS_Processor class*. Retrieved August 16, 2013, from http://msdn.microsoft.com/en-us/library/windows/desktop/aa394271(v=vs.85).aspx

Microsoft. (2013d). *Win32_PerfFormattedData_PerfOS_Memory class*. Retrieved August 16, 2013, from http://msdn.microsoft.com/en-us/library/windows/desktop/aa394268(v=vs.85).aspx

Microsoft. (2013e). *Win32_PerfFormattedData_PerfDisk_LogicalDisk class*. Retrieved August 16, 2013, from http://msdn.microsoft.com/en-us/library/windows/desktop/aa394261(v=vs.85).aspx

Milley, A. (2000). Healthcare and data mining. *Health Management Technology, 21*(8), 44–47.

Milojicic, D., Llorente, I. M., & Montero, R. S. (2011). Opennebula: A cloud management tool. *IEEE Internet Computing, 15*(2), 11–14. doi:10.1109/MIC.2011.44

Ming, L., Shucheng, Y., Yao, Z., Kui, R., & Wenjing, L. (2013). Scalable and Secure Sharing of Personal Health Records in Cloud Computing Using Attribute-Based Encryption. *IEEE Transactions on Parallel and Distributed Systems, 24*(1), 131–143. doi:10.1109/TPDS.2012.97

Miranda, M., Duarte, J., Abelha, A., Machado, J., & Neves, J. (2010). Interoperability in healthcare. In *Proceedings of European Simulation and Modelling Conference*. ESM.

Miranda, M., Salazar, M., Portela, F., Santos, M., Abelha, A., Neves, J., & Machado, J. (2012). Multi-agent Systems for HL7 Interoperability Services. In Procedia Technology (Vol. 5, pp. 725–733). Elsevier.

Miranda, M., Machado, J., Abelha, A., & Neves, J. (2013). In G. Fortino, C. Badica, M. Malgeri, & R. Unland (Eds.), *Healthcare Interoperability through a JADE Based Multi-Agent Platform* (Vol. 446, pp. 83–88). Intelligent Distributed Computing, VI: Springer. doi:10.1007/978-3-642-32524-3_11

Mirza, H., & El-Masri, S. (2013). National electronic medical records integration on Cloud computing system. *Studies in Health Technology and Informatics, 192*, 1219. PMID:23920993

Mirza, H., & El-Masri, S. (2013). National Electronic Medical Records integration on Cloud Computing System. *Studies in Health Technology and Informatics, 192*, 1219. PMID:23920993

Mitchell, J. C., Shmatikov, V., & Stern, U. (1998). Finite-state analysis of SSL 3.0. In *Proceedings of Seventh USENIX Security Symposium* (pp. 201-216). USENIX.

Mohammed, Y., Mostovenko, E., Henneman, A. A., Marissen, R. J., Deelder, A. M., & Palmblad, M. (2012). Cloud parallel processing of tandem mass spectrometry based proteomics data. *Journal of Proteome Research, 11*(10), 5101–5108. doi:10.1021/pr300561q PMID:22916831

Mohan, T. S. (2011). Migrating into a Cloud. In R. Buyya, J. Nroberg, & A. Goscinski (Eds.), *Cloud Computing: Principles and Paradigms* (pp. 43–56). Wiley. doi:10.1002/9780470940105.ch2

MongoDB. (n.d.). Retrieved from http://www.mongodb.org

Morris, D., & Brandon, J. (1993). *Reengineering your Business*. New York: McGraw-Hill.

Morris, G. M., Huey, R., Lindstrom, W., Sanner, M. F., Belew, R. K., Goodsell, D. S., & Olson, A. J. (2009). AutoDock4 and AutoDockTools4: Automated docking with selective receptor flexibility. *Journal of Computational Chemistry, 30*(16), 2785–2791. doi:10.1002/jcc.21256 PMID:19399780

Mouli, K. C., & Sesadri, U. (2013). Single to Multi Clouds for Security in Cloud Computing by using Secret Key Sharing. *Internatioonal Journal of Computers and Technology*, *10*(4), 1539–1545.

Mouwen, D. J., Capita, R., Alonso-Calleja, C., Prieto-Gomez, J., & Prieto, M. (2006). Artificial neural network based identification of Campylobacter species by Fourier transform infrared spectroscopy. *Journal of Microbiological Methods*, *67*(1), 131–140. doi:10.1016/j.mimet.2006.03.012 PMID:16632003

Muir, E. (2011). *Challenges of cloud computing in healthcare integration*. Retrieved from http://www.zdnet.com/news/challenges-of-cloud-computing-in-healthcare-integration/6266971

Murro, A. (2005). *Architecture and interface specifications*. Paper presented at Architecture Workshop. Brussels, Belgium.

Murty, R. N., Mainland, G., Rose, I., Chowdhury, A. R., Gosain, A., Bers, J., & Welsh, M. (2008). *Citysense: An urban-scale wireless sensor network and testbed*. Paper presented at the Technologies for Homeland Security. New York, NY.

Muth, T., Peters, J., Blackburn, J., Rapp, E., & Martens, L. (2013). ProteoCloud: A full-featured open source proteomics cloud computing pipeline. *Journal of Proteomics*, *88*, 104–108. doi:10.1016/j.jprot.2012.12.026 PMID:23305951

Nair, S. (2008). The Art of Database Monitoring. *Information Systems Control Journal*, (Ccm), 1–4.

Narayan, S., Gagné, M., & Safavi-Naini, R. (2010). Privacy preserving EHR system using attribute-based infrastructure. In *Proceedings of the 2010 ACM Workshop on Cloud Computing Security Workshop* (pp. 47-52). ACM.

NASSCOM. (2012). *Big Data: The Next Big Thing*. New Delhi, India: NASSCOM.

National Institute of Standards and Technology. (2010). Retrieved July 19, 2013 from http://healthcare.nist.gov/testing_infrastructure/

National Quality Forum. (2010). Retrieved July 19, 2013 from www.qualityforum.org/Projects/Measure_Harmonization.aspx

National Quality Forum. (2012). Retrieved July 17, 2013 from www.qualityforum.org/projects/care_coordination.aspx

Naylor, M. D., Brooten, D., Campbell, R., Jacobsen, B. S., Mezey, M. D., Pauly, M. V., & Schwartz, J. S. (1999). Comprehensive discharge planning and home follow-up of hospitalized elders: A randomized clinical trial. *Journal of the American Medical Association*, *281*(7), 613–620. doi:10.1001/jama.281.7.613 PMID:10029122

Nelson, M. R. (2010). The Cloud, the Crowd, and Public Policy. *Issues in Science and Technology*. Retrieved June 1, 2013, from http://www.issues.org/25.4/nelson.html

Ng, H. S., Sim, M. L., & Tan, C. M. (2006). Security issues of wireless sensor networks in healthcare applications. *BT Technology Journal*, *24*(2), 138–144. doi:10.1007/s10550-006-0051-8

Nguyen, T., Shi, W., & Ruden, D. (2011). CloudAligner: A fast and full-featured MapReduce based tool for sequence mapping. *BMC Research Notes*, *4*, 171. doi:10.1186/1756-0500-4-171 PMID:21645377

Niemenmaa, M., Kallio, A., Schumacher, A., Klemela, P., Korpelainen, E., & Heljanko, K. (2012). Hadoop-BAM: Directly manipulating next generation sequencing data in the cloud. *Bioinformatics (Oxford, England)*, *28*(6), 876–877. doi:10.1093/bioinformatics/bts054 PMID:22302568

NIKE+ FUELBAND. (n.d.). Retrieved from http://www.nike.com/

Nokia Energy Profiler Tool Home Page. (n.d.). Retrieved from http://www.forum.nokia.com/Library/Tools_and_downloads/Other/Nokia_Energy_Profiler/

Nygren, N. (2006). *Cooperative freight and fleet application*. Paper presented at CVIS W2 Open Workshop. Brussels, Belgium.

O'Malle, A. S., Grossman, J. M., Kemper, N. M., & Pham, K. H. (2010). Are Electronic Medical Records Helpful for Care Coordination? Experiences of Physician Practices. *Journal of General Internal Medicine*, *25*(3), 177–185. doi:10.1007/s11606-009-1195-2 PMID:20033621

O'Brien, M. J., Takahashi, M., Brugal, G., Christen, H., Gahm, T., & Goodell, R. M. ... Winkler, C. (1998). Digital imagery/telecytology. International Academy of Cytology Task Force summary: Diagnostic Cytology Towards the 21st Century: An International Expert Conference and Tutorial. *Acta Cytologica, 42*(1), 148-164.

O'Connor, B. D., Merriman, B., & Nelson, S. F. (2010). SeqWare Query Engine: storing and searching sequence data in the cloud. *BMC Bioinformatics*, *11*(Suppl 12), S2. doi:10.1186/1471-2105-11-S12-S2 PMID:21210981

Oemig, F., & Blobel, B. (2011). A formal analysis of HL7 version 2.x. *Studies in Health Technology and Informatics*, *169*, 704–708. PMID:21893838

Olhede, T., & Peterson, H. E. (2000). Archiving of care related information in XML-format. *Studies in Health Technology and Informatics*, *77*, 642–646. PMID:11187632

Olson, M. J. (2014). *Cloud computing services for seismic networks*. (Doctoral Dissertation). California Institute of Technology. Qmee. (2013). *Qmee infographic*. Retrieved August 13, 2013, from http://blog.qmee.com/qmee-online-in-60-seconds/

OSGi Alliance (OA). (2013). About the OSGi Alliance. *OSGi Alliance*. Retrieved October 23, 2013, from http://www.osgi.org/About/HomePage

OSGI. (2012). *OSGI Alliance*. Retrieved December 07, 2013, from http://www.osgi.org/Specifications/HomePage

Padhy, P. R., Patra, M. R., & Satapathy, S. C. (2012). Design and Implementation of a Cloud based Rural Healthcare Information System Model. *Universal Journal of Applied Computer Science & Technology, 2*(1), 149–157.

Palazzo, L., Sernani, P., Claudi, A., Dolcini, G., Biancucci, G., & Dragoni, A. F. (2013). *A Multi-Agent Architecture for Health Information Systems*. Retrieved from http://netmed2013.dii.univpm.it/sites/netmed2013.dii.univpm.it/files/papers/paper5.pdf

Paletta, M. (2012a). Self-Organizing Multi-Agent Systems by means of Scout Movement. *Recent Patents on Computer Science*, *5*(3), 197–210. doi:10.2174/2213275911205030197

Paletta, M. (2012b). MAS-based Agent Societies by Means of Scout Movement. *International Journal of Agent Technologies and Systems, 4*(3), 29–49. doi:10.4018/jats.2012070103

Paletta, M. (2012c). Intelligent Clouds – By means of using multi-agent systems environments. In L. Chao (Ed.), *Cloud Computing for Teaching and Learning: Strategies for Design and Implementation* (pp. 254–279). Hershey, PA: IGI Global. doi:10.4018/978-1-4666-0957-0.ch017

Paletta, M., & Herrero, M. P. (2010). *An awareness-based learning model to deal with service collaboration in cloud computing. Transactions on Computational Collective Intelligence I (LNCS)* (Vol. 6220, pp. 85–100). Berlin: Springer.

Pantazopoulos, D., Karakitsos, P., Iokim-Liossi, A., Pouliakis, A., Botsoli-Stergiou, E., & Dimopoulos, C. (1998). Back propagation neural network in the discrimination of benign from malignant lower urinary tract lesions. *The Journal of Urology*, *159*(5), 1619–1623. doi:10.1097/00005392-199805000-00057 PMID:9554366

Pantelopoulos, A., & Bourbakis, N. G. (2010). A survey on wearable sensor-based systems for health monitoring and prognosis. *IEEE Transactions on Systems, Man and Cybernetics. Part C, Applications and Reviews*, *40*(1), 1–12. doi:10.1109/TSMCC.2009.2032660

Papadias, D., Zhang, J., Mamoulis, N., & Tao, Y. (2003). *Query processing in spatial network databases*. Paper presented at the 29th VLDB Conference. Berlin, Germany.

Papakonstantinou, D., Poulymenopoulou, M., Malamateniou, F., & Vassilacopoulos, G. (2011). A cloud-based semantic wiki for user training in healthcare process management. In *Proceedings of the XXIII Conference of the European Federation for Medical Informatics* (MIE 2011) (vol. 169, pp. 93-97). Oslo, Norway: MIE.

Papazoglou, M. P., & Van den Heuvel, W. J. (2007). Service oriented architectures: Approaches, technologies and research issues. *The VLDB Journal*, *16*(3), 389–415. doi:10.1007/s00778-007-0044-3

Paquette, S., Jaeger, P. T., & Wilson, S. C. (2010). Identifying the security risks associated with governmental use of cloud computing. *Government Information Quarterly*, 27(3), 245–253. doi:10.1016/j.giq.2010.01.002

Pardamean, B., & Rumanda, R. R. (2011). Integrated Model of Cloud-Based E-Medical Record for Health Care Organizations. In *Proceedings of the 10th WSEAS International Conference on E-Activities* (pp. 157-162). WSEAS.

Partala, J., Keränen, N., Särestöniemi, M., Hämäläinen, M., Iinatti, J., Jämsä, T., et al. (2013). Security threats against the transmission chain of a medical health monitoring system. In *Proceedings of the 2013 IEEE 15th International Conference on e-Health Networking, Applications and Services* (pp. 218-223). IEEE.

Patel, R. P. (2012). Cloud computing and virtualization technology in radiology. *Clinical Radiology*, 67(11), 1095–1100. doi:10.1016/j.crad.2012.03.010 PMID:22607956

Pearson, S., & Charlesworth, A. (2009). Accountability as a Way Forward for Privacy Protection in the Cloud. In M. G. Jaatun, G. Zhao, & C. Rong (Eds.), *Cloud Computing* (pp. 131–144). Berlin: Springer-Verlag. doi:10.1007/978-3-642-10665-1_12

Peikes, D., Chen, A., Schore, J., & Brown, R. (2009). Effects of Care Coordination on hospitalization, quality of care, and health care expenditures among Medicare beneficiaries15 randomized trials. *Journal of the American Medical Association*, 301(6), 603–618. doi:10.1001/jama.2009.126 PMID:19211468

Peixoto, H., Santos, M., Abelha, A., & Machado, J. (2012). Intelligence in Interoperability with AIDA. In *Proceedings of 20th International Symposium on Methodologies for Intelligent Systems* (LNCS), (Vol. 7661). Berlin: Springer.

Pereira, R., Duarte, J., Salazar, M., Santos, M., Abelha, A., & Machado, J. (2012). Usability of an Electronic Health Record. *IEEM, 5*.

Pereira, R., Salazar, M., Abelha, A., & Machado, J. (2013). SWOT Analysis of a Portuguese Electronic Health Record. In Collaborative, Trusted and Privacy-Aware e/m-Services (Vol. 399, pp. 169–177). Springer.

Perera, I. (2009). Implementing Healthcare Information in Rural Communities in Sri Lanka: A Novel Approach with Mobile Communication. *Journal of Health Informatics in Developing Countries*, 3(2). PMID:21822397

Perez, R., Sailer, R., & van Doorn, L. (2006). vTPM: Virtualizing the trusted platform module. In *Proceedings of the 15th Conference on USENIX Security Symposium* (pp. 305-320). USENIX.

Peter, M., & Tim, G. (2009). *The NIST definition of Cloud Computing* (Version 15). Information Technology Laboratory. Retrieved August 20, 2013, from http://www.hexistor.com/blog/bid/36511/The-NIST-Definition-of-Cloud-Computing

Peterson, Z. N., Gondree, M., & Beverly, R. (2011). A position paper on data sovereignty: The importance of geolocating data in the cloud. In *Proceedings of the 8th USENIX confErence on Networked Systems Design and Implementation*. USENIX.

Pieters, W., & Cleeff, A. (2009). The precautionary principle in a world of digital dependencies. *IEEE Computer*, 42(6), 50–56. doi:10.1109/MC.2009.203

Pireddu, L., Leo, S., & Zanetti, G. (2011). SEAL: A distributed short read mapping and duplicate removal tool. *Bioinformatics (Oxford, England)*, 27(15), 2159–2160. doi:10.1093/bioinformatics/btr325 PMID:21697132

Poese, I., Uhlig, S., Kaafar, M. A., Donnet, B., & Gueye, B. (2011). IP geolocation databases: Unreliable? *ACM SIGCOMM Computer Communication Review*, 41(2), 53–56. doi:10.1145/1971162.1971171

Porres, J. M. (1974a). Quality control in microbiology: Utilization of reference laboratory data. *American Journal of Clinical Pathology*, 62(3), 407–411. PMID:4415417

Porres, J. M. (1974b). Quality control in microbiology: The need for standards. *American Journal of Clinical Pathology*, 62(3), 412–419. PMID:4472270

Pouliakis, A., & Karakitsos, P. (2011). *Concepts of software design for population based cervical cencer screening*. Paper presented at the 36th European Congress of Cytology. Istanbul, Turkey.

Pouliakis, A., Iliopoulou, D., & Karakitsou, E. (2012). Design and Implementation Issues of an Information System Supporting Cervical Cancer Screening Programs. *Journal of Applied Medical Sciences, 1*(1), 61–91.

Pouliakis, A., Margari, C., Margari, N., Chrelias, C., Zygouris, D., & Meristoudis, C. et al. (2013). Using classification and regression trees, liquid-based cytology and nuclear morphometry for the discrimination of endometrial lesions. *Diagnostic Cytopathology*. http://dx.doi.org/10.1002/dc.23077 doi:10.1002/dc.23077 PMID:24273089

Prud'Hommeaux, E., & Seaborne, A. (2008). SPARQL query language for RDF. *W3C Recommendation, 15*.

QT Software Homepage. (n.d.). Retrieved from http://qt.digia.com/

R Project. (n.d.). Retrieved from http://www.r-project.org/

Rabi, P. P., Manas, R. P., & Suresh, C. S. (2012). Design and Implementation of a Cloud based Rural Healthcare Information System Model. *Universal Journal of Applied computer Science and Technology, 2*(1), 149-157.

Radwan, A. S., Abdel-Hamid, A. A., & Hanafy, Y. (2012). Cloud-based service for secure electronic medical record exchange. In *Proceedings of the 22nd International Conference on Computer Theory and Applications* (ICCTA) (pp. 94-103). Alexandria, Egypt: ICCTA.

Ramos, L. (2007). *Performance Analysis of a Database Caching System In a Grid Environment*. FEUP.

Rao, G. S. V. R. K., Sundararaman, K., & Parthasarathi, J. (2010). Dhatri - A Pervasive Cloud initiative for primary healthcare services. In *Proceedings of the 14th International Conference on Intelligence in Next Generation Networks* (ICIN) (pp. 1-6). Berlin, Germany: ICIN.

Reese, G. (2009). *Cloud Application Architectures: Building Applications and Infrastructure in the Cloud*. Sebastopol, CA: O'Reilly Media.

Ren, J., Xie, L., Li, W. W., & Bourne, P. E. (2010). SMAP-WS: A parallel Web service for structural proteome-wide ligand-binding site comparison. *Nucleic Acids Research, 38*, W441-444. doi:10.1093/nar/gkq400 PMID:20484373

Renshaw, A. A. (2011). Quality improvement in cytology: Where do we go from here? *Archives of Pathology & Laboratory Medicine, 135*(11), 1387–1390. doi:10.5858/arpa.2010-0606-RA PMID:22032562

Richardson, H., Wood, D., Whitby, J., Lannigan, R., & Fleming, C. (1996). Quality improvement of diagnostic microbiology through a peer-group proficiency assessment program: A 20-year experience in Ontario: The Microbiology Committee. *Archives of Pathology & Laboratory Medicine, 120*(5), 445–455. PMID:8639047

Rich, B. (2013). *Oracle Database Reference, 11g Release 2 (11.2)*. Oracle.

Rich, M. W., Beckman, V., Wittenberg, C., Leven, C. L., Freedland, K. E., & Carney, R. M. A. (1995). Multidisciplinary intervention to prevent the readmissions of elderly patients with congestive heart failure. *The New England Journal of Medicine, 333*(18), 1190–1195. doi:10.1056/NEJM199511023331806 PMID:7565975

Ripley, B. D. (2001). The R project in statistical computing. *MSOR Connections, 1*(1), 23–25. doi:10.11120/msor.2001.01010023

Riquelme, E., Lorente, S., & Crespo, M. D. (2011). Implementing a quality management system according to iso model in a Microbiology laboratory. *Enfermedades Infecciosas y Microbiologia Clinica, 29*(1), 72–73. doi:10.1016/j.eimc.2010.04.018 PMID:21193248

Robinson, I., Webber, J., & Eifrem, E. (2013). *Graph Databases*. Sebastopol, CA: O'Reilly.

Rochwerger, B., Vazquez, C., Breitgand, D., Hadas, D., Villari, M., Massonet, P., & Galán, F. (2011). An Architecture for Federated Cloud Computing. In R. Buyya, J. Nroberg, & A. Goscinski (Eds.), *Cloud Computing: Principles and Paradigms* (pp. 391–411). Wiley. doi:10.1002/9780470940105.ch15

Rodrigues, R., Gonçalves, P., Miranda, M., Portela, F., Santos, M., & Neves, J. … Machado, J. (2012). Monitoring Intelligent System for the Intensive Care Unit using RFID and Multi-Agent Systems. In *Proceedings of IEEE International Conference on Industrial Engineering and Engineering Management (IEEM2012)*. IEEE.

Rodrigues, A. (2005). *Oracle 10g e 9i: Fundamentos Para Profissionais*. Lisboa: FCA.

Rodriguez-Martinez, M., Valdivia, H., Rivera, J., Seguel, J., & Greer, M. (2012). MedBook: A Cloud-Based Healthcare Billing and Record Management System. In *Proceedings of the 5th International Conference on Cloud Computing (CLOUD)* (pp.899-905). Honolulu, HI: IEEE Computer Society.

Rogers, R., Peres, Y., & Müller, W. (2010). Living longer independently - A healthcare interoperability perspective. *E&I Elektrotechnik und Informationstechnik, 127*(7-8), 206–211. doi:10.1007/s00502-010-0748-8

Rorive, S. N. D. H., Fossion, C., Delpierre, I., Arbaguia, N., Avni, F., Decaestecker, C., & Salmon, I. (2010). Ultrasound-guided fine-needle aspiration of thyroid nodules: Stratification of malignancy risk using follicular proliferation grading, clinical and ultrasonographic features. *European Journal of Endocrinology*. doi:10.1530/EJE-09-1103 PMID:20219856

Rosenthal, A., Mork, P., Li, M. H., Stanford, J., Koester, D., & Reynolds, P. (2010). Cloud computing: A new business paradigm for biomedical information sharing. *Journal of Biomedical Informatics, 43*(2), 342–353. doi:10.1016/j.jbi.2009.08.014 PMID:19715773

Rost, B., Yachdav, G., & Liu, J. (2004). The Predict-Protein server. *Nucleic Acids Research, 32*, W321-326. doi:10.1093/nar/gkh377

Rostrom, T., & Teng, C. C. (2011). Secure communications for PACS in a cloud environment. In *Proceedings of Engineering in Medicine and Biology Society* (pp. 8219–8222). IEEE. doi:10.1109/IEMBS.2011.6092027

Rozsnyai, S., Vecera, R., Schiefer, J., & Schatten, A. (2007). Event cloud-searching for correlated business events. In *Proceedings of E-Commerce Technology and the 4th IEEE International Conference on Enterprise Computing, E-Commerce, and E-Services,* (pp. 409-420). IEEE.

Rudnisky, C. J., Tennant, M. T., Weis, E., Ting, A., Hinz, B. J., & Greve, M. D. (2007). Web-based grading of compressed stereoscopic digital photography versus standard slide film photography for the diagnosis of diabetic retinopathy. *Ophthalmology, 114*(9), 1748–1754. doi:10.1016/j.ophtha.2006.12.010 PMID:17368543

Sackett, D., Rosenberg, W., Gray, J., Haynes, R., & Richardson, W. (1996). Evidence based medicine: What it is and what it isn't. *BMJ (Clinical Research Ed.), 312*(7023), 71–72. doi:10.1136/bmj.312.7023.71 PMID:8555924

Sadeghi, A. R., Stüble, C., & Winandy, M. (2008). Property-based TPM virtualization. In *Information Security* (pp. 1-16). Springer. Bowers, K. D., Juels, A., & Oprea, A. (2009). HAIL: A high-availability and integrity layer for cloud storage. In *Proceedings of the 16th ACM Conference on Computer and Communications Security* (pp. 187-198). ACM.

Sani, A. A., Polack, F., & Paige, R. (2010). Generating Formal Model Transformation Specification Using a Template-based Approach. In *Proceedings of the 3rd York Doctoral Symposium on Computing* (pp. 11-18). York, UK: University of York.

Santos, M. F., Portela, F., & Vilas-Boas, M. (2011). *INTCARE: Multi-agent approach for real-time intelligent decision support in intensive medicine*. Academic Press.

Saranummi, N. (2008). In the spotlight: Health information systems. *IEEE Reviews in Biomedical Engineering, 1*, 15–17. doi:10.1109/RBME.2008.2008217 PMID:22274895

Saranummi, N. (2009). In the spotlight: Health information systems—PHR and value based healthcare. *IEEE Reviews in Biomedical Engineering, 2*, 15–17. doi:10.1109/RBME.2009.2034699 PMID:22275039

Saranummi, N. (2011). In the spotlight: Health information systems - Mainstreaming mHealth. *IEEE Reviews in Biomedical Engineering, 4*, 17–19. doi:10.1109/RBME.2011.2176998 PMID:22273787

Sarna, D. E. Y. (2011). *Implementing and Developing Cloud Computing Applications*. Boca Raton, FL: CRC Press.

Schadt, E. E., Linderman, M. D., Sorenson, J., Lee, L., & Nolan, G. P. (2010). Computational solutions to large-scale data management and analysis. *Nature Reviews. Genetics, 11*(9), 647–657. doi:10.1038/nrg2857 PMID:20717155

Schaefer, G., Huguet, J., Zhu, S. Y., Plassmann, P., & Ring, F. (2006). Adopting the DICOM standard for medical infrared images. In *Proceedings of Engineering in Medicine and Biology Society* (pp. 236–239). IEEE. doi:10.1109/IEMBS.2006.259523

Schaffer, A. A., Simon, R., Desper, R., Richter, J., & Sauter, G. (2001). Tree models for dependent copy number changes in bladder cancer. *International Journal of Oncology*, *18*(2), 349–354. PMID:11172603

Schatz, M. C. (2009). CloudBurst: Highly sensitive read mapping with MapReduce. *Bioinformatics (Oxford, England)*, *25*(11), 1363–1369. doi:10.1093/bioinformatics/btp236 PMID:19357099

Schatz, M. C., Delcher, A. L., & Salzberg, S. L. (2010). Assembly of large genomes using second-generation sequencing. *Genome Research*, *20*(9), 1165–1173. doi:10.1101/gr.101360.109 PMID:20508146

Schatz, M. C., Langmead, B., & Salzberg, S. L. (2010). Cloud computing and the DNA data race. *Nature Biotechnology*, *28*(7), 691–693. doi:10.1038/nbt0710-691 PMID:20622843

Schmuck, F. B., & Haskin, R. L. (2002). *GPFS: A Shared-Disk File System for Large Computing Clusters*. Paper presented at the FAST. New York, NY.

Schumacher, R. (2003). *Oracle Performance Troubleshooting With Dictionary Internals SQL & Tuning Scripts*. Kittrell: Rampant TechPress.

Seti. (2013). *Seti@home official website*. Retrieved August 13, 2013, from http://setiathome.berkeley.edu/

Shallahamer, C. (2007). *Forecasting Oracle Performance*. Berkeley, CA: Apress.

Shannon, P., Markiel, A., Ozier, O., Baliga, N. S., Wang, J. T., & Ramage, D. et al. (2003). Cytoscape: A software environment for integrated models of biomolecular interaction networks. *Genome Research*, *13*(11), 2498–2504. doi:10.1101/gr.1239303 PMID:14597658

Sharma, G. (2012). Performance analysis of database on different Cloud computing environments. *International Journal of Advanced Computer Science and Information Technology*, *2*(2), 5.

Sherman, M. E., Dasgupta, A., Schiffman, M., Nayar, R., & Solomon, D. (2007). The Bethesda Interobserver Reproducibility Study (BIRST), a Web-based assessment of the Bethesda 2001 System for classifying cervical cytology. *Cancer*, *111*(1), 15–25. doi:10.1002/cncr.22423 PMID:17186503

Silva, P., Quintas, C., Duarte, J., Santos, M., Neves, J., Abelha, A., & Machado, J. (2012). Hospital database workload and fault forecasting. In *Step Towards Fault Forecasting in Hospital Information Systems*. Academic Press.

Simoncini, L. (2009). Resilient computing: An engineering discipline. In Proceedings of Parallel & Distributed Processing, (pp. 1-1). IEEE.

Singh, H., Naik, A. D., Rao, R., & Petersen, L. A. (2008). Reducing diagnostic errors through effective communication: Harnessing the power of information technology. *Journal of General Internal Medicine*, *23*, 489–494. doi:10.1007/s11606-007-0393-z PMID:18373151

Siwpersad, S. S., Gueye, B., & Uhlig, S. (2008). Assessing the geographic resolution of exhaustive tabulation for geolocating Internet hosts. In *Proceedings of Passive and Active Network Measurement* (pp. 11–20). Springer. doi:10.1007/978-3-540-79232-1_2

Sniderman, A. D., LaChapelle, K. J., Rachon, N. A., & Furberg, C. D. (2013). The Nessecity for Clinical Reasoning in the Era of Evidence-Based Medicine. *Mayo Clinic Proceedings*, *88*(10), 1108–1114. doi:10.1016/j.mayocp.2013.07.012 PMID:24079680

Sobhy, D., El-Sonbaty, Y., & Abou Elnasr, M. (2012). MedCloud: Healthcare cloud computing system. In *Proceedings of the 7th International Conference for Internet Technology and Secured Transactions* (ICITST) (pp. 161-166). London: ICITST.

Sohn, J., Do, K. A., Liu, S., Chen, H., Mills, G. B., & Hortobagyi, G. N. et al. (2013). Functional proteomics characterization of residual triple-negative breast cancer after standard neoadjuvant chemotherapy. *Annals of Oncology*. doi:10.1093/annonc/mdt248 PMID:23925999

Solomon, D., Davey, D., Kurman, R., Moriarty, A., O'Connor, D., & Prey, M. et al. (2002). The 2001 Bethesda System: Terminology for reporting results of cervical cytology. *Journal of the American Medical Association*, *287*(16), 2114–2119. doi:10.1001/jama.287.16.2114 PMID:11966386

Soman, A. K. (2011). *Cloud-based Solutions for Healthcare IT*. Science Publishers. doi:10.1201/b10737

Song, Z., & Roussopoulos, N. (2001). K-Nearest neighbor search for moving query point. In *Proceedings of ACM SIGMOD*. Santa Barbara, CA: ACM.

Starr, P. (1982). *The social transformation of American medicine*. New York, NY: Basic Books.

Stein, L. D. (2010). The case for cloud computing in genome informatics. *Genome Biology*, *11*(5), 207. doi:10.1186/gb-2010-11-5-207 PMID:20441614

Stergiou, N., Georgoulakis, G., Margari, N., Aninos, D., Stamataki, M., & Stergiou, E. et al. (2009). Using a web-based system for the continuous distance education in cytopathology. *International Journal of Medical Informatics*, *78*(12), 827–838. doi:10.1016/j.ijmedinf.2009.08.007 PMID:19775933

Stewart, J. A., Day, M., Print, C., & Favato, G. (2009). Compliance in the supply chain: implications of Sarbanes-Oxley for UK businesses. *ICFAI Journal of Supply Chain Management*, *6*(1), 8–19.

Stewart, J. III, Miyazaki, K., Bevans-Wilkins, K., Ye, C., Kurtycz, D. F., & Selvaggi, S. M. (2007). Virtual microscopy for cytology proficiency testing: Are we there yet? *Cancer*, *111*(4), 203–209. doi:10.1002/cncr.22766 PMID:17580360

Stonebraker, M. (2010). SQL databases v. NoSQL databases. *Communications of the ACM*, *53*(4), 10–11. doi:10.1145/1721654.1721659

Strohm, R. (2012). *Oracle Real Application Clusters Administration and Deployment Guide, 11g Release 2 (11.2)*. Oracle.

Subbe, C. P., Kruger, M., Rutherford, P., & Gemmel, L. (2001). Validation of a Modified Early Warning Score in medical admissions. *QJM*, *94*(10), 521–526. doi:10.1093/qjmed/94.10.521 PMID:11588210

Szalay, A., Bunn, A., Gray, J., Foster, I., & Raicu, I. (2006). *The importance of data locality in distributed computing applications*. Paper presented at the NSF Workflow Workshop. New York, NY.

Tao, Y., & Papadias, D. (2003). Time-parameterized queries in spatio-temporal databases. In *Proceedings of ACM SIGMOD*. San Diego, CA: ACM.

Taylor, C. R. (2011). From microscopy to whole slide digital images: A century and a half of image analysis. *Applied Immunohistochemistry & Molecular Morphology*, *19*(6), 491–493. doi:10.1097/PAI.0b013e318229ffd6 PMID:22089486

TClouds. (2011). *Trustworthy Clouds*. Retrieved December 07, 2013, from http://www.tclouds-project.eu/

Terry, K. (2013). *Health IT Startups Make VCs Swoon*. Retrieved December 2, 2013, from http://www.informationweek.com/healthcare/leadership/health-it-startups-make-vcs-swoon/240147655

Theodoridis, S., & Koutroumbas, K. (2009). *Pattern recognition* (4th ed.). London: Academic Press.

Thrall, M., Pantanowitz, L., & Khalbuss, W. (2011). Telecytology: Clinical applications, current challenges, and future benefits. *Journal of Pathology Informatics*, *2*, 51. doi:10.4103/2153-3539.91129 PMID:22276242

Timmermans, J., Ikonen, V., Stahl, B. C., & Bozdag, E. (2010). The ethics of cloud computing: A conceptual review. In Proceedings of Cloud Computing Technology and Science (CloudCom), (pp. 614-620). IEEE Press.

Timmermans, S., & Mauck, A. (2005). The promises and pitfalls of evidence-based medicine. *Health Affairs*, *24*(1), 18–28. doi:10.1377/hlthaff.24.1.18 PMID:15647212

Toouli, G., Georgiou, A., & Westbrook, J. (2012). Changes, disruption and innovation: An investigation of the introduction of new health information technology in a microbiology laboratory. *Journal of Pathology Informatics*, *3*, 16. doi:10.4103/2153-3539.95128 PMID:22616028

Torres-Cabala, C., Bibbo, M., Panizo-Santos, A., Barazi, H., Krutzsch, H., Roberts, D. D., & Merino, M. J. (2006). Proteomic identification of new biomarkers and application in thyroid cytology. *Acta Cytologica*, *50*(5), 518–528. doi:10.1159/000326006 PMID:17017437

Tsilalis, T., Archondakis, S., Meristoudis, C., Margari, N., Pouliakis, A., & Skagias, L. et al. (2012). Assessment of static telecytological diagnoses' reproducibility in cervical smears prepared by means of liquid-based cytology. *Telemedicine Journal and e-Health*, *18*(7), 516–520. doi:10.1089/tmj.2011.0167 PMID:22856666

Twitter. (n.d.). Retrieved from https://twitter.com

Tygar, J. D., & Yee, B. S. (1991). *Dyad: A system for using physically secure coprocessors*. Academic Press.

Underwood, A., & Green, J. (2011). Call for a quality standard for sequence-based assays in clinical microbiology: Necessity for quality assessment of sequences used in microbial identification and typing. *Journal of Clinical Microbiology*, 49(1), 23–26. doi:10.1128/JCM.01918-10 PMID:21068275

UPMC'S 'Big Data' Technology Shows Promise in Breast Cancer Research. (2013, June 19). Retrieved November 22, 2013, from http://www.upmc.com/media/newsreleases/2013/pages/upmc-big-data-tech-breast-cancer-research.aspx

Uppal, D. S., & Powell, S. M. (2013). Genetics/genomics/proteomics of gastric adenocarcinoma. *Gastroenterology Clinics of North America*, 42(2), 241–260. doi:10.1016/j.gtc.2013.01.005 PMID:23639639

Valarmathi, J., Lakshmi, K., Menaga, R. S., Abirami, K. V., & Uthariaraj, V. R. (2012). SLA for a Pervasive Healthcare Environment. In *Advances in Computing and Information Technology* (pp. 141–149). Springer. doi:10.1007/978-3-642-31513-8_15

van Leeuwen, W., & van Belkum, A. (2013). The European Journal of Clinical Microbiology and Infectious Diseases: Quality and quantity in 2013. *European Journal of Clinical Microbiology & Infectious Diseases*, 32(1), 1–2. doi:10.1007/s10096-012-1804-6 PMID:23263838

Vaquero, L. M., Rodero-Merino, L., Caceres, J., & Lindner, M. (2008). A break in the clouds: Towards a cloud definition. *ACM SIGCOMM Computer Communications Review*, 39(1), 50–55. doi:10.1145/1496091.1496100

Varlatzidou, A., Pouliakis, A., Stamataki, M., Meristoudis, C., Margari, N., & Peros, G. et al. (2011). Cascaded learning vector quantizer neural networks for the discrimination of thyroid lesions. *Analytical and Quantitative Cytology and Histology*, 33(6), 323–334. PMID:22590810

Varley, I. T., Aziz, A., Aziz, C.-S. A., & Miranker, D. (2009). *No relation: The mixed blessings of non-relational databases*. Academic Press.

Varshney, U. (2007). Pervasive healthcare and wireless health monitoring. *Mobile Networks and Applications*, 12(2-3), 113–127. doi:10.1007/s11036-007-0017-1

Vasilakos, A. V., & Lisetti, C. (2010). Special section on affective and pervasive computing for healthcare. *IEEE Transactions on Information Technology in Biomedicine*, 14, 183–185. doi:10.1109/TITB.2010.2043299 PMID:20684047

Vicentino, W., Rodriguez, G., Saldias, M., & Alvarez, I. (2009). Guidelines to implement quality management systems in microbiology laboratories for tissue banking. *Transplantation Proceedings*, 41(8), 3481–3484. doi:10.1016/j.transproceed.2009.09.012 PMID:19857776

Vieira, M. A. M., Viera, L. F. M., Ruiz, L. B., Loureiro, A. A. F., Fernandes, A. O., & Nogueira, J. M. S. (2003). Scheduling nodes in wireless sensor networks: A Voronoi approach. In *Proceedings of Local Computer Networks* (pp. 423–429). IEEE. doi:10.1109/LCN.2003.1243168

Virtuoso. (n.d.). Retrieved from http://virtuoso.open-linksw.com

Vista Monograph. (2008, July 1). *Department of Veterans Administration*. Retrieved September 11, 2013, from http://www.va.gov/VISTA_MONOGRAPH

VMware Workstation Homepage. (n.d.). Retrieved from http://www.vmware.com/workstation

Vogels, W. (2008). A head in the clouds the power of infrastructure as a service. In *Proceedings of the 1st Workshop on Cloud Computing and Applications*.

Volkamer, A., Kuhn, D., Grombacher, T., Rippmann, F., & Rarey, M. (2012). Combining global and local measures for structure-based druggability predictions. *Journal of Chemical Information and Modeling*, 52(2), 360–372. doi:10.1021/ci200454v PMID:22148551

Vooijs, G. P., Davey, D. D., Somrak, T. M., Goodell, R. M., Grohs, D. H., & Knesel, E. A., Jr. … Wilbur, D. C. (1998). Computerized training and proficiency testing. International Academy of Cytology Task Force summary: Diagnostic Cytology Towards the 21st Century: An International Expert Conference and Tutorial. *Acta Cytologica, 42*(1), 141-147.

Voorsluys, W., Broberg, J., & Buyya, R. (2011). Introduction to Cloud Computing. In R. Buyya, J. Nroberg, & A. Goscinski (Eds.), *Cloud Computing: Principles and Paradigms* (pp. 1–41). Wiley. doi:10.1002/9780470940105.ch1

Vriesema, J. L., van der Poel, H. G., Debruyne, F. M., Schalken, J. A., Kok, L. P., & Boon, M. E. (2000). Neural network-based digitized cell image diagnosis of bladder wash cytology. *Diagnostic Cytopathology, 23*(3), 171–179. doi:10.1002/1097-0339(200009)23:3<171::AID-DC6>3.0.CO;2-F PMID:10945904

W3C. (2012). OWL 2 Web Ontology Language Document Overview (2nd Ed.). *W3C Recommendation.* Retrieved October 24, 2013, from http://www.w3.org/TR/owl2-overview/

Walker, K., Neuburger, J., Groene, O., Cromwell, D. A., & Vand der Mulen, J. (2013). Public Reporting of Surgeon outcomes: Low Numbers of Procedures Lead to False Complacency. *The Lancet.* http://dx.doi.org.10.1016/S0140-6736(13)61491-9

Wallace, P. S., & MacKay, W. G. (2013). Quality in the molecular microbiology laboratory. *Methods in Molecular Biology (Clifton, N.J.), 943,* 49–79. doi:10.1007/978-1-60327-353-4_3 PMID:23104281

Wall, D. P., Kudtarkar, P., Fusaro, V. A., Pivovarov, R., Patil, P., & Tonellato, P. J. (2010). Cloud computing for comparative genomics. *BMC Bioinformatics, 11,* 259. doi:10.1186/1471-2105-11-259 PMID:20482786

Wang, Q., Wang, C., Li, J., Ren, K., & Lou, W. (2009). Enabling public verifiability and data dynamics for storage security in cloud computing. In Proceedings of Computer Security–ESORICS 2009 (pp. 355-370). Springer. Li, C., Raghunathan, A., & Jha, N. K. (2010). Secure virtual machine execution under an untrusted management OS. In Proceedings of Cloud Computing (CLOUD), (pp. 172-179). IEEE.

Wang, S., Brown, K., Capretz, M. A., Hines, P., & Boyd, J. (2009). A process oriented semantic healthcare service composition. In Proceedings of Science and Technology for Humanity (TIC-STH), (pp. 479-484). IEEE.

Wang, X., & Tan, Y. (2010). Application of cloud computing in the health information system. In *Proceedings of International Conference on Computer Application and System Modeling* (ICCASM) (vol. 1, pp. 179-182). Shanxi, China: ICCASM.

Warnes, G. R., Bolker, B., Bonebakker, L., Gentleman, R., Huber, W., Liaw, A.,... Moeller, S. (2009). Gplots: Various R programming tools for plotting data. *R Package Version, 2*(4).

Waxer, N., Ninan, D., Ma, A., & Dominguez, N. (2013). How cloud computing and social media are changing the face of health care. *The Physician Executive Journal, 39*(2), 58-60, 62.

Webb, G. (2012). Making the cloud work for healthcare: Cloud computing offers incredible opportunities to improve healthcare, reduce costs and accelerate ability to adopt new IT services. *Health Management Technology, 33*(2), 8–9. PMID:22397112

Weber-Jahnke, J., Peyton, L., & Topaloglou, T. (2012). eHealth system interoperability. *Information Systems Frontiers, 14*(1), 1–3. doi:10.1007/s10796-011-9319-8

Weerawarana, S., Curbera, F., Leymann, F., Storey, T., & Ferguson, D. (2005). *Web Services Platform Architecture.* Upper Saddle River, NJ: Prentice Hall.

Weicher, M., Chu, W., Lin, W. C., Le, V., & Yu, D. (1995). *Business Process Reengineering Analysis and Recommendations.* Baruch College. Retrieved from http://www.netlib.com/bpr1.htm

Weiss, A. (2007). Computing in the Clouds. *Networker, 11*(4), 16–25. doi:10.1145/1327512.1327513

Wetterstrand, K. (2013). *DNA Sequencing Costs.* National Human Genome Reserach Institute. Retrieved December 1, 2013, from: http://www.genome.gov/sequencingcosts/

Whitby, J. L., Black, W. A., Richardson, H., & Wood, D. E. (1982). System for laboratory proficiency testing in bacteriology: organisation and impact on microbiology laboratories in health care facilities funded by the Ontario Government. *Journal of Clinical Pathology, 35*(1), 94–100. doi:10.1136/jcp.35.1.94 PMID:7061723

Widya, I., van Beijnum, B. J., & Salden, A. (2006). QoC-based Optimization of End-to-End M-Health Data Delivery Services. In *Proceedings of Quality of Service* (pp. 252–260). IEEE. doi:10.1109/IWQOS.2006.250476

Wikipedia. (2010). Retrieved July 13, 2013 from http://hbr.org/2010/12/column-good-decisions-bad-outcomes/ar/1

Wikipedia. (2011). Retrieved July 22, 2013 from http://en.wikipedia.org/wiki/Diagnosis-related_group

Wikipedia. (2013a). Retrieved July 17, 2013 from http://en.wikipedia.org/wiki/Edwin_Hubble

Wikipedia. (2013b). Retrieved November 29, 2013 from http://en.wikipedia.org/wiki/Copernican_heliocentrism

Williamson, J. W. (1971). Evaluating quality of patient care: A strategy relating outcome and process assessment. *Journal of the American Medical Association*, *218*(4), 564–569. doi:10.1001/jama.1971.03190170042009 PMID:5171005

Williamson, J. W. (1978). *Assessing and Improving Outcomes in Health Care: The Theory and Practice of Health Accounting*. Cambridge, MA: Ballinger.

Wilson, D. (2012). *How to Improve Helthcare with Cloud Computing*. Hitachi Data Systems. Retrieved from http://docs.media.bitpipe.com/io_10x/io_108673/item_650544/cloud%20computing%20wp.pdf

Wilson, M. E., Faur, Y. C., Schaefler, S., Weitzman, I., Weisburd, M. H., & Schaeffer, M. (1977). Proficiency testing in clinical microbiology: The New York City program. *The Mount Sinai Journal of Medicine, New York*, *44*(1), 142–163. PMID:300463

Withings. (n.d.). Retrieved from www.withings.com

Wolberg, W. H., Tanner, M. A., Loh, W. Y., & Vanichsetakul, N. (1987). Statistical approach to fine needle aspiration diagnosis of breast masses. *Acta Cytologica*, *31*(6), 737–741. PMID:3425134

Wootton, R. (2001). Telemedicine and developing countries & successful implementation will require. *Journal of Telemedicine and Telecare*, *7*(1), 1–6. doi:10.1258/1357633011936589 PMID:11576471

World Health Organisation. (2005). *58th World Health Assembly Report*. WHO Tech Report.

Wright, A. M., Smith, D., Dhurandhar, B., Fairley, T., Scheiber-Pacht, M., & Chakraborty, S. et al. (2013). Digital slide imaging in cervicovaginal cytology: A pilot study. *Archives of Pathology & Laboratory Medicine*, *137*(5), 618–624. doi:10.5858/arpa.2012-0430-OA PMID:22970841

Wright, D. D., & Kane, R. L. (1982). Predicting the outcome of primary care. *Medical Care*, *20*(2), 180–187. doi:10.1097/00005650-198202000-00005 PMID:7078280

Wu, C. S., & Khoury, I. (2012). E-Healthcare Web Service Broker Infrastructure in Cloud Environment. In Proceedings of Services (SERVICES), (pp. 317-322). IEEE.

Wu, R., Ahn, G. J., & Hu, H. (2012). Towards HIPAA-compliant healthcare systems. In *Proceedings of the 2nd ACM SIGHIT International Health Informatics Symposium* (pp. 593-602). ACM.

Wu, R., Ahn, G. J., Hu, H., & Singhal, M. (2010). Information flow control in cloud computing. In *Proceedings of 6th International Conference on Collaborative Computing: Networking, Applications and Worksharing* (CollaborateCom) (pp. 1-7). IEEE.

Xively. (n.d.). Retrieved from https://xively.com/

Yamamura, Y., Nakajima, T., Ohta, K., Nashimoto, A., Arai, K., & Hiratsuka, M. et al. (2002). Determining prognostic factors for gastric cancer using the regression tree method. *Gastric Cancer*, *5*(4), 201–207. doi:10.1007/s101200200035 PMID:12491077

Yao, J., & Warren, S. (2005). Applying the ISO/IEEE 11073 standards to wearable home health monitoring systems. *Journal of Clinical Monitoring and Computing*, *19*(6), 427–436. doi:10.1007/s10877-005-2033-7 PMID:16437294

Yao, Y., & Gehrke, J. (2002). The cougar approach to in-network query processing in sensor networks. *SIGMOD Record*, *31*(3), 9–18. doi:10.1145/601858.601861

Yim, E. K., & Park, J. S. (2006). Role of proteomics in translational research in cervical cancer. *Expert Review of Proteomics, 3*(1), 21–36. doi:10.1586/14789450.3.1.21 PMID:16445348

Yu, W. D., Joshi, B., & Chandola, P. (2011). A service modeling approach to service requirements in SOA and cloud computing — Using a u-Healthcare system case. In *Proceedings of 13th IEEE International Conference on e-Health Networking Applications and Services* (Healthcom) (pp. 233 - 236). IEEE Xplore.

Yuksel, M., & Dogac, A. (2011). Interoperability of medical device information and the clinical applications: An HL7 RMIM based on the ISO/IEEE 11073 DIM. *IEEE Transactions on Information Technology in Biomedicine, 15*(4), 557–566. doi:10.1109/TITB.2011.2151868 PMID:21558061

Yuriyama, M., & Kushida, T. (2010). *Sensor-cloud infrastructure-physical sensor management with virtualized sensors on cloud computing.* Paper presented at the Network-Based Information Systems (NBiS). New York, NY.

Zephyr. (n.d.). Retrieved from http://www.zephyranywhere.com/

Zhang, R., & Liu, L. (2010). Security models and requirements for healthcare application clouds. In Proceedings of Cloud Computing (CLOUD), (pp. 268-275). IEEE.

Zhang, W., Wang, X., Lu, B., & Kim, T. H. (2013). Secure encapsulation and publication of biological services in the cloud computing environment. *BioMed Research International, 170580.*

Zhang, L., Gu, S., Liu, Y., Wang, B., & Azuaje, F. (2012). Gene set analysis in the cloud. *Bioinformatics (Oxford, England), 28*(2), 294–295. doi:10.1093/bioinformatics/btr630 PMID:22084254

Zhang, S. (2011). Computer-aided drug discovery and development. *Methods in Molecular Biology (Clifton, N.J.), 716,* 23–38. doi:10.1007/978-1-61779-012-6_2 PMID:21318898

Zhou, L., Zhu, Y., Lin, Y., & Bentley, Y. (2012). Cloud Supply Chain: A Conceptual Model. In *Proceedings of European, International Working Seminar on Production Economics.* Innsbruck, Austria: Academic Press.

About the Contributors

Anastasius Moumtzoglou is a Former Executive Board Member of the European Society for Quality in Health Care, President of the Hellenic Society for Quality & Safety in Health Care, holds a BA in Economics, MA in Health Services Management, MA in Macroeconomics, and a PhD in Economics. He teaches the module of quality at the graduate and postgraduate level. He has also written three Greek books, which are the only ones in the Greek references. The first deals with "Marketing in Health Care," the following with "Quality in Health Care," and the third with "Quality and Patient Safety in Health Care." He has edited the books *E-Health Systems Quality and Reliability: Models and Standards* and *E-Health Technologies & Improving Patient Safety: Exploring Organizational Factors*. He is also the Editor-in-Chief of the *International Journal of Reliable & Quality in Healthcare* (IJRQEH). He has served as the scientific coordinator in research programs in Greece and participated as a researcher in European research programs. He has been declared a "Person of Quality," with respect to Greece, for 2004.

Anastasia N. Kastania, PhD, received her BSc in Mathematics and her PhD degree in Medical Informatics from the National & Kapodistrian University of Athens, Greece. She works in the Athens University of Economics and Business, Greece since 1987. Research productivity is summarized in various articles (monographs or in collaboration with other researchers) in international journals, international conferences proceedings, international book series, and international books chapters. She has more than 20 years of teaching experience in university programs, and she is the writer of many didactic books. She also has 10 years of experience as researcher in national and European research projects. Research interests are telemedicine and e-health, e-learning, bioinformatics, tele-epidemiology, mathematical modeling and statistics, Web engineering, quality engineering, and reliability engineering.

* * *

António Abelha is an Auxiliary Professor of the Department of Informatics of the University of Minho, in Braga, Portugal. He got his PhD in Informatics, in 2004, and he is a researcher of the Computer Science and Technology Center (in Portuguese CCTC). His research interests span the domain of Biomedical Informatics, Databases, and Artificial Intelligence. He is the author of more than 100 papers in international books, journals, and conference proceedings.

Jalel Akaichi received his PhD in Computer Science from the University of Sciences and Technologies of Lille (France) and then his Habilitation degree from the University of Tunis (Tunisia), where he is currently an Associate Professor in the Computer Science Department. Jalel Akaichi has published in international journals and conferences, and has served on the program committees of several international conferences and journals. He is currently the Chair of the Master Science in Business Intelligence. Jalel Akaichi visited and taught in many institutions such as the State University of New York, Worcester Polytechnic Institute, INSA-Lyon, University of Blaise Pascal, University of Lille 1, etc.

Stavros Archondakis (MD, PhD) is a certified Pathologist, Director of Cytopathology Department of 401 Athens Army Hospital. He graduated from Thessaloniki Medical School and National Military Medical School in 1996. Since 2007, he has been assessor of the Hellenic Accreditation System (ESYD) for the accreditation of medical laboratories according to ISO 15189:2012. He speaks English and French. He is member of Hellenic Society of Clinical Cytopathology, Society of Medical Studies, and Society for Quality Management in the Health Sector. He is the author of 29 medical books, some of them awarded by the Greek Anticancer Society. He has participated with posters and oral presentations in more than 200 congresses and seminars. He has authored more than 25 articles in Greek and foreign medical journals. He possesses more than 800 hours of teaching experience in medical and paramedical schools.

Keerthana Boloor received her MS and PhD in Computer Engineering from North Carolina State University, USA in 2009 and 2012, respectively. She is a two-time recipient of IBM PhD Fellowship for the years 2010-2011 and 2011-2012. Keerthana is currently a Software Engineer at Google, New York. Before this, she was an Advisory Software Engineer with the Watson Technologies Group at IBM Research, Yorktown Heights, NY. Her research interests include distributed computing, service-oriented architectures, and everything cloud.

Luciana Cardoso concluded her MS degree in Biomedical Engineering – Medical Informatics at University of Minho in 2013. During that year, she developed a Biomedical Multi-Agent Platform for Interoperability. This platform and its implementation in a real environment were the main subjects of her Master Thesis. She has been publishing in several areas related to Medical Informatics, more specifically, Ambient Intelligence and the usability of Electronic Health Record. Her current research focuses on the interoperability in Hospital Information Systems through multi-agent systems.

Ali Chehab received his Bachelor degree in EE from the American University of Beirut (AUB) in 1987, the Master's degree in EE from Syracuse University, and the PhD degree in ECE from the University of North Carolina at Charlotte, in 2002. From 1989 to 1998, he was a lecturer in the ECE Department at AUB. He rejoined the ECE Department at AUB as an assistant professor in 2002 and became an associate professor in 2008. His research interests are VLSI Testing and Information Security and Trust.

Roma Chauhan is Assistant Professor in the Department of Information Technology at IILM Graduate School of Management, Greater Noida, India. She, before joining academics and research, had comprehensive experience with IT corporate giants as a software developer and consultant. She has conducted IT training programs for faculty, staff, and students at her institute. She is active in professional service, serving conference program committees, organizing workshops, and industry engagements. Her areas of interest includes information retrieval, data mining, knowledge management, and Semantic Web. She is Indian national who is amicable to international culture and practices. She is an innovative self-starter, who rarely needs supervision, and she enjoys learning new things from diverse cultural and social settings.

Rahul Ghosh is an Advisory Software Engineer at IBM, USA. He received his MS and PhD in Electrical and Computer Engineering from Duke University, USA in 2009 and 2012, respectively. Prior to this, he received his BE in Electronics and Telecommunication Engineering from Jadavpur University, India in 2007. Rahul's research interests include stochastic processes, queuing systems, Markov chains, performance and dependability analysis of large-scale computer systems. During his PhD, Rahul also worked as a research intern at IBM T.J. Watson Research Center. His PhD thesis research was focused on developing scalable analytic models for Cloud services. Rahul is a co-author of more than 20 peer-reviewed conference and journal papers and has filed 3 US patents with his co-inventors.

Piero Giacomelli owns a degree in Mathematics from the University of Padua. He has worked in many different industrial sectors, such as aerospace, ISP, textile, and plastic manufacturing, and e-health association, both as a software developer and as an IT manager. He has also been involved in many EU research-funded projects in FP7 EU programs, such as CHRONIOUS, I-DONT-FALL, FEARLESS, and CHROMED. In recent years, he has published some papers on scientific journals and has been awarded two best paper awards by the International Academy, Research, and Industry Association (IARIA). He published *HornetQ Messaging Developer's Guide* and *Apache Mahout Cookbook* with Packt Publishing.

Li Guo is Lecturer at the School of Computing, Engineering, and Computer Science at the University of Central Lancashire. He has PhD from the University of Edinburgh (2007) and has worked as research associate at Imperial College London. His research interests are in Cloud Computing, distributed sensor informatics, big data analysis, and intelligent multi-agent systems, and has more than 40 peer-reviewed publications in these areas. He has contributed to many EPSRC and EU research projects and was the chief architect of the Imperial College Cloud (IC Cloud) system currently in use in a wide variety of Digital Economy projects, and was also chief architect for EU FP6 project-GridEcon providing computational facilities for data analysis services from a variety of sources and devices.

Yike Guo has been working in the area of data intensive analytical computing since 1995. During last 15 years, he has been leading the data mining group to carry out many research projects, including UK e-science projects, such as Discovery Net on Grid based data analysis for scientific discovery, MESSAGE on wireless mobile sensor network for environment monitoring, BAIR on system biology for diabetes study, iHealth on modern informatics infrastructure for healthcare decision making, UBIOPRED on large informatics platform for translational medicine research, Digital City Exchange on sensor information-based urban dynamics modelling. He was the Principal Investigator of the Discovery Science Platform grant from UK EPSRC, where he is leading the team to build the IC Cloud system for large-scale collaborative scientific research. He is now the Principal Investigator of the eTRIKS project, a 23M Euro project in building a Cloud-based translational informatics platform for global medical research.

Benoit Hudzia is a Distributed System Researcher and Cloud/System Architect currently working on designing the next-generation Cloud technology for Stratoscale. Benoit has authored more than 20 academic publications and also is the holder of numerous patents in the domain of virtualization, OS, Cloud, distributed systems, etc. His code and ideas are included in various SAP commercial solutions as well as Open source solutions such as Qemu/KVM Hypervisor, Linux Kernel, Openstack. His research currently focus on bringing together the flexibility of virtualization, Cloud, and high-performance computing. This framework aims at providing memory, I/O, and CPU resource disaggregation of physical server while enabling dynamic management and aggregation capabilities to Linux native application as well as to Linux/KVM VMs using commodity hardware.

Wassim Itani was born in Beirut, Lebanon in 1978. He received his BE in Electrical Engineering, with distinction, from Beirut Arab University (BAU) in 2001 and his ME in Computer and Communications Engineering from the American University of Beirut (AUB) in 2003. Currently, he is a Research Associate in the Department of Electrical and Computer Engineering at AUB and an Assistant Professor at BAU. Wassim's research interests include wireless and body sensor networks security and privacy, Cloud Computing trust and security protocols, and cryptographic protocols performance evaluation.

Petros Karakitsos graduated from the Medical School of Athens University in 1982; in 1988, he received specialization in Cytopathology and a PhD degree from the same university. Now he is Professor of Cytopathology and Director of the Department of Cytopathology at the Medical School of the University of Athens ("Attikon" University Hospital). He is responsible for the specialized for Cytopathology eLearning platform of the Department. He is member of 4 Greek and 4 international Scientific Societies. He has contributed chapters to 10 medical books and 2 educational CDs. Principal investigator in 22 research programs (artificial intelligence in pathology, cervical screening, molecular pathways in colon carcinogenesis, implication of molecular markers in HPV-related oncogenesis, ThinPrep cytology, e-Learning and e-Health) having yielded, up to now, 156 papers in peer-reviewed journals and more than 200 presentations or invited lectures in international scientific congresses, with 12 scientific awards.

Efrossyni Karakitsou is within the School of Applied Mathematical and Physical Sciences of the National Technical University of Athens, and with the Biomedical Engineering Laboratory of the same university. She is experienced in information and data processing as well as in software development for the creation of support systems related to cytopathology practice. She has contributed three chapters in honorary books, and numerous publications in international and national conferences as well as in scientific journals. Her research interests include bioinformatics technologies, information and data processing for knowledge discovery, neural networks, genetic algorithms, and distributed computing systems.

Ayman Kayssi was born in Lebanon in 1967. He studied electrical engineering and received the BE degree, with distinction, in 1987 from the American University of Beirut (AUB), and the MSE and PhD degrees from the University of Michigan, Ann Arbor, in 1989 and 1993, respectively. In 1993, he joined the Department of Electrical and Computer Engineering (ECE) at AUB, where he is currently a full professor. His research interests are in information security and integrated circuit design and test. He is a senior member of IEEE and a member of ACM.

Vahé Kazandjian is Principal for ARALEZ HEALTH LLC, a Baltimore, Maryland-based global consulting company for healthcare performance improvement and accountability. He was the architect of the first multi-national hospital quality assessment project, the Maryland Quality Indicator Project (QIP) which he directed from 1990-2000. Dr. Kazandjian is Professor (Adjunct) The Johns Hopkins University, Bloomberg School of Public Health; Associate Professor (Adjunct), The University of Maryland, School of Medicine; and Professor (Adjunct) The Uniformed Health Services University, School of Medicine, Maryland. Since 2002, he serves as Advisor to the World Health Organization (WHO) to assist in hospital and healthcare systems performance assessment project in European countries. Since 2011, he has conducted evaluation programs for indicator-based programs, such as those funded by WHO in Poland, Hungary, and Croatia. Dr. Kazandjian is the author of 4 healthcare books on quality of care improvement and author/co-author of more than 70 peer-reviewed articles and book chapters.

Andreas Kliem is a researcher at the Complex and Distributed IT Systems Group of Technische Universität Berlin in Berlin, Germany. In 2010, he received his diploma in computer science for his work on dynamic online compression for distributed data flow programs. Andreas's current research interests center around middleware-platforms for Sensor Management, Internet of Things, Cyber-Physical Systems, QoS and non-functional requirements, and pervasive Cloud Computing Approaches (Sensor Virtualization, Resource Sharing). He is involved in several research projects related to the E-health and AAL application domain and also works as a technology advisor for other research institutions such as Fraunhofer FOKUS.

Christine Kottaridi is biologist, has a PhD in Applied Microbiology-Virology: "Molecular Detection and Study of the Evolution of Echo Viruses," and a MSc in "Biology Applications in Medicine" with Master thesis "The Role of Single and Multiple HPV Infections in Cervical Cancer." Her Postdoctoral Research in Diagnostic Cytopathology Laboratory, University of Athens, Medical School involves: a) study and evaluation of methods necessary to the prognosis of a successive vaccination against HPV 28/11/2008–31/12/2010 Ministry of Health; b) hospital-based surveillance of Rotavirus Gastroenteritis in children younger than 5 years old 20/02/2009–30/10/2010 GlaxoSmithKlein Hellas S.A.; c) a decision support system based on advanced clinical theranostics protocols for the cost-effective, personalised management of HPV-related diseases, 2013-2015, SYNERGASIA-2011, http://www.hpvguard.org. She has 30 published papers in peer-reviewed journals. Her research interests are focused to evaluation of experimental protocols concerning molecular and cellular mechanisms of pathogen emergence, public health, virus evolution, epidemiology, and surveillance.

Yiannis Koumpouros (BSc, MSc, MBA, PhD) is a Lecturer in the Technological Educational Institute of Athens, Department of Informatics, specialized in health informatics, e-health, telemedicine, and strategic management. He is an expert for the European Commission in the e-health sector and evaluator of numerous research and development projects, senior manager in business operations with wide expertise in design and implementation of strategic, conceptual, and complex changes in an international framework. He has significant experience in introducing organizational, process, and IT solutions for business performance improvement. He has top-level managerial experience in private and public healthcare sector (as chairman of hospitals) and has taught in several universities for almost 10 years. He has served as project and R&D manager in IT fields with European experience, chairman of several Permanent Committee of Experts (Ministry of Development, General Secretariat of Trade) for issues related to Electronic Scientific Equipments and Medical Equipments. He was a regular member of the Consultative Technical Council (Ministry of Internal Public Administration and Decentralisation) for subjects on new technologies and IT in the wider public administration, etc.

Chun-Hsiang Lee received a BSc degree in Industrial and System Engineering in 2001, and BSc and MSc degrees in Management Information System from Chung Yung Christian University, Taiwan, in 2001 and 2003, respectively. From 2003 to 2008, he was a research assistant at Science & Technology Policy Research and Information Centre of National Applied Research Laboratories, Taiwan. His research has mainly focused on applying text mining and quantitative analysis approaches on Scientometrics. From 2009, he joined Department of Computing, Imperial College London, UK, where he is a full-time PhD student working on Augmented Reality application on the mobile device in combination with Cloud services.

Yang Li is a researcher and PhD student at the Department of Computing, Imperial College London, UK. He received MSc in Computing from Imperial College London and BSc in Mathematics from University College London, UK. His research interests are Cloud Computing, Cloud storage, Cloud Computing applications for healthcare, and big data platforms.

José Machado is an Associate Professor with Habilitation of the Department of Informatics of the University of Minho, in Braga, Portugal. He got his PhD in Informatics, in 2002, and is now the Director of the Computer Science and Technology Center (in Portuguese CCTC). His research interests span the domain of Biomedical Informatics, Databases, and Artificial Intelligence. He is the author of more than 150 papers in international books, journals, and conference proceedings.

Fernando Marins obtained in 2013 his MS degree in Medical Informatics, concluding Biomedical Engineering in University of Minho. His Master's Thesis is titled "Monitoring and Prevention in Interoperability Healthcare Platforms." Consequently, his current research includes monitoring and prevention in Hospital Information Systems, through interoperability, multi-agent systems, data mining, proactive monitoring, and fault forecasting models. He has been publishing several papers not only based on his main research but also in other subjects, Namely in the areas of the usability of Electronic Health Record and Ambient Intelligence in Intensive Care Units.

Antonia Mourtzikou obtained a MSc in Biochemistry, a MSc in Clinical Chemistry, and a MSc in National Health System Management. She is a EurClinChem and has worked as a staff Clinical Biochemist since 1985 in "Asclepeion" Voulas Hospital. From 2010, she works in the Laboratory of Diagnostic Cytology in "Attikon" University Hospital. She is PhD candidate.

Mauricio Paletta is an Assistant Professor at the Universidad Nacional Experimental de Guayana and the Universidad Católica Andrés Bello (Guayana), Venezuela. He has a PhD in Computer Science at the Universidad Politécnica de Madrid, Spain. He was the co-founder of a Research Center in Computer Science at the UNEG (in Spanish: Centro de Investigación en Informática y Ciencia de la Computación – CITEC), and for more than two years, he has coordinated the research line named "intelligent and emergence computing" attached to the CITEC. His research interests include agents and multi-agent systems, emergence computing and object-oriented technology, and more recently, collaborative and Cloud computing systems.

Ioannis Papapanagiotou received the Dipl.Ing. degree in Electrical and Computer Engineering from the University of Patras, Greece in 2006. The MSc degree and a dual major PhD degree in Computer Engineering and Operations Research from North Carolina State University in 2009 and 2012, respectively. He has been awarded the best paper awards in IEEE GLOBECOM 2007 and IEEE CAMAD 2010. He is also the recipient of the IBM PhD Fellowship, Academy of Athens, and A. Metzelopoulos scholarships. He is currently an Assistant Professor in the department of Computer and Information Technology at Purdue University. Before this, he was working in the Emerging Technology Institute in IBM, an in-house incubator team directly reporting to the CTO and working in the areas of mobile and Cloud computing.

Filipe Portela holds a PhD in Information Systems and Technologies. He is inserted in the R&D Centre ALGORITMI and is developing his research work in the topic "Pervasive Intelligent Decision Support in Critical Health Care." Currently, he is an invited professor in the department of information systems, school of engineering, University of Minho, Portugal. This research was started with the INTCare research project in cooperation with the ICU of Centro Hospitalar do Porto and already has some important publications in intelligent system, pervasive environment, intensive medicine, data mining knowledge discovery, and decision support areas. He is the author of more than 50 papers in international books, journals, and conference proceedings.

Abraham Pouliakis is a Physicist, holds a MSc in Electronics and Radio Communications, and a PhD degree from the Medical School (University of Athens) related to the Application of Neural Networks in Cytopathology Diagnosis. Since 1993, he has participated in numerous national, European, and European Space Agency research projects related to information and communication technology, artificial intelligence applied in medicine, collaborative systems, e-learning, and e-health. Currently, he is research associate and responsible for quality control and assurance in the Department of Cytopathology, University of Athens, School of Medicine. He has 32 publications in international peer reviewed scientific magazines, more than 90 presentations in international and Greek conferences, and is co-author of 3 book chapters. His research interests are related to information and communication technology, image/signal processing, and artificial intelligence, including their applications in the fields of industry and health.

César Quintas is a technical member of the Information System team of the Centro Hospitalar do Porto, one of the major Portuguese hospitals. He is now a PhD student in Biomedical Engineering in the area of Medical Informatics.

Manuel Filipe Santos holds a PhD in Computer Science – Artificial Intelligence. Currently, he is associate professor in the department of information systems, school of engineering, University of Minho, Portugal. He is the Investigator Responsible in research projects (grid data mining and intelligent decision support systems for intensive care). He is the head of the Intelligent Data Systems group in the R&D Centre Algoritmi. He has around 100 publications in conference proceedings, chapters in books, and journals. His main interests are knowledge discovery from databases and data mining, intelligent decision support systems, and machine learning.

Jonathan Sinclair is a Senior Software Engineer currently working on architecting distributed middleware for RepKnight Ltd in the area of real-time distributed open-source intelligence. He has completed his PhD with Queen's University Belfast, having researched legal compliance auditing for distributed computer systems as a Research Associate with SAP Research Belfast. He obtained his MEng degree in Computer Science from Queen's University Belfast in 2009. His research interests include topics such as GRC (Governance, Risk, and Compliance), Security and Privacy, Service Level Agreements, and Argumentation.

Aris Spathis received his BSc in Biology in 2005 from the School of Science of the National and Kapodistrian University of Athens, and his PhD in 2009 from the School of Medicine of the National and Kapodistrian University of Athens. He has been a research associate of the Department of Cytopathology of the University General Hospital "ATTIKON" in Athens from 2005. His main focus is molecular analysis of liquid-based cytology preserved clinical samples with regard to cancer development and progression. He has 20 peer-reviewed publications and several announcements in international and Hellenic congresses, focused on HPV, colorectal cancer, and lymphomas.

Marilena Stamouli received the Diploma in Biology (1986) from the University of Athens, Greece, and the MS degree in Health Management (2010) from the University of Pireus, Greece. From 1987 until today, she works at the Biopathology Laboratory of the Naval and Veterans Hospital of Athens, as tenured civilian scientific personnel, and she is supervisor of the Biochemistry Laboratory since 2011. Her main research interests include biochemistry, autoimmunity, haemoglobinopathies, molecular diagnostic methods, and laboratory quality control. She has published 18 related articles in scientific journals and 57 articles in proceedings of peer-reviewed scientific conferences. She has also attended many scientific seminars and workshops. She is a member of the Greek Society of Clinical Chemistry-Clinical Biochemistry, of the Hellenic Society of Immunology, and of the European Register of Specialists in Clinical Chemistry and Laboratory Medicine (EurClinChem). She is a MS degree candidate in Quality Assurance from the Hellenic Open University.

A. Stewart graduated from The Queen's University of Belfast with a B.Sc (Hons) in 1982 and earned a PhD in 1987. He is now a lecturer at The Queen's University of Belfast having previously been a Research Fellow at The University of Oxford, CWI (Amsterdam) and INRIA (Paris – Rocquencourt). His main research interests are hoare logic, parallel models of computation, BSP, (parallel) algorithms, service-based computation, and Clouds. He is currently developing a power-domain model of orchestrations in which the non-determinism resulting from service uncertainty is analysed by means of game theory.

Chao Wu is a research associate in Department of Computing, Imperial College London. He got his Doctor degree from Zhejiang University. His research interests are in the areas of social networking, Cloud Computing, folksonomy system, data visualization, etc.

Index